ORBISON

Changing Concepts in Cardiovascular Disease

Changing Concepts in Cardiovascular Disease

edited by

Henry I. Russek, M.D.

Visiting Professor in Cardiovascular Disease,
Hahnemann Medical College and Hospital,
Philadelphia, Pennsylvania
and
Senior Attending Cardiologist, St. Barnabas Hospital,
New York, N.Y.

Burton L. Zohman, M.D.

Clinical Professor of Medicine, State University of New York
Downstate Medical Center College of Medicine,
Brooklyn, N.Y.
and
Senior Attending Cardiologist, St. Barnabas Hospital,
New York, N.Y.

The Williams & Wilkins Company *Baltimore*

Copyright ©, 1972
The Williams & Wilkins Company
428 E. Preston Street
Baltimore, Md. 21202, U.S.A.

Made in the United States of America

Library of Congress Catalog Card Number 73-185334
SBN 683-07455-5

Composed and printed at the
Waverly Press, Inc.
Mt. Royal and Guilford Aves.
Baltimore, Md. 21202, U.S.A.

Preface

Science is an endless frontier that provides opportunities and consequences often difficult to imagine. The magnitude of its potential is recognized by the realization that, only a few decades ago, the greatest scientific minds of the time failed to foresee nuclear energy, antibiotics, radar, the electronic computer, rocketry, or transplantation of the human heart. Although cardiovascular disease still remains the most formidable and challenging of all health problems, possibilities just beyond the present capabilities of science may soon provide the answers to its effective prevention and control.

The epic of recent achievements in medical and surgical cardiology has evolved not only from a close alliance and constructive interaction between internist and surgeon but also from the prudent application of fundamental researches in physiology, anatomy, pathology, and biochemistry. Despite these spectacular gains, there has been no clear evidence of favorable trends in mortality or longevity in the United States. Obviously, improved patient care can only be achieved by a program of continuing education which enables the practicing physician to apply changing and new concepts skillfully on a clinical level. The real measure of medical progress, to be sure, cannot be determined solely from the activities observed in university medical centers since these do not necessarily reflect the practices prevailing in the thousands of smaller community hospitals across the nation.

Although standard textbooks may provide an authoritative source for established principles of diagnosis and treatment, the physician must turn elsewhere for knowledge of the rapidly advancing frontiers in research and discovery. Scientific meetings and medical journals unfortunately have often failed to fulfill their needed role in graduate medical education. These avenues of scientific communication have become inundated with investigations which often appear to have no relevance to cardiovascular practice or are lost to the busy practitioner in the complex format of scientific presentation. A common meeting ground for the physiologist, pharmacologist, cardiologist, and cardiovascular surgeon is therefore invaluable for defining the significance of new discovery and its impact upon rational management in cardiovascular disease. Moreover, in the present era in which clinical impression and uncontrolled observation find no forum for their expression, there is a growing necessity for the cross-fertilization that follows the free exchange of impressions and ideas, however nebulous, among trained clinicians and investigators. The American College of Cardiology–St. Barnabas Hospital Symposium on "New Frontiers in Cardiovascular Disease" which was held at the Americana Hotel in New York City, December 11 to 13, 1970, and this textbook of its edited proceedings therefore represent a concerted effort to fulfill these needs in the cardiovascular field.

The contributors to this volume, in sharing their knowledge and accomplishments without personal gain, have served the highest tradition of the medical profession. By placing new concepts and techniques in historical perspective and surveying horizons for future achievement, they have also brought into clear focus the continuity of all medical progress. The American College of Cardiology and St. Barnabas Hospital wish to express their sincere thanks to each of the members of this faculty for outstanding service and cooperation.

We wish to express our deep appreciation to Dr. William Likoff and Dr. George Griffith, Chairmen of the National Program Committee for Continuing Medical Education of the American College of Cardiology for their encouragement and support.

As in previous offerings, the success of this symposium was in no small measure the result of the excellent administrative management provided by Mr. William D. Nelligan, Executive Director of the American College of Cardiology, and his able associates, Dr. John C. Bish and Miss Mary Anne McInerny, whose planning and performance reflected their usual pattern of excellence. To them we extend our warm thanks.

Finally, we wish to express our appreciation to the following organizations for educational grants in partial support of this program:

Ives Laboratories
Ayerst Laboratories
Merck Sharp & Dohme
William S. Merrell Company
Wallace Pharmaceuticals
Warner-Chilcott Laboratories
Bristol Laboratories
Ciba Pharmaceutical Company

Pfizer Laboratories
Eli Lilly & Company
Smith Kline & French Laboratories
McNeil Laboratories
Schering Corporation
Burroughs Wellcome & Company
Hoechst Pharmaceuticals
Endo Laboratories

Their valuable assistance in helping to improve the quality of medical care again demonstrates a sincere dedication to the public interest.

Henry I. Russek, M.D.
Burton L. Zohman, M.D.

A Tribute to Wilhelm Raab

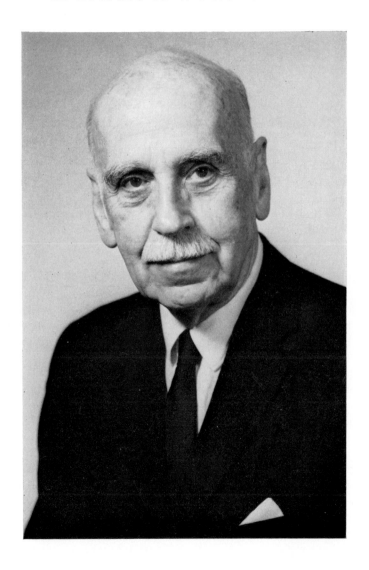

Wilhelm Raab, M.D., was born in Vienna, Austria, on January 14, 1885, and received his early medical training in Prague, Czechoslovakia. In 1929, as the recipient of a Rockefeller fellowship, he spent a year with the famous physiologist Walter B. Cannon at Harvard Medical School in Boston. This experience determined his life-long interest in the Sympathetic Nervous System. Upon his return to Vienna, where he was made Associate Professor of Medicine, Dr. Raab taught Endocrinology and, among other things, conducted his study on the effect of dietary habits on the incidence of atherosclerosis and hypertension, which established the contributing roles of dietary fats and smoking as early as 1932. His involvement with the causative role of epinephrine in heart disease started also in the same year, when he injected himself with a heavy dose of the substance in order to study its effect on lipid metabolism and promptly developed a typical episode of angina pectoris accompanied by the classical electrocardiographic changes. A direct outgrowth of this observation were his studies with Dr. Scherf and Dr. Schönbrunner on the treatment of angina by Roentgen irradiation of the adrenals and, later, by depression of thyroid function by means of propylthiouracil.

In 1937 after the Nazis took over Austria, Dr. Raab found the climate in Vienna more and more dangerous, and in 1939 he came to the University of Vermont as Chairman of the Division of Experimental Medicine which was created especially for him. Although his teachings on the unfavorable role of dietary fats were not received with enthusiasm in a state whose major business then was dairy farming, he was able to build up a modest laboratory and staff, and to develop fully his concept that angina pectoris and myocardial infarction depend not only on the blood supply to the myocardium but to a large extent on its oxygen consumption. The oxygen consumption in turn, he showed, greatly depends on epinephrine and other catecholamines produced in the heart by sympathetic nervous stimulation or brought to it through the blood stream. I had known Dr. Raab in Vienna, and after World War II was over, he invited me to join him in Burlington in 1946; and since that time I have been working with him on the electrocardiographic aspects of catecholamine effects and on the role of electrolytes in the myocardial repolarization processes which underly them

Dr. Raab had a brilliant and versatile mind, which enabled him to bring together many apparently irrelevant observations to form a single unifying concept. But his versatility was not limited to medicine. He was a brilliant racconteur and impersonator, an excellent amateur artist and photographer, a poet, and a first class violinist. He was fluent in seven languages, including Russian, which he learned on short notice in preparation for his lecture and studies in the Soviet Union. Any of these gifts could probably have formed the basis of a career had he chosen to develop them. But it is his personal warmth and concern for events surrounding him which endeared him most to his friends and associates.

Dr. Raab's observations on the decreased sympathetic tone and cardiac work in athletes led him to explore the possibility of preventing heart attacks by means of physical exercise. This culminated in the creation of the "Preventive Heart Reconditioning Foundation." Only a few months before his death on September 21, 1970, he organized a Seminar in Preventive Myocardiology in Stowe, Vermont, the results of which are now in print. Other books by Dr. Raab are *Preventive Myocardiology*, 1970; *Prevention of Ischemic Heart Disease*, 1966; *Hypokinetic Disease* (with H. Kraus), 1961; and *Hormonal and Neurogenic Cardiovascular Disorders*, 1963.

Eugene Lepeschkin

Contributors

Forrest H. Adams, M.D., Professor of Pediatrics and Head, Division of Cardiology, Department of Pediatrics, University of California, Los Angeles; President, Elect, American College of Cardiology

Ezra A. Amsterdam, M.D., Chief, Coronary Care. Section of Cardiovascular Medicine, Departments of Medicine and Pharmacology, University of California at Davis, School of Medicine

Charles P. Bailey, M.D., Director of Thoracic and Cardiovascular Surgery, St. Barnabas Hospital, New York

Christiaan N. Barnard, Ph.D., M.D., Professor of Surgical Science and Head of the Department of Cardiothoracic Surgery and Organ Transplantation, University of Cape Town, South Africa

Marius S. Barnard, M.Ch., Associate Professor of Surgical Science, University of Cape Town, South Africa

Louis F. Bishop, M.D., Senior Attending Cardiologist, St. Barnabas Hospital, New York

Joseph A. Bonanno, M.D., Assistant Clinical Professor of Medicine, Section of Cardiovascular Medicine, Department of Internal Medicine, University of California at Davis, School of Medicine

Norman Brachfeld, M.D., Associate Professor of Medicine, New York Hospital, Cornell Medical Center, New York

John F. Briggs, M.D., Clinical Professor of Medicine, The University of Minnesota Medical School, Minneapolis

Otto A. Brusis, M.D., Assistant Professor in Community Medicine, University of Vermont College of Medicine, Vermont

George E. Burch, M.D., Henderson Professor and Chairman, Department of Medicine, Tulane University School of Medicine, New Orleans

Hugo Carrasco, M.D., Fellow in Research, Cedars of Lebanon Hospital, Los Angeles

Jacques J. Col, M.D., Cardiovascular Center, Good Samaritan Hospital Dayton, Ohio

Theodore Cooper, M.D., Director, National Heart and Lung Institute, National Institutes of Health, Bethesda, Maryland

Eliot Corday, M.D., Clinical Professor of Medicine, University of California, Los Angeles, and Chairman, Cardiac Care Committee, Cedars of Lebanon Hospital Division of Cedars-Sinai Medical Center, Los Angeles

Anthony N. Damato, M.D., Chief, Cardiovascular Program, United States Public Health Service Hospital, New York

Abner J. Delman, M.D., Adjunct Attending in Medicine and Cardiology, Montefiore Hospital and Medical Center, New York

Leonard S. Dreifus, M.D., Associate Clinical Professor of Medicine, Hahnemann Medical College, Philadelphia

Rene G. Favaloro, M.D., Department of Thoracic Surgery, Cleveland Clinic, Cleveland

Frank S. Folk, M.D., Associate Attending Thoracic and Cardiovascular Surgeon, St. Barnabas Hospital, New York

Donald S. Frederickson, M.D., Director of Intramural Research and Chief, Molecular Disease Branch, National Heart and Lung Institute, Bethesda, Maryland

Ray W. Gifford, Jr., M.D., Head, Department of Hypertension and Renal Disease, Cleveland Clinic, Cleveland

T. D. Giles, M.D., Department of Medicine, Tulane University School of Medicine, New Orleans

Julius Grollman, M.D., Assistant Professor of Medicine, UCLA School of Medicine, Los Angeles

William S. Gualtiere, Ph.D., Exercise Research Director, Work Physiology Unit, Department of Rehabilitative Medicine, Montefiore Hospital and Medical Center, New York

Dwight Emary Harken, M.D., Clinical Professor of Surgery, Harvard Medical School (Emeritus), Boston; Chief, Thoracic Surgery, Mount Auburn Hospital, Cambridge, Massachusetts

Teruo Hirose, M.D., Senior Attending Surgeon in Thoracic and Cardiovascular Surgery and Director of the Cardiovascular Laboratory, St. Barnabas Hospital, New York

James L. Hughes, III, M.D., Cardiovascular Fellow, Section of Cardiovascular Medicine, Department of Internal Medicine, University of California at Davis, School of Medicine

Albert A. Kattus, Jr. M.D., Professor of Medicine and Chief, Division of Cardiology, University of California, Los Angeles School of Medicine, Los Angeles

Tzu-Wang Lang, M.D., Senior Resident Scientist, Cedars of Lebanon Hospital, Los Angeles

John H. Laragh, M.D., Professor of Clinical Medicine, Columbia University College of Physicians and Surgeons, New York

Marianne J. Legato, M.D., Attending Physician in Cardiology, Roosevelt Hospital, New York

Robert I. Levy, M.D., Head, Section on Lipoproteins and Chief, Clinical Service, Molecular Disease Branch, National Heart and Lung Institute, Bethesda, Maryland

William Likoff, M.D., Clinical Professor of Medicine, Hahnemann Medical College and Hospital, Philadelphia; Chairman, National Program Committee for Continuing Medical Education, American College of Cardiology

Harold M. Lowe, M.D., Director, Department of Cardiovascular-Pulmonary Diseases, Mercy Hospital, Sacramento

Jose Lozano, M.D., Fellow in Research, Cedars of Lebanon Hospital, Los Angeles

James R. Malm, M.D., Professor of Clinical Surgery, Columbia University College of Physicians and Surgeons, New York

Edward J. Mansour, M.D., Cardiovascular Fellow, Section of Cardiovascular Medicine, Department of Internal Medicine, University of California at Davis, School of Medicine

Dean T. Mason, M.D., Professor of Medicine and Physiology and Chief, Cardiopulmonary Section, University of California at Davis, School of Medicine

Rashid A. Massumi, M.D., Professor of Medicine, Chief, Electrophysiology and Heart Station, Section of Cardiovascular Medicine, Department of Internal Medicine, University of California at Davis, School of Medicine

Arthur M. Master, M.D., Emeritus Clinical Professor of Medicine, Mount Sinai School of Medicine of the City University of New York and Consultant Cardiologist, Mount Sinai Hospital, New York

Richard R. Miller, M.D., Fellow in Cardiovascular Medicine, Department of Medicine, University of California at Davis, School of Medicine

John H. Moyer, III, M.D., Professor and Chairman, Department of Internal Medicine, Hahnemann Medical College and Hospital, Philadelphia

John Ross, Jr., M.D., Professor of Medicine and Director, Cardiovascular Division, University of California, San Diego School of Medicine, La Jolla

Henry I. Russek, M.D., Senior Attending Cardiologist, St. Barnabas Hospital, New York, and Visiting Professor in Cardiovascular Disease. Hahnemann Medical College and Hospital, Philadelphia

Antone F. Salel, M.D., Fellow in Cardiovascular Medicine, Department of Medicine, University of California at Davis, School of Medicine

Roy J. Shephard, M.D., Ph.D., Professor of Applied Physiology, University of Toronto, School of Hygiene

Sol Sherry, M.D., Professor and Chairman, Department of Medicine, Temple University School of Medicine, Philadelphia

Neil J. Stone, M.D., Molecular Disease Branch, National Heart and Lung Institute, Bethesda, Maryland

John K. Vyden, M.B.B.S., Director, Peripheral Vascular Disease Section, Cedars of Lebanon Hospital, Los Angeles

Yoshio Watanabe, M.D., Department of Medicine, Hahnemann Medical College, Philadelphia

Sylvan Lee Weinberg, M.D., Chairman, Cardiovascular Center and Director, Coronary Care Unit, Good Samaritan Hospital, Dayton, Ohio

Paul D. White, M.D., Emeritus Clinical Professor of Medicine, Harvard Medical School and Consultant in Medicine, Massachusetts General Hospital, Boston

Robert Zelis, M.D., Assistant Chief, Section of Cardiovascular Medicine, Chief, Clinical Physiology and Cardiovascular Diagnosis, Departments of Medicine and Physiology, University of California at Davis, School of Medicine

Burton L. Zohman, M.D., Clinical Professor of Medicine, State University of New York, Downstate Medical Center College of Medicine. New York; Senior Attending Cardiologist, St. Barnabas Hospital, New York

Lenore R. Zohman, M.D., Director, Work Physiology Unit, Department of Rehabilitation Medicine, Montefiore Hospital and Medical Center; Associate Professor of Rehabilitative Medicine, Albert Einstein College of Medicine, New York

Contents

"The Wisdom of the Creator is in Nothing
Seen More Glorious Than the Heart"

1

New Explorations of the Ultrastructure and Function of the Myocardium

MARIANNE J. LEGATO, M.D.

One of the most rapidly expanding areas in modern physiology is the exploration of cardiac structure and function on a cellular level. The fundamental problem of how the individual cell engenders and supports the essential events of excitation, contraction, and relaxation has been of special interest in the past decade. As a result, we are now advancing some new concepts of how the subcellular systems of the myofiber produce and coordinate the activity of the heart.

It is very important to understand that the myocardium does not have a homogenous cell population. There is a wide spectrum of variation both in cell structure and function.

We will discuss first the ordinary working ventricular myofiber. Figure 1.1 is an electron micrograph illustrating the edges of two adjacent ventricular cells, separated by the extracellular space (ECS). The phenomenon of excitation, as in all cells, is mediated by the cell membrane or sarcolemma (S). The sarcolemma has two components, an electron-dense, structured basement membrane (BM) and the amorphous, less dark, so-called perimembrane (PM).

The sarcolemma has two important derivatives in the cell. The first is the intercalated disc (ID), a complex intercellular junction unique to cardiac tissue. Figure 1.2 is a micrograph showing two ventricular cells. Their sarcolemmae have invaginated to form an extensive, intimate, and highly complex junction which locks the two units together. Figure 1.3, a high power view of the intercalated disc (ID), shows the two specialized areas of this intercellular connection, the zona occludens (ZO) and a multi-layered "desmosomal" (D) area. The zona occludens is the place at which adjacent cell membranes come into the closest physical contact, and it has always been postulated to be a low resistance junction across which the

1

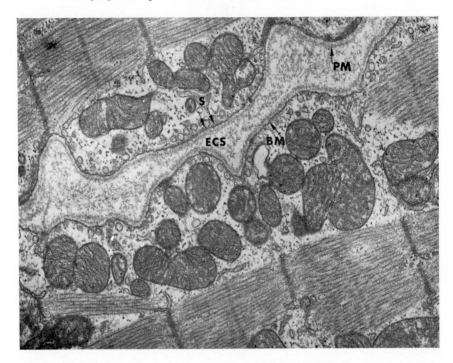

FIG. 1.1. This is an electron micrograph of portions of two adjacent ventricular myocardial cells. The two components of the cell membrane or sarcolemma (S) are illustrated: the thin, electron-dense basement membrane (BM) and the thick, amorphous, and lighter staining perimembrane (PM). ECS, extracellular space. × 20,000.

depolarizing impulse is rapidly transmitted from cell to cell, facilitating the orderly, sequential spread of excitation throughout the myocardium.

At frequent intervals in the ventricular cell, the sarcolemma sends invaginating fingers downward into the substance of the cell to form the second sarcolemmal derivative (Fig. 1.4), a system of tubules filled with the amorphous substance of the sarcolemmal perimembrane. They anastomose widely throughout the substance of the myofiber and are known collectively as the transverse tubular system (TT). The transverse tubular system is an extension of the cell membrane over which depolarization can be rapidly propagated throughout the substance of the myofiber, and it carries the extracellular compartment downward to all levels of the cell.

The actual contractile event in the cardiac cell takes place as a result of the interaction of the filaments of the sarcomeric unit. In Figure 1.5 the sarcomere, with its characteristic pattern of alternating dark and light bands, makes up the bulk of the working ventricular cell. The thin filaments, which are composed primarily of the protein actin, are anchored in the dark Z bands which delimit the sarcomere at each end. The thin fila-

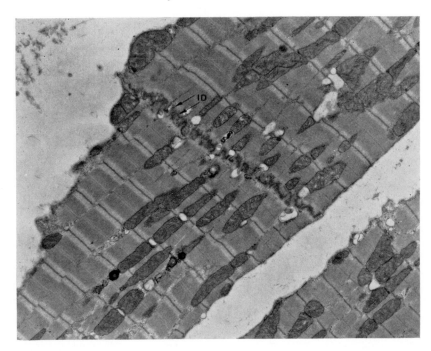

FIG. 1.2. This micrograph shows two cells joined in the intercellular link unique to cardiac tissue, the intercalated disc (ID). × 4,600.

ments interdigitate in the central portion of the sarcomere with the thick filaments; the latter are composed of the protein myosin. The portion of the sarcomere where thin filaments exist alone is called the I band (I); where thin and thick filaments interdigitate in the central portion of the sarcomere is called the A band (A). Figure 1.6, a schematic drawing of the sarcomeric unit, illustrates the substructure of thick and thin myofilaments. The thin filament is composed of two strands, intertwined in the pattern of a double helix, much like a double strand of beads, one wound about the other. The thick filaments are made up of clusters of subunits shaped very much like golf clubs, with their thin or bare areas toward the center of the filament and their round globular heads clustered at either end. In the interaction between the thin and thick filaments, cross bridges form between the two, one end of the bridge being attached at the pitch of the actin helix and the other to a globular head of the myosin filament. The formation of the bridge pulls the thin filaments centrally, thus shortening the Z to Z distance of the sarcomere. The active formation and breakage of these cross bridges is what produces the sliding of the thin filament along the thick toward the center of the sarcomere, so that shortening is achieved. During the resting state, the active sites on the thin filament are blocked by a protein called

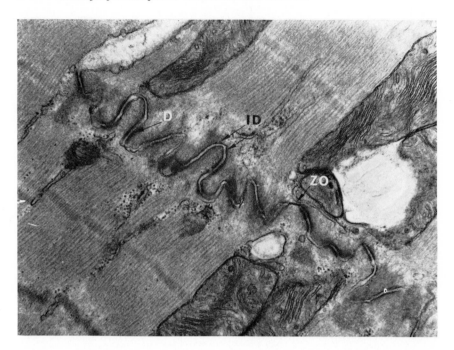

Fig. 1.3. This micrograph illustrates the specialized portions of the intercalated disc, the zona occludens (ZO) and the desmosomal area of the disc (D). ID, intercalated disc.

troponin which, by virtue of its configuration, prevents actin's active sites from interaction with those on the myosin filament. When calcium is presented to the area of the myofilament, it attaches to troponin, producing a configurational change in that protein. This exposes the active site on the thin filament so that it can interact with the active site on the thick filament. Calcium then is the pivotal factor not only in the initiation of the contractile event but in the degree of sarcomeric shortening, and hence of total muscle shortening that is achieved. In a very definite sense, then, calcium controls muscle inotropism. When calcium is removed from the myofilaments, troponin configuration returns to its original state, the active sites on the thin filaments are masked, and sarcomeric shortening ceases. Muscular relaxation is essentially achieved by the removal of calcium from the area of the myofilaments to an inactive site or storage depot in the muscle.

The central importance of the calcium ion in the coupling of excitation to contraction and in the generation and control of systolic force in the muscle has focused attention on a subcellular system remarkable for its specialized ability to transport and store calcium in the heart cell, the sarcoplasmic reticulum. In Figure 1.7, the sarcoplasmic reticulum (SR) is seen as a com-

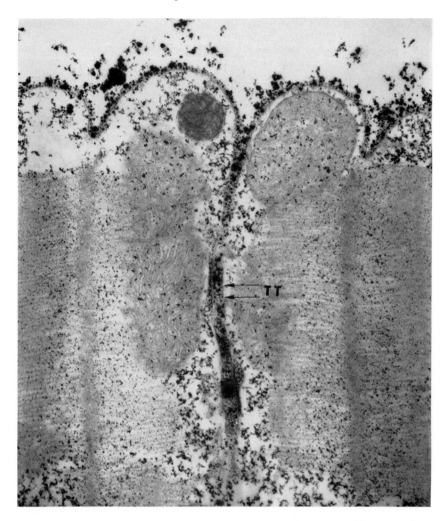

FIG. 1.4. This micrograph shows a transverse tubule (TT) formed by a sarcolemmal invagination. The extracellular space has been labeled with the electron-dense precipitate of sodium pyroantimonate, which fills the lumen of the transverse tubule. × 25,000.

plex network of tubules which envelops each sarcomeric unit in the myofiber. At the level of the I band, it comes into intimate relationship with the transverse tubular system (T) in a specialized cuff of tissue called the lateral sac (LS). Figure 1.8, an artist's sketch of the preceding micrograph, shows the intimate relationship between the SR network and the transverse tubular system. When one lateral sac is present, the resulting configuration of large T tubular vesicle and closely applied thin lateral sac of the sarco-

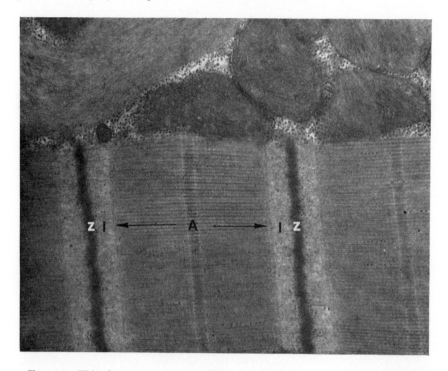

Fɪɢ. 1.5. This electron micrograph illustrates the component parts of the sarco-mere or contractile unit of the myocardium. The sarcomere is delimited at either end by the electron-dense Z band (Z) into which the thin filaments insert. The portion of the sarcomere where the thin filaments exist alone is called the I band (I). The A band (A) contains both thick and thin filaments. × 28,500.

plasmic reticulum is called a diad. Where two lateral sacs are present, each one contributed from the sarcoplasmic reticular network of adjacent sarco-meres, the resulting configuration is called a triad (Fig. 1.9).

The lateral sacs of the sarcoplasmic reticulum contain large concentra-tions of calcium ion, and they probably function as storage areas or depots for this ion in muscle.

The tubular network of the sarcoplasmic reticulum itself has been shown to have a capacity to bind and actively transport calcium out of the sur-rounding medium. Presumably, it pumps calcium out of the area of the myofilaments at the end of the contractile event and returns it to the storage area of the lateral sacs. To the best of our knowledge, at least in the ven-tricular working myocardial cell, the individual cellular components react in the following way to produce the events of excitation, contraction, and relaxation (Fig. 1.10):

1. Depolarization: The sarcolemma and T system

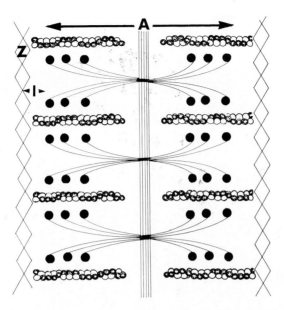

F_{IG}. 1.6. This is an artist's sketch of the sarcomere, illustrating the fact that the thin filament, which inserts into the lattice-like Z band (Z), has the structure of a double helix. The thin filaments, before they pass centrally to interdigitate with the thick filaments in the sarcomeric Z band (A), make up the I band (I) of the sarcomere. The substructure of the thick filament is illustrated; note the globular heads which are the active sites on myosin where cross bridge attachment occurs during the contractile event (see text).

2. Excitation-contraction coupling: Ca^{++} release from the lateral sacs
3. Contraction: Ca^{++} in the region of the sarcomere
4. Relaxation: Removal of Ca^{++} from myofilaments by SR tubular network

As recently as 2 years ago, our discussion would have ended here. As our knowledge of the ultrastructure of different cell populations in the heart grows, however, it becomes more and more apparent that this rather simplistic view of cell component function must be modified when it comes to, for example, the Purkinje cell or even the ordinary atrial cell.

Almost all mammalian atrial cells are entirely without any vestige of a transverse tubular system. Peculiar to this population of myofibers, however, is a specialized modification of the sarcoplasmic reticulum. Figure 1.11 is an electron micrograph of a small area of a human atrial cell which shows the typical ballooning out of the sarcoplasmic reticular tubule (SR) on either side of a small central tubule (arrows), the source of which we do not know. This configuration may well be analogous to the triadic structure seen in ventricular cells, but this remains to be more completely explored.

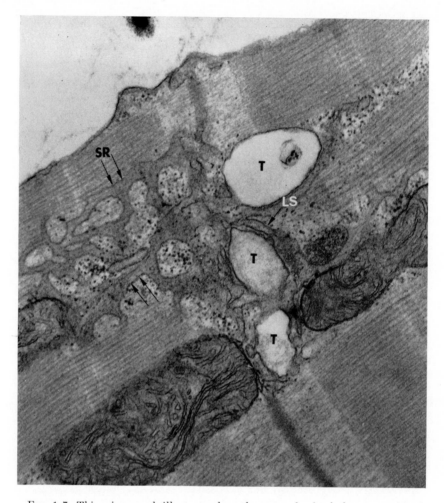

Fig. 1.7. This micrograph illustrates how the network of tubules composing the sarcoplasmic reticulum (SR) comes into close apposition to the sarcolemmal derivative, the transverse tubule (T). LS, lateral sac. × 40,000.

Purkinje cell ultrastructure is, in a way, the most interesting and unique of all. In work done in collaboration with Dr. J. Thomas Bigger of the Columbia-Presbyterian Medical Center, New York, we identified Purkinje tissue in the false tendon of the dog's right ventricle by obtaining from it the action potential characteristic of this cell population prior to fixation of tissue.

Cells so identified (Fig. 1.12), when examined in the electron microscope, have no transverse tubular system, and the question of how excitation is coupled to contraction in these cells is not clear. There are, in true Purkinje

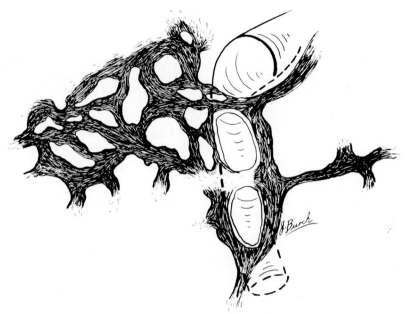

FIG. 1.8. This is an artist's sketch of the relationship between the sarcoplasmic reticular network and transverse tubule illustrated in Figure 1.7.

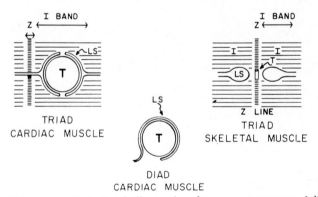

FIG. 1.9. This is an artist's sketch illustrating the component parts of diadic and triadic figures in both cardiac and skeletal muscle. LS, lateral sac; T, transverse tubule.

cells, only what are called peripheral coupling sites, where the lateral sac of the sarcoplasmic reticulum is closely apposed to the sarcolemma, but it is apparent that the calcium released from such a configuration in response to excitation would have to diffuse downward from the cell surface through the entire substance of the myofibril to reach the level of the myofilaments for the initiation of the contractile event.

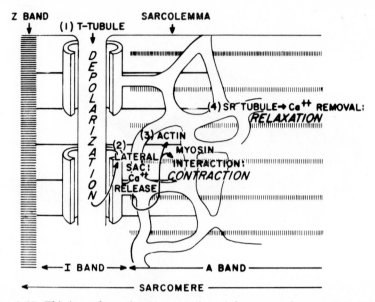

FIG. 1.10. This is a schematic representation of the proposed sequential steps involved in excitation, contraction, and relaxation in the ordinary working ventricular cell.

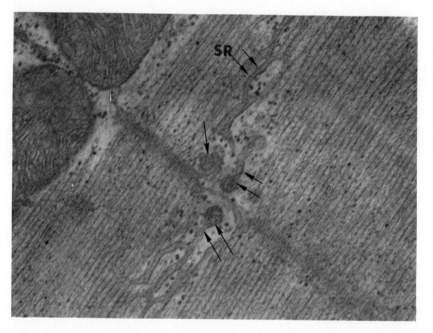

FIG. 1.11. This micrograph of a portion of an atrial cell shows the configuration which may be analogous to the triad of the ventricular cell. Note the much smaller size of the central tubule which is flanked on either side by the ballooned-out terminations (arrows) of the sarcoplasmic reticular network (SR). × 40,000.

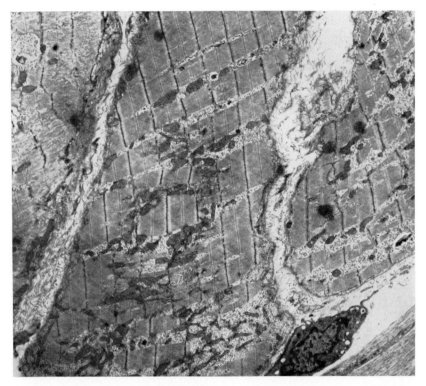

Fig. 1.12. This micrograph shows portions of three Purkinje cells and illustrates the absence of a T system in these myofibers. There are, therefore, no diadic or triadic units in this tissue. (Compare to Figure 1.2.)

The intercalated disc of Purkinje tissue is another area of special interest. One sees a zona occludens very rarely. As mentioned above, this is postulated to be the low resistance junction across which the depolarizing impulse is rapidly transmitted from cell to cell. And yet, in this tissue, which has the most rapid speed of conduction in the heart, there are very infrequent zonae occludentes in the intercalated disc. The desmosomal areas are much more numerous, and it seems reasonable to postulate that the desmosomal area, and not the zona occludens, is actually the spot across which the depolarizing impulse spreads with the greatest ease from cell to cell.

How the myocardial cell achieves normal growth in pre-adult life, how it replaces deteriorated sarcomeric units, and how it hypertrophies in disease states are subjects of special interest in this laboratory.

The Z band, the delimiting unit of the sarcomere, until now has been thought to perform a purely mechanical function in the cardiac cell, serving to anchor thin filaments in place in the sarcomeric unit.

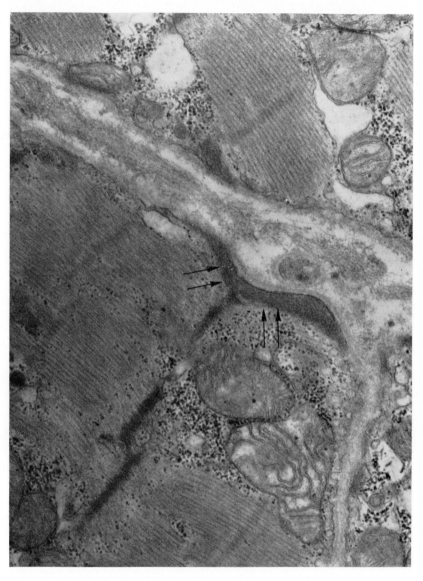

FIG. 1.13. This photomicrograph of human atrial tissue illustrates the arms of accumulated Z material which extend from the Z band (arrows) in either direction at the periphery of the cell, just under the sarcolemma. × 40,000.

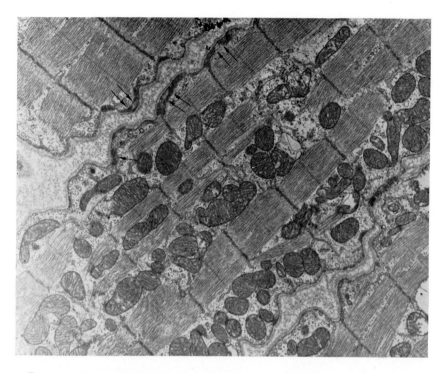

Fig. 1.14. Subsarcolemmal arches of Z substance (arrows) are clearly apparent in this electron micrograph of portions of three human atrial cells. × 1,250.

When we examined human myocardium from 22 patients obtained at the time of open heart surgery, with the collaboration of Dr. Marcia B. Bull, we found areas of accumulation or hypertrophy of Z substance in association with the cell membrane or sarcolemma and its derivative, the intercalated disc.

In Figure 1.13, immediately subjacent to the sarcolemma, we frequently observed Z bands which extended an arm in either direction to meet and apparently merge with a similar extension from an adjacent sarcomeric Z band (arrows).

The result was a series of arches of accumulated Z substance (Fig. 1.14) immediately under the sarcolemma (arrows). Similar areas of Z substance accumulation were identified at the desmosomal areas of the intercalated discs.

High power views of these subsarcolemmal areas revealed that the accumulations of Z substance were actually composed of a homogeneous mass of fine filaments embedded in an amorphous matrix (Fig. 1.15). These filaments had the same dimension as sarcomeric thin filaments but were more electron dense, or darker staining, than the usual thin filament.

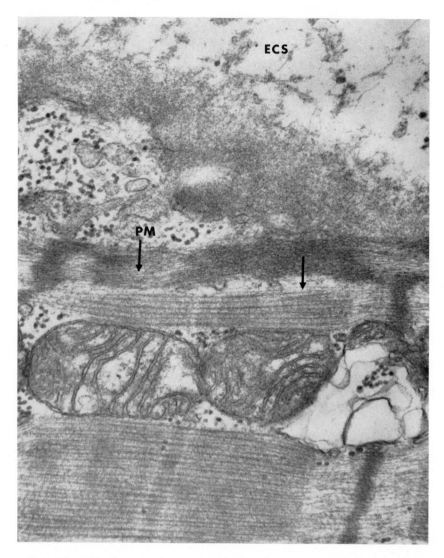

Fig. 1.15. This electron micrograph shows the homogeneous filaments (PM) embedded in amorphous Z substance which are apparent under the sarcolemma of this sarcomere from a human atrial cell. Note the fully differentiated thick and thin filaments that are being spun off the parent group of primary myofilaments (arrow). ECS, extracellular space. × 50,000.

At the periphery of the Z accumulation were myofilaments structurally indistinguishable from mature sarcomeric thick and thin filaments. These apparently new myofilaments or primary myofilaments (PM) were being laid down in register with the remainder of the sarcomeric unit. In addition

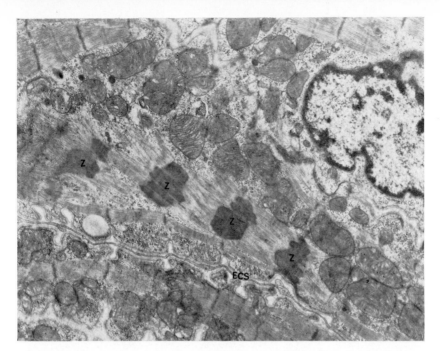

FIG. 1.16. This electron micrograph illustrates a portion of an atrial cell from a child with Tetralogy of Fallot. Bilaterally symmetrical areas of Z substance accumulation 10 to 15 times the size of the normal Z band are apparent (Z) deep within the cell. × 2,000.

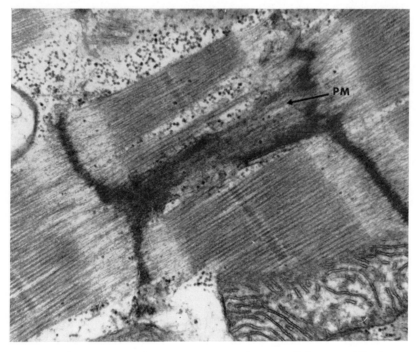

FIG. 1.17. This is a photomicrograph of a deeply intracellular area of Z substance which is differentiating into primary myofilaments (PM). Note the fully formed thick and thin filaments which are adjacent to the parent unit. × 3,000.

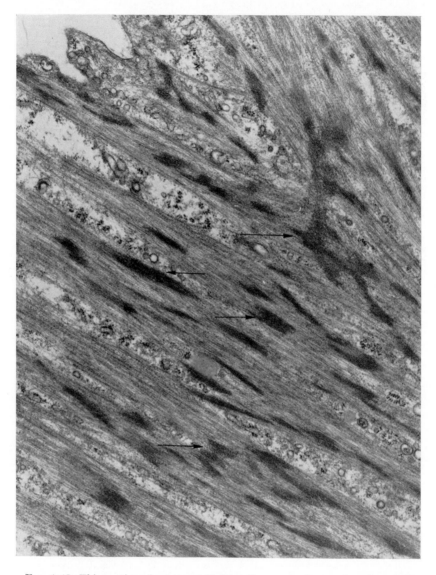

Fig. 1.18. This portion of a rat ventricular cell grown in tissue culture is remarkable for the abundant plaques of Z substance (arrows) distributed throughout the cytoplasm. × 12,000.

to subsarcolemmal accumulations of Z substance there were deeply intracellular areas of accumulated Z material (Fig. 1.16). These varied from subtle, fusiform swellings to complex and very symmetrical areas 10 to 15 times as large as the normal Z band diameter (Z).

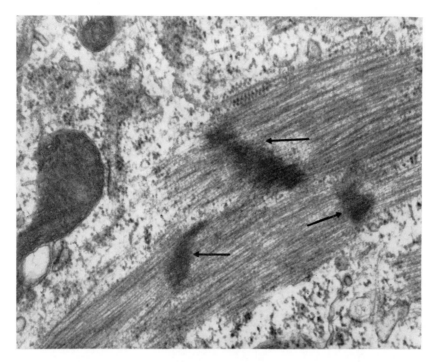

F_{IG}. 1.19. In this high power view of one of the areas of Z accumulations seen in a rat ventricular tissue culture cell, it is clear that the two separating areas of Z substance are connected by primary myofilaments which are identical to those seen in human myocardium (see text). × 52,000.

In other areas, Z accumulations extended across the sarcomere (Fig. 1.17) and clearly contained filaments exactly like those produced at the periphery of the cell (PM). Fully differentiated thick and thin filaments were being spun off the mass of accumulated Z substance.

The Z band then, is intimately involved in the production of new sarcomeric units. To support this thesis, we examined the pattern of myofilament production in rat ventricular cells grown in tissue culture. The abundance of Z substance present in these early cells, which were actively engaged in myofilament production, was clearly apparent (Figs. 1.18 and 1.19, arrows). Configurations exactly analogous to those found in human myocardium, in which Z accumulations were separating and/or being consumed in the midline to produce filaments, were everywhere in the myoblast. An exactly similar pattern of Z substance hypertrophy and conversion into primitive filaments was a frequent finding in the myocardium of 24-hour-old dogs, whose actively growing myocardium bridged the gap between the primitive situation of tissue culture and adult, presumably fully grown, heart muscle cells.

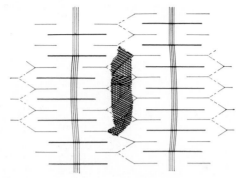

Fig. 1.20. Stage I: early hypertrophy of Z substance.

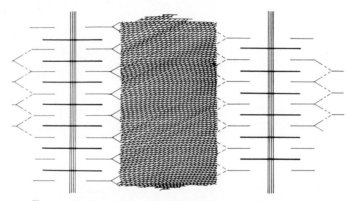

Fig. 1.21. Stage II: maximal hypertrophy of Z substance.

The actual mechanism of how the normal Z band proliferates and is transformed into, or at least is a major contributor to the formation of, a new sarcomeric unit is envisioned by us to be as follows.

Huxley has pointed out that the Z disc essentially consists of two halves, each one a mirror image of the other. This is necessary to assure the proper alignment of the thin filaments in the sarcomere so that their movement will occur in the proper, which is to say opposite, direction. It is obvious that, if all thin filaments moved in the same direction, no sarcomeric and hence no total muscle shortening could ever occur.

The concept of the Z disc as composed of two matched halves, together with the extraordinary and consistent symmetry of the accumulated masses of Z substance, suggested that Z band proliferation begins at the midline and that the matched halves of the Z disc grow at exactly the same rate at any given level in the Z band (Fig. 1.20).

In Figure 1.21, Z band hypertrophy is maximal. If proliferation did not begin centrally but peripherally, the I bands and even the A bands of adjacent sarcomeres would be consumed as Z substance began to accumulate.

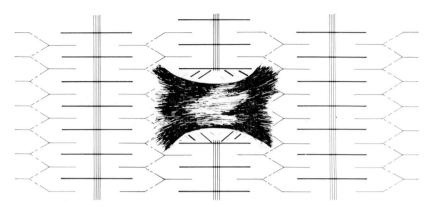

F*IG*. 1.22. Stage III: differentiation of Z substance into primary myofilaments.

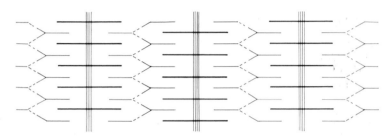

F*IG*. 1.23. Stage IV: production of finished sarcomere.

This is never seen. It is as though the Z disc pushes the adjacent I band as it grows and, when it reaches its maximal size, is then converted or transformed into true filaments, producing a new sarcomeric unit (Figs. 1.22 and 1.23).

The Z band, then, far from being only a mechanical anchor in the cell, is actually the generative source of new sarcomeric units which are added to the normally growing or hypertrophying cell, or to a cell in which repair of pre-existing units is essential.

To summarize, we have tried to give some insight into the fundamental anatomy of the mammalian myocardial cell population and into the function of subcellular systems. It is becoming more and more apparent that no one theory of how the cell achieves and supports excitation, contraction, and relaxation will be adequate for the heterogeneous population of the heart. Moreover, pre-existing concepts of the function of subcellular components, such as the sarcomeric Z band, must always be open to constant revision and expansion if our understanding of the heart at a cellular level is to continue to progress at the remarkable rate at which it has moved over the past decade of investigation.

This work is supported by a grant-in-aid from the New York Heart Association.

2

Factors Regulating the Oxygen Consumption of the Heart

JOHN ROSS, JR., M.D.

One of the areas in which an understanding of physiological principles can contribute importantly to appropriate clinical therapy is the control of cardiac oxygen consumption. In recent years, a considerable body of new information has been gathered, and it is the purpose of this brief review to consider the relative importance of four key determinants of myocardial oxygen utilization ($M\dot{V}O_2$) in several therapeutic settings.

In analyzing the role of these factors, it should be recalled at the outset that the left ventricle exhibits a basal O_2 utilization, which can be measured experimentally in the potassium-arrested heart or after calcium removal. This basal O_2 usage, averaging 1.5 ml. of O_2 per 100 g. of left ventricle (LV) per minute,[1, 2] comprises somewhat less than 20 per cent of the 7 to 8 ml. per 100 g. LV of O_2 used per minute by the beating heart.[3] There is also a small energy cost for electrical and chemical excitation, the so-called activation energy, as yet unmeasured in the intact heart. In addition to these factors, four major determinants of $M\dot{V}O_2$ that assume importance clinically can be identified, all being related primarily to events surrounding the mechanical function of the heart in the resting subject and during various forms of physiological stress. It is of interest that these major determinants are closely related to the factors which affect the performance of the left ventricle, the preload, the afterload, the inotropic state, and the heart rate.[4]

These four determinants of $M\dot{V}O_2$, shown in Figure 2.1, include the heart rate, the wall tension, the myocardial inotropic state, and fiber shortening against a load (the Fenn effect).

HEART RATE

It has been known for many years that $M\dot{V}O_2$ varies directly with the heart rate in the intact circulation over a wide range of rates.[5, 6] Recently this relationship was re-examined in an experimental preparation which

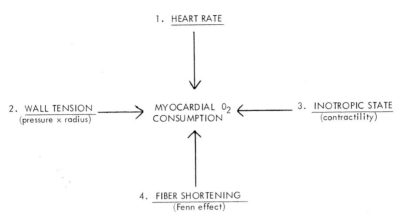

FIG. 2.1. Four major determinants of the oxygen consumption (MV̇O₂) of the intact heart.

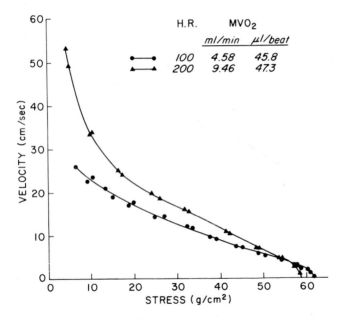

FIG. 2.2. Force-velocity relations in the isovolumetric canine left ventricle at heart rates (H.R.) of 100 to 200 beats per minute. Velocity = calculated contractile element velocity; stress = force per unit area. Myocardial oxygen consumption per 100 g. of left ventricular weight is expressed as both milliliters per minute and microliters per beat. Peak tension was held relatively constant by regulating ventricular volume, and it is apparent that the velocity of shortening was elevated at the higher heart rate, indicating an increase in inotropic state. (Reproduced by permission from Boerth, R. C., Covell, J. W., Pool, P. E., and Ross, J., Jr.: Circ. Res. 24: 725–734, 1969.[9])

allowed control of two other major determinants of MVO₂, the peak wall tension and the amount of fiber shortening. With the latter two factors held constant in the isovolumetrically contracting left ventricle of the dog, the heart rate was varied.[7] As shown in Figure 2.2, the force-velocity relation was shifted upward and to the right at a constant peak tension, the increased velocity at low levels of tension indicating an enhanced inotropic state. Concomitantly, upon changing the average heart rate from 100 to 200 per minute, the MVO₂ more than doubled, indicating that there also was a modest increase in oxygen consumption per beat.[7] This finding was attributed to the effect of doubling the number of contractions per minute and to the added affect of increased inotropic state (mediated through the force-frequency relation) as discussed further below. Therefore, the heart rate is an extremely important determinant of oxygen usage, a doubling of heart rate resulting in more than a doubling of the MVO₂ (Fig. 2.3).

MYOCARDIAL WALL TENSION

A number of investigators have demonstrated the relation between MVO₂ and the wall tension developed by the left ventricle, increasing wall tension

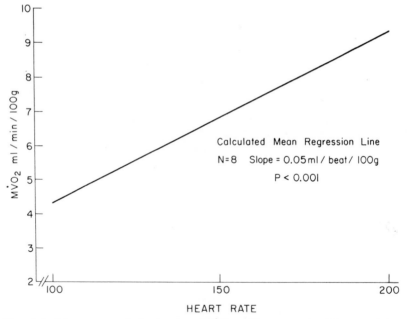

FIG. 2.3. The average relation between MVO₂ and heart rate in eight experiments in the isovolumetrically contracting canine left ventricle. It can be seen that a doubling of the heart rate results in a somewhat more than doubling of the MVO₂ (see text). (Reproduced by permission from Boerth *et al.*[9])

causing a substantial augmentation of $M\dot{V}O_2$.[8, 9] Indeed, earlier workers had already demonstrated clearly the relation between systolic arterial pressures and cardiac oxygen utilization,[10, 11] and until recently it was considered that the product of systolic pressure and heart rate,[12] or the area under the pressure pulse (the tension-time index),[13] always correlated closely with the $M\dot{V}O_2$. While this relation holds under many conditions, particularly in isolated heart preparations in which inotropic state is constant, other studies had suggested that in the intact circulation another factor must be operative as well.[14-16]

THE INOTROPIC STATE

Accordingly, using an experimental preparation in which the other major determinants of $M\dot{V}O_2$ could be controlled, the effects of variations in the inotropic state of the myocardium on $M\dot{V}O_2$ were examined.[17] With heart rate, systemic arterial pressure, and stroke volume held relatively constant, agents having a positive inotropic effect on the myocardium such as calcium and the catecholamines were shown to effect a pronounced augmentation of $M\dot{V}O_2$. In this hemodynamically controlled preparation, the major expression of the positive inotropic effect on the left ventricle was an increased velocity of contraction (increased LV dp/dt and ejection rate) and, since the duration of systole was shortened, the augmentation in $M\dot{V}O_2$ was accompanied by a significant reduction in the tension-time index.[17] Subsequently, it was also shown that, in the normal heart, digitalis[18] and other positive inotropic agents[19] exerted a similar effect, whereas agents having a negative inotropic influence resulted in a decrease in $M\dot{V}O_2$.[20] These variations in the inotropic state, which can affect the $M\dot{V}O_2$ by more than 100 per cent when other factors are controlled, are summarized in Figure 2.4.

SHORTENING AGAINST A LOAD (THE FENN EFFECT)

It is well established that when cardiac work is increased by augmenting the cardiac output with systemic pressure maintained relatively constant, the $M\dot{V}O_2$ increase is small compared with that induced when the cardiac work is increased by elevating aortic pressure and maintaining the cardiac output constant.[13, 15] Nevertheless, studies in skeletal muscle by Fenn,[22] also now confirmed in principle in isolated cardiac muscle by studies which compared isometric with isotonic contractions at the same tension levels,[23] indicated that there is an added energy cost of shortening against load. Recently, such studies have been extended to the whole heart, using a preparation which allowed the production of isovolumetric left ventricular contractions or contractions that shortened isotonically against the same wall tension.[24] It was shown that shortening, or volume work, contributes about 15 per cent to the oxygen cost of an average cardiac contraction,[25] demonstrating the operation of the Fenn effect in the intact ventricle.

CLINICAL SIGNIFICANCE

What are the clinical implications of these effects on the $M\dot{V}O_2$? Since the interplay between the four determinants can be complex in any given therapeutic setting, it is well to consider first their role in some relatively simple

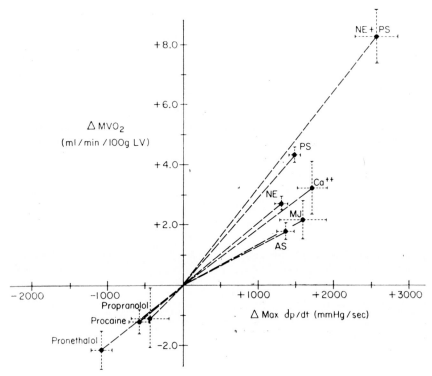

Fig. 2.4. Changes in myocardial oxygen consumption (Δ $M\dot{V}O_2$) in a positive and negative direction induced by various inotropic agents in the isovolumetric canine left ventricle in which heart rate and wall tension were held constant. Changes in the inotropic state of the myocardium in a positive and negative direction are indicated by the changes in maximal rate of rise of the left ventricular pressure pulse (Δ max dp/dt). Depression of the myocardium was induced acutely by large doses of either propranolol, procaine amide, or pronethalol, whereas positive inotropic stimulation was provided by acetylstrophanthidin (AS), calcium, paired electrical stimulation of the heart (PS), norepinephrine (NE), or a combination of the latter two. It can be seen that enhancement of the inotropic state can cause a large increase of $M\dot{V}O_2$, whereas depression of the inotropic state causes a reduction in $M\dot{V}O_2$. (Reproduced by permission from Graham, T. P., Ross, J., Jr., Covell, J. W., Sonnenblick, E. H., and Clancy, R. L.: Circ. Res. 21: 123–138, 1967.[21])

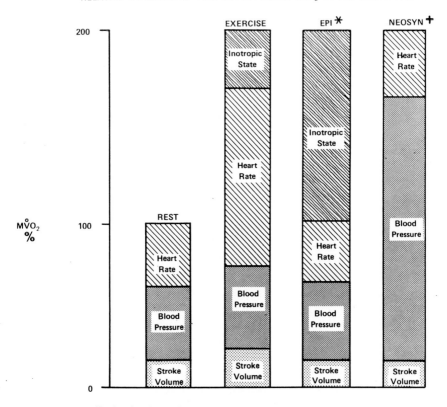

RELATIVE INFLUENCE OF FACTORS AFFECTING MV̇O₂ IN THE NORMAL HEART

Basal and activation O₂ consumption not shown
* Heart Rate and Blood Pressure controlled
+ Heart Rate and Stroke Volume controlled

Fig. 2.5. The estimated relative contributions of the four major determinants of MV̇O₂ under several conditions (see text). EPI, epinephrine; NEOSYN, neosynephrine.

examples. Figure 2.5 shows diagrammatically estimated contributions of these four factors to the MV̇O₂, the oxygen requirements of the non-beating heart having been omitted. In the left-hand bar, in the basal or resting state a certain proportion of the MV̇O₂ can be assigned to the heart rate, a portion to the blood pressure, and a small percentage to shortening or stroke volume. In the normal subject under these conditions, sympathetic tone to the myocardium and circulating catecholamine levels are minimal and, since the intrinsic effect of inotropic state on MV̇O₂ is difficult to estimate, no value has been given to this determinant in the resting state. One of the center bars shows a situation in which stimulation of the inotropic state of the myocardium alone by epinephrine has caused a marked augmentation of $\text{M}\dot{\text{V}}\text{O}_2$, while heart rate and blood pressure remained constant or were held relatively unchanged. In the right-hand bar, a marked increase in blood pressure (wall tension) alone, as could occur during a physiological stress such as isometric exercise or during the infusion of an alpha adrenergic stimulating agent such as neosynephrine under conditions of relatively constant heart rate, has markedly augmented $\text{M}\dot{\text{V}}\text{O}_2$. Finally, in the remaining center bar, the more complex effect of a mild level of supine muscular exercise is illustrated. In this example, the increase of $\text{M}\dot{\text{V}}\text{O}_2$ has been brought about primarily by an increase in heart rate but also through stimulation of the myocardial inotropic state by increased sympathetic nerve discharge and by circulating catecholamines, as well as by a mild increase in blood pressure and stroke volume.

Given these relations, it can be recognized readily how beta adrenergic receptor blockade with propranolol during exercise can limit the heart rate increase and the effects of enhanced inotropic state mediated by the sympathetic nervous system, thereby reducing the mechanical and metabolic activity of the myocardium and alleviating or preventing angina pectoris. Stimulation of the carotid sinus nerves[26] may also affect $\text{M}\dot{\text{V}}\text{O}_2$ and relieve angina during exercise by slowing the heart rate and reducing the level of inotropic state, as well as by modifying exercise-induced elevations of blood pressure through reflex withdrawal of sympathetic tone to the peripheral arterioles.

Another therapeutic situation in which the interaction between two or more determinants of $\text{M}\dot{\text{V}}\text{O}_2$ may be of importance is the administration of digitalis to the failing heart. As mentioned, digitalis like other positive inotropic agents causes a pronounced augmentation of oxygen utilization in the normal canine heart.[20] However, this observation was at variance with studies in the isolated supported heart which suggested that digitalis did not affect oxygen utilization.[27] Accordingly, we postulated that in the failing and dilated heart the interplay between two factors, the wall tension and the inotropic state, could counterbalance one another after digitalis administration. This proved to be the case, as shown in Figure 2.6. In the normal dog heart with heart rate and blood pressure controlled, the administration of acetylstrophanthidin produced an increase in $\text{M}\dot{\text{V}}\text{O}_2$ with little change in the left ventricular end-diastolic pressure or the calculated systolic wall tension. However, when cardiac failure and dilatation, with left ventricular end-diastolic pressures in excess of 25 mm. Hg, were induced by barbiturate infusion, digitalis increased the inotropic state (reflected by an increased LV dp/dt and a substantial decrease in the left ventricular end-diastolic pressure), but no change or slight fall in the $\text{M}\dot{\text{V}}\text{O}_2$ occurred.[20] Therefore, the effects of stimulating the inotropic state on $\text{M}\dot{\text{V}}\text{O}_2$

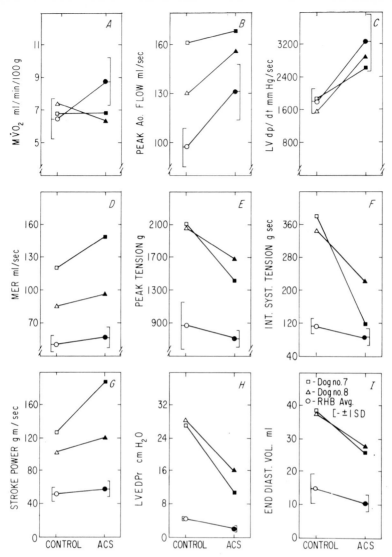

FIG. 2.6. The effects of digitalis preparation, acetylstrophanthidin (ACS) in normal and acutely failing canine left ventricles. The open symbols represent the control state prior to digitalis administration, and the closed symbols represent the conditions after digitalis administration. The average values in a group of normal animals (panel A) show the increase in myocardial oxygen consumption (MV̇O₂) with an increased speed of left ventricular contraction (peak flow rate), LV dp/dt, and mean ejection rate (MER) while peak and integrated systolic wall tension changed only slightly in the normal heart; likewise, there was only a small change in the left ventricular end-diastolic (DIAST.) pressure and volume in the normal group. In contrast, two animals with acute heart failure (triangles and squares) exhibited no change or a fall in MV̇O₂ after digitalis administration, despite increases in the speed of contraction produced by this agent. In contrast to the normal group, however, a large fall in systolic wall tension occurred (panels E and F), accompanied by a large drop in diastolic left ventricular end-diastolic pressure (LVEDPr) (panel H). This effect presumably counterbalanced the influence of increased inotropic state on MV̇O₂ (see text). (Reproduced by permission from Covell, J. W., Braunwald, E., Ross, J., Jr., and Sonnenblick, E. H.: J. Clin. Invest. 45: 1535–1542, 1966.[20])

undoubtedly were offset by the marked reduction in systolic wall tension that occurred.

Acute myocardial infarction provides another clinical setting in which interaction between these variables could be of considerable importance. It can be suspected that with acute myocardial infarction there are regions of inadequately perfused tissue directly adjacent to the area of damage in which the balance between oxygen supply and demand could be critical to the ultimate survival of that tissue. Therefore, it seemed possible that altering the oxygen requirements of myocardium surrounding an infarct might increase or decrease the size of the involved area.[28] This supposition recently has been demonstrated to be correct in the normal dog heart, in which experimental ligation of the anterior descending coronary artery was produced. Before and during the occlusion, the area of infarction was measured by the extent and degree of ST segment elevation at multiple epicardial sites over the surface of the left ventricle. After recovery from the initial ligation, the experiment was then repeated during isoproterenol infusion (which increased $M\dot{V}O_2$ by augmentation of heart rate and the inotropic state), and a substantial increase in the area of ST segment involvement and in the average height of ST elevation was observed (Fig. 2.7).[29] That this intervention had caused an increase in the size of the infarcted area was confirmed by demonstrating a reduction of the intracellular enzyme creatine phosphokinase (CPK) in the myocardium underlying the abnormal epicardial sites 24 hours later, and a close correlation was shown between the amount of ST segment change and degree of CPK reduction.[29, 30] Therefore, it may be surmised that increased oxygen requirements in marginally perfused areas had caused an extension of the myocardial infarction. In addition, it was shown in normal dog hearts that administration of the beta adrenergic blocking agent propranolol reduced the size of the involved area.[29] Caution should be exercised in extending such observations to patients with acute myocardial infarction, however, since in the failing or dilated heart (as discussed above), the ventricular wall tension may be elevated and positive inotropic agents such as digitalis can exert opposite effects on $M\dot{V}O_2$ under such circumstances (Fig. 2.6).[20, 31] Patients with acute myocardial infarction frequently have associated left ventricular failure,[32] and clearly it will be necessary to evaluate such agents in the clinical setting. Nevertheless, it seems reasonable to expect that measures to improve the balance between oxygen supply and demand in surviving myocardium could well prove beneficial in patients with acute myocardial infarction.

From these examples, it is apparent that the interaction between the major determinants of $M\dot{V}O_2$ and cardiac performance can be of great importance in various cardiac disease states. The operation of the physiological variables discussed is relatively straightforward, and their application

DOG E7

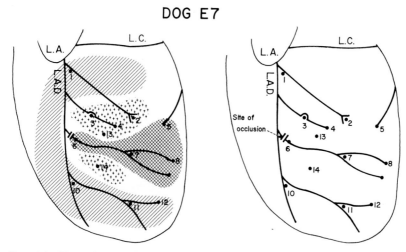

F<small>IG</small>. 2.7. Example of studies by Maroko and co-workers[29] using 12 epicardial ECG leads on the surface of the canine left ventricle at numbered sites, making use of anatomic landmarks as shown in the right-hand panel. L.A.D., left anterior descending coronary artery; L.C., left circumflex coronary artery. The site of occlusion of a branch of the anterior descending coronary is shown. A control map prior to occlusion is obtained, the average ST segment elevation is calculated, and the number of sites involved is determined. The surface mapping is then repeated 15 minutes after the coronary occlusion. The ligature is then released and, when control conditions again obtain, the occlusion is repeated during an isoproterenol infusion, an intervention designed to increase $M\dot{V}O_2$. In the left-hand panel, the double-cross hatched area shows the extent of ischemic ST segment change during the first period of occlusion, sites 5, 6, 7, and 8 showing significant ST segment elevation. A repeat occlusion during the isoproterenol infusion now shows involvement not only in sites 5 through 8 but also in those contained in the area encompassed by the crosses, indicating an increase in the area of myocardial injury. That the isoproterenol infusion did not affect normal myocardium was indicated by the fact that, in the diagonally shaded area, sites 1, 10, 11, and 12 remained without ST segment elevation throughout all of the interventions.

can considerably enhance the understanding of the effects of various forms of therapy.

SUMMARY

Four major determinants of myocardial oxygen consumption ($M\dot{V}O_2$) are discussed. Each of these factors, the heart rate, wall tension, myocardial inotropic state, and fiber shortening against a load (the Fenn effect) can independently affect the $M\dot{V}O_2$. The interactions between these factors and the determinants of ventricular performance are considered in relation to the therapy of angina pectoris, to the use of digitalis in the failing heart, and to the survival of myocardial tissue in acute experimental myocardial infarction.

This research was supported in part by National Heart and Lung Institute Program Project Grant HE 12373 and National Heart and Lung Institute Contract PH 68-43-1332.

REFERENCES

1. Klocke, F. J., Kaiser, G. A., Ross, J., Jr., and Braunwald, E.: Mechanism of increase of myocardial oxygen uptake produced by catecholamines. Amer. J. Physiol. 209: 913–918, 1965.

2. Kohn, R. M.: Myocardial oxygen uptake during ventricular fibrillation and electromechanical dissociation. Amer. J. Cardiol. 11: 483–486, 1963.

3. Bing, R. J.: The coronary circulation in health and disease as studied by coronary sinus catheterization. Bull. N. Y. Acad. Med. 27: 407, 1951.

4. Messer, J. W., and Neill, W. A.: The oxygen supply of the human heart. Amer. J. Cardiol. 9: 384–394, 1962.

5. Ross, J., Jr.: The assessment of myocardial performance in man by hemodynamic and cineangiographic techniques. Amer. J. Cardiol. 23: 511–515, 1969.

6. Braunwald, E., Ross, J., Jr., and Sonnenblick, E. H.: Mechanisms of contraction of the normal and failing heart. New Engl. J. Med. Medical Progress Series. Little, Brown and Company, Boston, 1968.

7. Laurent, D., Bolene-Williams, C., Williams, F. L., and Katz, L. N.: Effects of heart rate on coronary flow and cardiac oxygen consumption. Amer. J. Physiol. 185: 355, 1956.

8. Maxwell, G. M., Castillo, C. A., White, D. H., Jr., Crumpton, C. W., and Rowe, G. G.: Induced tachycardia: its effect upon the coronary hemodynamics, myocardial metabolism and cardiac efficiency of the intact dog. J. Clin. Invest. 37: 1413, 1958.

9. Boerth, R. C., Covell, J. W., Pool, P. E., and Ross, J., Jr.: Increased myocardial oxygen consumption and contractile state associated with increased heart rate in dogs. Circ. Res. 24: 725–734, 1969.

10. Monroe, R. G., and French, G. N.: Left ventricular pressure-volume relationships and myocardial oxygen consumption in the isolated heart. Circ. Res. 9: 362, 1961.

11. Graham, T. P., Jr., Covell, J. W., Sonnenblick, E. H., Ross, J., Jr., and Braunwald, E.: Control of myocardial oxygen consumption: relative influence of contractile state and tension development. J. Clin. Invest. 47: 375–385, 1968.

12. Rohde, E.: Uber den Einfluss der mechanischen Bedingungen auf die Tatigkeit und den Sauerstoffverbrauch das Warmbluterherzens. Arch. Exp. Pathol. Pharmacol. 68: 401, 1912.

13. Evans, C. L., and Matsuoka, Y.: The effect of various mechanical conditions on the gaseous metabolism and efficiency of the mammalian heart. J. Physiol. 49: 378, 1915.

14. Katz, L. N., and Feinberg, H.: The relation of cardiac effort to myocardial oxygen consumption and coronary flow. Circ. Res. 6: 656, 1958.

15. Sarnoff, S. J., Braunwald, E., Welch, G. H., Jr., Case, R. B., Stainsby, W. N., and Macruz, R.: Hemodynamic determinants of oxygen consumption of the heart with special reference to the tension-time index. Amer. J. Physiol. 192: 148, 1958.

16. Granata, L., Olsson, R. A., Huves, A., and Gregg, D. E.: Coronary inflow and

oxygen usage following cardiac sympathetic nerve stimulation in unanesthetized dogs. Circ. Res. 16: 114, 1965.

17. Krasnow, N., Rollett, E. L., Yurchak, P. M., Hood, W. B., Jr., and Gorlin, R.: Isoproterenol and cardiovascular performance. Amer. J. Med. 37: 514, 1964.

18. Ross, J., Jr., Sonnenblick, E. H., Kaiser, E. H., Frommer, G. A., and Braunwald, E.: Electroaugmentation of ventricular performance and oxygen consumption by repetitive application of paired electrical stimuli. Circ. Res. 16: 332–341, 1965.

19. Sonnenblick, E. H., Ross, J., Jr., Covell, J. W., Kaiser, G. A., and Braunwald, E.: Velocity of contraction as a determinant of myocardial oxygen consumption. Amer. J. Physiol. 209: 919, 1965.

20. Covell, J. W., Braunwald, E., Ross, J., Jr., and Sonnenblick, E. H.: Studies on digitalis. XVI. Effects on myocardial oxygen consumption. J. Clin. Invest. 45: 1535–1542, 1966.

21. Graham, T. P., Jr., Ross, J., Jr., Covell, J. W., Sonnenblick, E. H., and Clancy, R. L.: Myocardial oxygen consumption in acute experimental cardiac depression. Circ. Res. 21: 123–138, 1967.

22. Fenn, W. O.: A quantitative comparison between the energy liberated and the work performed by the isolated sartorius muscle of the frog. J. Physiol. (London) 58: 175–203, 1923.

23. Coleman, H. N.: Effect of alterations in shortening and external work on oxygen consumption of cat papillary muscle. Amer. J. Physiol. 214: 100–106, 1968.

24. Covell, J. W., Fuhrer, J. S., Boerth, R. C., and Ross, J., Jr.: The production of isotonic contractions in the intact canine left ventricle. J. Appl. Physiol. 27: 577–581, 1969.

25. Burns, J. W., and Covell, J. W.: A comparison of the energy cost of external and tension generation work in the canine left ventricle. Fed. Proc. 29: no. 2, 450 (abstract) 1970.

26. Braunwald, E., Epstein, S. E., Glick, G., Wechsler, A. S., and Braunwald, N. S.: Relief of angina pectoris by electrical stimulation of the carotid-sinus nerves. New Engl. Med. 277: 1278, 1967.

27. Sarnoff, S. J., Gilmore, J. P., Wallace, A. G., Skinner, N. S., Jr., Mitchell, J. H., and Daggett, W. M.: Effects of acetyl strophanthidin therapy on cardiac dynamics, oxygen consumption and efficiency in the isolated heart with and without hypoxia. Amer. J. Med. 37: 3, 1964.

28. Braunwald, E., Covell, J. W., Maroko, P. R., and Ross, J., Jr.: Effects of drugs and of counterpulsation on myocardial oxygen consumption: observations on the ischemic heart. Amer. Heart Assoc. Monograph 27, pp. 220–228, Suppl. IV to Circulation, Vols. 39 and 40, Nov. 1969.

29. Maroko, P. R., Kjekshus, J. K., Sobel, B. E., Watanabe, T., Covell, J. W., Ross, J., Jr., and Braunwald, E.: Factors influencing infarct size following experimental coronary artery occlusions. Circulation 43: 67–81, 1971.

30. Kjekshus, J. K., and Sobel, B. E.: Depressed myocardial creatine phosphokinase activity following experimental myocardial infarction. Circ. Res. 27: 403, 1970.

31. Watanabe, T., Covell, J. W., Maroko, P. R., Braunwald, E., and Ross, J. Jr.: Effects of increased arterial pressure and digitalis on the severity of myocardial ischemia in the normal and failing heart (in preparation).

32. Karliner, J. S., and Ross, J., Jr.: Left ventricular performance after acute myocardial infarction. Progr. Cardiovasc. Dis. 13: no. 4, 374, 1971.

3

The Metabolic Basis and Management of Inherited Premature Ischemic Heart Disease

ROBERT I. LEVY, M.D. AND NEIL J. STONE, M.D.

Ischemic heart disease (IHD) is the leading cause of death in the United States. In the 10-year period between 1953 and 1963, it was the only cause of cardiovascular mortality which failed to decline.[1] Of even more concern is the fact that each year over 165,000 Americans die prematurely (before age 65) of IHD. These premature deaths and the even larger group of patients with premature IHD morbidity thus create a problem area of major medical proportions and socioeconomic importance.

The current attack on IHD has attempted to focus attention on those "risk factors" associated with accelerated or premature IHD and sudden death (attributable to IHD about 60 per cent of the time).[2] It is generally felt that, by so doing, not only can the subjects at increased risk be identified early but the basic pathogenesis of IHD might be unraveled. Inherent to this approach is the concept of decreasing risk through medical intervention. This latter concept thereby provides a rationale for therapeutic intervention trials designed to decrease mortality.

Atherosclerosis is clearly the predominant cause of IHD, often involving the major ramifications of the epicardial portions of the coronary tree. Other causes of premature IHD are as follows. (1) Congenital abnormalities of the coronary arteries.[3] Major anomalies include those of anomalous origin, hypoplasia, atresia, and even absence of one coronary artery, usually the right. When one major orifice serves all coronary vessels, the development of atherosclerosis will make the patient particularly vulnerable. Minor anomalies consist of multiple highly variable locations of coronary ostia from the sinus of Valsalva that, although apparently benign, may influence the course of coronary artery obstruction and the development of collaterals in a deleterious fashion. Abnormal communications may produce functioning arteriovenous fistulas with subsequent IHD. (2) Less well understood or less well proven factors such as diabetic microcirculation changes,[3] and vasculitides and embolic phenomena relating to the coronary circulation. (3) Situations in which increased myocardial demand outstrips available coronary blood flow, as in aortic valve disease, mitral insufficiency, hypertension, and left ventricular hypertrophy.

RISK FACTORS

Numerous risk factors have been identified as occurring frequently with premature atherosclerotic IHD. Comprehensive reviews of risk factors and IHD are available.[4-7] All major investigators agree that subjects with **elevated cholesterol concentrations** run an increased risk. This is especially true of those with high cholesterols below age 50. Cornfield's analysis of statistics from the prospective Framingham study suggested that the risk of IHD was proportional to the cube of the serum cholesterol concentration.[8] This translated into a postulated 35 per cent decline in risk if a 15 per cent fall in serum cholesterol concentration could be achieved. Although essentially all epidemiological studies in man have identified cholesterol as a risk factor, no study has reported any absolute cutoff for serum cholesterol that could be used to identify susceptibles.

The Framingham data also suggest **elevations in both systolic and diastolic blood pressure** (BP) as risk factors for IHD.[19] Study of a Chicago labor force also noted that **hypertension** was associated with an increased rate of new heart attacks and sudden death.[10] In Los Angeles, an increased rate of angina pectoris has been documented in hypertensives over age 40 when compared to matched controls, although no difference in heart attack rate was seen in men under 60.[11] Seasonal changes in BP have been reported in a prospective study,[12] and it has been suggested that these changes explain differences between studies.

Epstein has demonstrated the striking differentials that can be obtained using only serum cholesterol and BP as risk factors. He calculated that, of the 30 out of 100 American men who will develop IHD prior to age 65, 20 will have either high cholesterol or BP elevations.[5] With the Framingham data in hand, it can be shown that the combination of hypertension and high cholesterol in any subject is more than additive as a risk factor.

Subjects with **diabetes** have been shown to have occurrence rates of IHD almost twice that of nondiabetics.[10] The Framingham data suggest that not only do diabetics have an increased rate of IHD but they appear to be susceptible to a lethal outcome.[19] It has been suggested that microangiopathy affecting vasa vasorum of the coronary arterial wall can produce ischemic injury resulting in the diabetic predilection for IHD.[13] Obesity is an important risk factor for diabetes and hyperlipidemia but not for IHD.[14, 15] The alleged differences in mortality rates between obese and non-obese individuals seem to reflect only the association that increased weight has with increased cholesterol and BP.[11] **Hyperuricemia**[19] and hemoglobin levels of greater than 17 g. per ml[14] have been reported by some to identify those at risk for IHD.

Interest in **familial factors** resulted in a recent study from Tecumseh, Michigan. It was shown that fatal IHD was commonest when parental death from IHD occurred before age 65 and rarest when due to other causes. Both cholesterol and sugar elevations were prominent in the group experiencing early, fatal IHD.[16]

There are other environmental factors that appear to enhance the risk of IHD without promoting atherosclerosis. The greatly increased risk in IHD mortality from **cigarette smoking** has been shown to be transient, non-cumulative, and unrelated to cigar smoking.[19] **Physical activity** appears to exert a protective effect on those who develop IHD. Studies of West Coast longshoremen revealed physical activity to be independent of other risk factors such as high BP and cigarette smoking.[17] Indirect measurements of stress such as coffee and tea consumption, marital status, and family size did not correlate with IHD.[19] Methodological problems have made those studies which relate personality traits or occupational stress to IHD of questionable scientific validity.[18] Selye has emphasized the importance of **stress** in its own right as a relevant cause for cardiac necroses, mediated by catecholamines.[19] Studies which reveal that 25 per cent of patients dying from IHD have no demonstrable acute occlusion at autopsy might be considered as evidence in support of this contention.[20]

Cholesterol as a Risk Factor

Although cholesterol has been identified as a major risk factor, it has become evident that the finding of an elevated plasma concentration of cholesterol does not define a specific disease entity. Hypercholesterolemia, like fever, is an outward sign of a heterogenous group of disorders that differ in many ways. All of the blood fats including cholesterol circulate in the blood bound to protein. Translation of hypercholesterolemia into hyperlipoproteinemia is now considered essential for the specific diagnosis and management of affected subjects.[21, 22] Of note is the fact that only certain types of hyperlipoproteinemia carry an increased risk of IHD.

Insight into the various mechanisms of hyperlipoproteinemia helps clarify the differences between the five types.[23] In Type I, there is an inability to clear dietary fat with a normal fat intake, and chylomicrons accumulate in the fasting plasma. In Type II, there is a defect in the metabolism of beta lipoproteins. This defect may represent increased synthesis of beta lipoproteins as occurs in porphyria or nephrosis, or decreased beta lipoprotein catabolism as occurs in familial Type II or myxedema. In Type III, abnormal beta lipoprotein forms are present in the plasma. In Type IV, there is a defect in the metabolism of endogenous glyceride. Prebeta lipoproteins (glycerides) accumulate in the plasma, often in the face of normal cholesterol concentrations. It is not clear whether familial Type IV results from increased glyceride production or decreased glyceride clearance (or even whether it represents a homogenous disorder). In Type V, the assimilation of plasma glycerides of exogenous and endogenous origin is delayed, and chylomicrons and prebeta lipoproteins accumulate.

Each of the five types is associated with specific clinical manifestations and secondary disorders. When primary, each is associated with a specific mode of inheritance, prognosis, and responsiveness to therapy. Types I and V do not appear to be associated with any increased risk of vascular disease despite often enormous elevations in glyceride and cholesterol concentrations. One might speculate that the large size of the particles accumulating in the plasma of these patients make them unlikely vehicles to penetrate the blood vessel lumen. Types II, III, and IV clearly appear to be associated with an increased risk of IHD, although the degree of risk, prognosis, responsiveness to intervention, inheritance, and epidemiological importance vary.

Type IV

Type IV hyperlipoproteinemia has been reported to occur frequently in subjects with IHD.[15, 24-27] The disorder is defined in terms of an age-adjusted increase in plasma triglyceride in fasting subjects who have neither chylomicronemia nor increased concentrations of beta lipoprotein.[23] Xanthomatosis is rarely found. Prevalent laboratory findings include hyperuricemia and abnormal glucose tolerance. It must be kept in mind that Type IV commonly is secondary to stress, alcoholism, obesity, and diabetes. When inherited, it appears to be transmitted as a Mendelian dominant trait with delayed expression or penetrance. Diagnosis of familial Type IV before age 25 cannot be made with certainty. Further study of this type is needed as it is not definitely proven that Type IV per se implies increased IHD risk and, in fact, what level of glyceride should be considered abnormal.

Type III

Type III hyperlipoproteinemia is a relatively uncommon form of hypercholesterolemia. Although it is occasionally secondary to myxedema or a dysproteinemia, it is usually familial. Demonstration of an abnormal beta lipoprotein which floats in the ultracentrifuge at serum density (d < 1.006) is the definitive diagnostic sign. Type III appears to be clearly associated with an increased risk of IHD,[23] as well as peripheral vessel disease.[28]

Males with Type III frequently present with claudication or angina between ages 25 and 35. Female patients seem to develop the signs and symptoms of this disorder some 15 to 25 years later. Tuboeruptive xanthomas of the elbows, knees, and buttocks as well as palmar xanthoma are frequent early signs of Type III. Type III subjects sometimes have hyperuricemia and glucose intolerance. An increased incidence of mild systolic hypertension in Type III subjects over age 40 seems best explained as secondary to the premature atherosclerosis. Although clearly familial, the exact mode of inheritance of Type III is not clear; it is infrequently diagnosed before age 20.

Type II

The clinical hallmark of Type II is xanthomatosis and/or accelerated atherosclerosis.[23] It is the most prevalent of the familial hyperlipoproteinemias; more than 200 of the 380 kindred with familial hyperlipoproteinemia diagnosed at the National Institutes of Health Clinical Center in the last 5 years have had Type II. The diagnosis is made by the demonstration of increased concentrations of plasma beta lipoproteins based upon age-corrected norms.[23] Early diagnosis is simple, and it can even be made with some certainty from umbilical cord blood.[29] In patients below age 20, a cholesterol concentration above 230 mg.% should make the diagnostician strongly suspect familial Type II.

The need for early diagnosis of Type II has gained impetus from the numerous reports which suggest an increased risk of sudden death and early mortality from IHD.[23, 30, 31] In a recent survey of affected Type II relatives of Type II propositi with xanthomatosis or IHD, the males had a mean age of IHD onset of 43 years, and almost three-quarters were dead of IHD by age 60.[31] The mean age of onset for females was 58 years, demonstrating the expected female lag in IHD incidence.

The reason why familial Type II has not previously been recognized as a pediatric problem is probably related to the **long latent period** between disease onset and complications. Only one of 117 children below age 20 in the NIH series of Type II patients had IHD.[29] That Type II is a pediatric problem is evident from the fact that in the third decade of life better than 20 per cent of affected Type II males have IHD.[16, 23] It is mandatory, therefore, to sample an affected subject's younger siblings and children; 50 per cent will have the same abnormality.

Diagnostic difficulties are less often encountered in the Type II homozygote. The cholesterol levels in childhood are in the range of 600 to 800 mg.%, and superficial planar xanthomas as well as tendon lesions occur over the extensor tendons of the hands, elbows, and heels. Fatal coronary disease before the second decade of life is not uncommon.[23]

MANAGEMENT[32, 33]

If typing merely allowed the differentiation of three different biochemical abnormalities associated with increased risk of IHD, it would be useful. That it helps define groups of patients that can effectively be treated by specific dietary and/or drug intervention makes it imperative.

Type II subjects respond best to a diet very low in cholesterol and high in polyunsaturated fats. With such treatment, cholesterol levels will fall by 15 to 25 per cent. In Type II, however, diet alone does not normalize the plasma lipids. The addition to diet of cholestyramine, a bile acid sequestrant, has allowed us to normalize cholesterol concentrations in essentially all heterozygous Type II subjects. With this therapy, resolution of external xanthomas occur. The effect of successful treatment on IHD risk awaits controlled study.

In Type III, reduction to ideal weight and then a diet balanced in fat and carbohydrate and low in cholesterol often will allow a normalization of blood lipids. Clofibrate is additive to diet and usually allows the maintenance of low normal lipids in these subjects. With therapy, xanthomatosis completely disappears,[23] and peripheral blood flow improves both objectively and subjectively.[28]

In Type IV, weight reduction often allows the complete normalization of blood lipids.[15] Maintenance diets somewhat restrictive in alcohol and carbohydrates help to sustain this effect. Neither cholestyramine nor clofibrate appears to be clearly efficacious in Type IV.

Cholesterol then is a major risk factor for IHD. The cutoff concentration for a safe or normal cholesterol is not clear. Some subjects with elevated blood lipids (outside the 90 per cent limits for the population) are clearly at a high risk for IHD. Of these types, Type II seems to be most important, especially to those interested in the early diagnosis and prevention of premature IHD. Although the prevalence of Type II remains to be established, its mode of inheritance and easy chemical diagnosis make its early detection possible. Detection is important since blood lipids in all of the types of hypercholesterolemia may be normalized with specific therapy. The effect of this lipid lowering on IHD, however, remains to be proven.

The identification of risk factors for IHD may make it possible to decrease and perhaps prevent premature IHD. The effectiveness of preventive therapy for those with both severe and mild hypertension has already been shown, as has the value of being a nonsmoker.[4] We now can effectively diagnose and treat specific types of hyperlipoproteinemia at risk for IHD. That such treatment will decrease the risk of IHD remains presumptive. If proven, we will have made effective inroads into premature IHD.

REFERENCES

1. Fredrickson, D. S.: Atherosclerosis and other forms of arteriosclerosis. In Wintrobe, M. M., Thorn, G. W., Adams, R. D., Bennett, I. L., Jr., Braunwald, E., Isselbacker, K. J., and Petersdorf, R. G. (eds.): *Harrison's Principles of Internal Medicine.* McGraw-Hill Book Company; New York, 1970.
2. Kuller, I., Lillienfeld, A., and Fisher, R.: Epidemiological study of sudden and unexpected deaths due to arteriosclerotic heart disease. Circulation 34: 1056, 1966.
3. Moore, C. B.: Unusual manifestations of coronary artery disease. Med. Clin. N. Amer. 51: 941, 1967.
4. Atherosclerosis Study Group and Epidemiology Study Group: Primary Prevention of the Atherosclerotic Diseases. Circulation 42: A-55, 1970.
5. Epstein, F. H.: Multiple risk factors and the prediction of coronary heart disease. Bull. N. Y. Acad. Med. 44: 916, 1968.
6. Epstein, F. H.: The epidemiology of coronary heart disaese. J. Chron. Dis. 18: 735, 1965.
7. Symposium on Atherosclerosis. Amer. J. Med. 46: 655, 1969.
8. Cornfield, J.: Joint dependence of risk of coronary heart disease on serum cholesterol and systolic blood pressure: a discriminant function analysis. Fed. Proc. 21 (Suppl. 11): 58, 1962.
9. Kannel, W. B., Castelli, P. P., and McNamara, P. M.: The coronary profile: 12 year follow-up in the Framingham study. J. Occup. Med. 9: 611, 1967.
10. Stamler, J., Lindberg, H. A., Berkson, D. M., Shaffer, A., Miller, W., and Poindexter, A.: Prevalence and incidence of coronary heart disease in strata of the labor force of a Chicago industrial corporation. J. Chron. Dis. 11: 405, 1960.
11. Chapman, J. M., and Massey, F. J., Jr.: The interrelationship of serum cholesterol, hypertension, body weight and risk of coronary heart disease. Results of the first ten years' follow-up in the Los Angeles Heart Study. J. Chron. Dis. 17: 933, 1964.
12. Paul, O., Lepper, M. H., and Phelan, W. H., *et al.:* A longitudinal study of coronary heart disease. Circulation 28: 20, 1963.
13. Herman, M. V., and Gorlin, R.: Premature coronary artery disease and the preclinical diabetic state. Amer. J. Med. 38: 481, 1965.
14. Dunn, J. P.: Risk factors in coronary artery disease, hypertension, and diabetes. Amer. J. Med. Sci. 259: 309, 1970.
15. Levy, R. I., and Glueck, C. J.: Hypertriglyceridemia, diabetes mellitus and coronary vessel disease. Arch. Intern. Med. 123: 220, 1969.
16. Deutecher, S., Ostrander, L. D., and Epstein, F. H.: Familial factors in premature coronary heart disease—a preliminary report from the Tecumseh community health study. Amer. J. Epidemiol. 91: 233, 1970.
17. Paffenbarger, R. S., Laughlin, M. E., Gima, A. S., and Black, R. A.: Work activity of longshoremen as related to death from coronary heart disease and stroke. New Engl. J. Med. 282: 1109, 1970.
18. Doyle, J. T.: Etiology of coronary disease: risk factors influencing coronary disease. Mod. Concepts Cardiovasc. Dis. 35: 81, 1966.
19. Selye, H.: The evolution of the stress concept. Amer. J. Cardiol. 26: 289, 1970.
20. Kagan, A., Liusic, A. M., and Sternby, N., *et al.:* Coronary artery thrombosis and the acute attack of coronary heart disease. Lancet 2: 1199, 1968.
21. Fredrickson, D. S., Levy, R. I., and Lees, R. S.: Fat transport in lipoproteins—an integrated approach to mechanisms and disorders. New Engl. J. Med. 276: 34, 94, 148, 215, 273, 1967.

22. Levy, R. I., and Fredrickson, D. S.: Diagnosis and management of hyperlipoproteinemia. Amer. J. Cardiol. 22: 576, 1968.
23. Fredrickson, D. S., and Levy, R. I.: Familial hyperlipoproteinemia. In Stanbury, J. B., Wyngaarden, J. B., and Fredrickson, D. S. (eds.): *Metabolic Basis of Inherited Disease*, Ed. 3. McGraw-Hill Book Company, New York, in press.
24. Blankenhorn, D. H., Chin, H. P., and Lau, F. Y. K.: Ischemic heart disease in young adults. Ann. Intern. Med. 69: 21, 1968.
25. Heinle, R. A., Levy, R. I., Fredrickson, D. S., and Gorlin, R.: Lipid and carbohydrate abnormalities in patients with angiographically documented coronary artery disease. Amer. J. Cardiol. 24: 178, 1969.
26. Kuo, P. T.: Current metabolic-genetic interrelationships in human atherosclerosis. With therapeutic considerations. Ann. Intern. Med. 68: 449, 1968.
27. Brown, D. F., and Doyle, J. T.: Pre-beta lipoproteinemia. Its bearing on the dietary management of serum lipid disorders as related to ischemic heart disease. Amer. J. Clin. Nutr. 20: 324, 1967.
28. Zelis, R., Mason, D. T., Braunwald, E., and Levy, R. I.: Effects of hyperlipoproteinemias and their treatment on the peripheral circulation. J. Clin. Invest. 49: 1007, 1970.
29. Kwiterovitch, P. O., Levy, R. I., and Fredrickson, D. S.: Early detection and treatment of familial Type II hyperlipoproteinemia. Circulation 42: III-11, 1970.
30. Jensen, J., Blankenhorn, O., and Kornerup, V.: Coronary disease in familial hypercholesterolemia. Circulation 36: 77, 1967.
31. Slack, J.: Risks of ischaemic heart-disease in familial hyperlipoproteinaemic states. Lancet 2: 1380, 1969.
32. Fredrickson, D. S., Levy, R. I., Jones, E., Bonnell, M., and Ernst, N.: The dietary management of hyperlipoproteinemia: a handbook for physicians. U. S. Dept. of Health, Education, and Welfare, Public Health Service, Washington, D. C., U. S. Government Printing Office, 1970, 83 pp.
33. Levy, R. I., and Fredrickson, D. S.: The current status of hypolipidemic drugs. Postgrad. Med. 47: 130, 1970.

4

Physiological Basis of Antianginal Therapy: The Nitrites, Beta Adrenergic Receptor Blockade, Carotid Sinus Nerve Stimulation, and Coronary Artery-Saphenous Vein Bypass Graft

DEAN T. MASON, M.D., EZRA A. AMSTERDAM, M.D.,
RICHARD R. MILLER, M.D., ANTONE F. SALEL,
M.D., AND ROBERT ZELIS, M.D.

It has been the traditional view that the relief of angina pectoris is accomplished by enhancement of blood flow to the ischemic myocardium.[1-4] Although certain studies in patients have suggested improved flow in apparently ischemic areas,[5] the diseased arteries in patients with coronary atherosclerosis often are not capable of responding to vasodilator drugs. Further, drug-induced dilation may not be possible in ischemic muscle since hypoxia itself is the most potent stimulus for coronary vasodilation.[6] However, the ischemic pain is often relieved by the antianginal agents without an increase in coronary blood flow.[7-10] The pathophysiological basis of myocardial ischemia is best considered as a discrepancy between myocardial oxygen demands and the availability of oxygen to the heart.[11, 12] Thus, angina can be diminished by reducing myocardial oxygen consumption as well as it would be by improving coronary blood flow. Consistent with this view is the finding that the extent of myocardial ischemia wnich develops following experimental coronary occlusion is directly related to the level of oxygen requirements of the heart existing at the time of interruption of blood flow.[13]

It is now acknowledged that the oxygen consumption of the heart is critically governed by the interplay among three major hemodynamic-related factors[14-17] (Fig. 4.1). Most important is (1) the intramyocardial tension which is the product of transmural ventricular systolic pressure and the radius of the ventricle divided by its wall thickness. The other two

Determinant	Nitrites	Beta-Adrenergic Blockade	Carotid-Sinus-Nerve Stimulation
Intramyocardial systolic tension	↓ ↓	↓	↓ ↓
Heart rate	↑	↓ ↓	↓ ↓
Cardiac contractility	↑	↓ ↓	↓ ↓

Fig. 4.1. Effects of the major antianginal measures on the hemodynamic-related determinants of myocardial oxygen consumption. (Reproduced by permission from Mason, D. T., Spann, J. F., Jr., Zelis, R., and Amsterdam, E. A.: New Engl. J. Med. 281: 1225, 1969.[12])

principal variables directly related to myocardial oxygen demands are (2) the heart rate and (3) the contractile state of the heart. One of the central concepts developed in this article is that the clinical benefit derived from the nitrites in the treatment of angina pectoris results largely and perhaps exclusively from the actions of these substances in reducing myocardial oxygen consumption rather than in increasing coronary blood flow.

THE NITRITES

The precise mechanisms of action of the nitrites in the relief of myocardial ischemic pain have been the subject of considerable debate despite their efficacy for over a full century following their introduction into clinical medicine by Brunton.[18] The nitrites as a group are generally considered to include the inorganic nitrite ion and the organic nitrites and nitrates, each of which possesses the same fundamental effect of directly relaxing smooth muscle of arterioles and veins. The most important agent of this group clinically is the organic nitrate glyceryl trinitrate (nitroglycerin). Although nitroglycerin produces coronary vasodilation in normal man, it does not appear regularly to increase coronary flow in patients with coronary artery disease. Although many aspects of the nitrites continue to excite controversy, advances in the past few years concerning the actions of these agents on the peripheral circulation have provided important information and new concepts concerning their pharmacodynamic effects in the treatment of angina pectoris.

Sublingual Nitroglycerin

The possibility was considered that one of the major therapeutic actions of nitroglycerin is to diminish the needs of the heart for oxygen, and that this effect might be dependent upon the drug's action upon the peripheral circulation. Accordingly, the effects of this drug on the arterioles and veins of the human forearm were determined when the agent was administered sublingually in the manner employed in clinical practice.[19] Forearm blood flow was measured with a strain gauge plethysmograph (Fig. 4.2), and venous tone was determined both by an acute occlusion technique (Fig. 4.2) and by several equilibration techniques (Fig. 4.3) in which absolute changes in venous pressure were related to venous volume. Nitroglycerin produced an increase in the distensibility of the venous system (decline in venous tone) (Fig. 4.2 to 4.4),[19] thereby causing pooling of blood in the peripheral veins and diminishing the return of blood to the heart. Also, the drug produced a mild decrease in systemic arterial pressure with an elevation of forearm blood flow and thus a fall in calculated forearm vascular resistance (Figs. 4.2 and 4.4).[19]

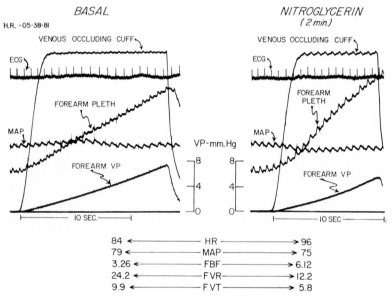

Fig. 4.2. Two segments of the recording of forearm blood flow and venous tone obtained by the acute venous occlusion method in a normal subject. The tracing on the left was recorded during the control period and that on the right 2 minutes after the sublingual administration of 0.9 mg. of nitroglycerin. PLETH refers to the forearm plethysmographic tracing; VP, forearm venous pressure. The figures below the tracing are the values of the variables that were measured or calculated. HR, heart rate; MAP, mean arterial pressure; FBF, forearm blood flow; FVR, forearm vascular resistance; FVT, forearm venous tone. Note that after nitroglycerin the rise in the plethysmographic tracing of forearm circumference was more rapid than during the control period, while the rise in forearm venous pressure was almost unchanged, indicating that venodilation had occurred. (Reproduced by permission from Mason, D. T., and Braunwald, E.: Circulation 32: 755, 1965.[19])

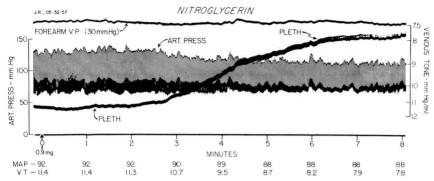

FIG. 4.3. Plethysmographic (PLETH.) tracing in a normal subject in whom forearm venous tone was determined by an equilibration method in which venous pressure was held constant while venous volume was allowed to vary. Forearm circumference (venous volume) was measured continuously before and after the administration of nitroglycerin. Note that following nitroglycerin the forearm circumference increased, while forearm venous pressure (V.P.) was held constant at 30 mm. Hg, signifying that dilation of the capacitance vessels had occurred. ART. PRESS., phasic systemic arterial pressure. (Reproduced by permission from Mason and Braunwald.[19])

The finding that sublingual nitroglycerin results in dilation of forearm veins and peripheral pooling of blood suggests the possibility that this drug might reduce ventricular size and intramyocardial tension and thereby decrease myocardial oxygen requirements. In this manner, nitroglycerin favorably reduces toward normal the ratio between myocardial oxygen demand and the reduced supply of oxygen to the heart. Consonant with this concept is that sublingual nitroglycerin decreases both end diastolic and end systolic dimensions of the intact human heart.[20] In addition, the direct arteriolar dilator action of the drug lowers systemic arterial pressure. This effect further reduces myocardial oxygen consumption by decreasing systolic intraventricular pressure and by lowering the resistance to ventricular ejection and thus allowing greater emptying of the chamber. The direct action on the veins producing venous pooling and diminishing ventricular preload (reduced end diastolic volume) appears to dominate over that on the arterioles of decreasing ventricular afterload (diminished systemic vascular resistance), since the cardiac output and stroke volume are reduced in normal subjects (Fig. 4.5). The nitrites do not possess direct actions on ventricular contractility and thus do not influence myocardial oxygen consumption by this mechanism,[21] although reflex cardiac stimulation induced by the depressor action of the drugs can indirectly increase contractility, an action which in itself increases myocardial oxygen needs and tends to diminish somewhat the greater effect of reduced ventricular loading of lowering overall myocardial oxygen requirements[22] (Fig. 4.1).

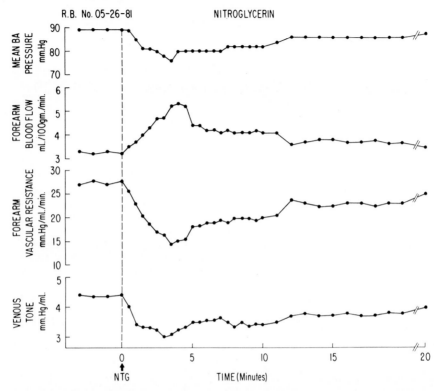

FIG. 4.4. Serial changes of brachial arterial (BA) pressure, forearm blood flow, forearm vascular resistance, and venous tone before and after sublingual nitroglycerin in a normal subject.

It is concluded that the effectiveness of sublingual nitroglycerin in relieving ischemic pain is importantly related to the peripheral vasodilator action of the drug which results in reductions of ventricular loading and oxygen needs (Fig. 4.1), despite the absence of accompanying decrease in coronary vascular resistance and improvement in diminished coronary blood flow. In other patients with angina pectoris, it is possible that the beneficial action is related to a combination of peripheral and coronary vasodilator effects when the coronary vessels and available collateral channels are capable of at least some dilation.[4, 5, 23] These considerations concerning the actions of nitroglycerin and angina pectoris are applicable to myocardial ischemia whether it is due to coronary artery disease or, in contrast, to ventricular hypertrophy which has exceeded the supply capacity of a normal coronary vascular bed such as in aortic stenosis[24] and in idiopathic hypertrophic cardiomyopathies. Thus, a peripheral circulatory

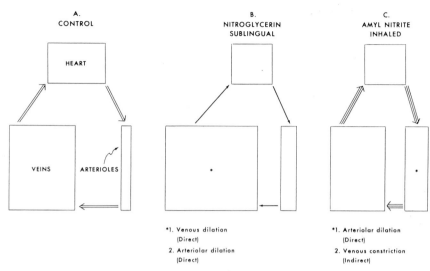

A.
CONTROL

B.
NITROGLYCERIN
SUBLINGUAL

C.
AMYL NITRITE
INHALED

HEART

VEINS   ARTERIOLES

*1. Venous dilation
   (Direct)
 2. Arteriolar dilation
   (Direct)

*1. Arteriolar dilation
   (Direct)
 2. Venous constriction
   (Indirect)

Fig. 4.5. Diagrammatic representation of the actions of sublingual nitroglycerin and inhaled amyl nitrite on the peripheral circulation. The over-all calibre of the systemic arteriolar vessels, the volume of the systemic venous bed, and cardiac size are shown relative to those prior to the administration of the agents (normal subject). The heart size diminishes after sublingual nitroglycerin because of the drug's greater reduction of preload than decrease of afterload, while heart size decreases following inhalation of amyl nitrite because of the agent's greater reduction of afterload than increase of preload. The predominant direct action of the nitrites are indicated by the asterisks.

mechanism is described which is immediately available for the relief of angina pectoris in response to nitroglycerin and is operative even in the absence of action of the agent on the coronary blood vessels.

Other observations are in agreement with the direct peripheral vasodilator action of sublingual nitroglycerin, particularly its powerful dilator effect on the systemic veins which produces systemic venous pooling and reduces venous return to the heart. Thus, this venodilator action of nitroglycerin should be useful in the relief of acute pulmonary edema in patients with congestive heart failure.[25] Consistent with this drug-effected reduction of ventricular preload is the finding that sublingual nitroglycerin rapidly reduces the abnormally elevated end diastolic pressure in the left ventricle while relieving angina.[2] In addition, nitroglycerin-induced decline in systemic venous return provides an explanation for the syncopal episodes which are occasionally seen with nitroglycerin,[26] the decrease caused by the agent of the prominent a wave of the apex cardiogram in patients with angina,[27] and the action of the drug of intensifying obstruction to left ventricular outflow in idiopathic hypertrophic subaortic stenosis.[28]

Inhaled Amyl Nitrite

The effects of inhaling amyl nitrite differ strikingly from those observed after sublingual nitroglycerin. These differences are due to the rapid entrance of the nitrite into the circulation, thereby producing marked direct arteriolar dilation and large decrease in arterial pressure (Fig. 4.6), combined with powerful reflex sympathetic activity induced by baroreceptor stimulation and hyperventilation.[19] Thus, arterial pressure falls precipitously while forearm blood flow increases, indicating a marked fall in vascular resistance (Figs. 4.6 and 4.7, A). These changes are opposed by the activity of the sympathetic nervous system since, after adrenergic blockade, amyl nitrite results in even greater reductions in arterial pressure and calculated vascular resistance (Fig. 4.7, B). Accompanying the marked arterial depressor action of inhaled amyl nitrite is powerful reflex venous constriction which overrides the direct effect of venodilation of the nitrite (Figs. 4.7, A and 4.8, A).[19] Thus, the cardiac output is elevated as a consequence of marked decline of the resistance to ventricular emptying (diminished afterload) coupled with both the reflex constricting effect on the veins enhancing venous return and sympathetic stimulation of cardiac contractility. That this venoconstriction is reflex in origin is shown by the finding that the response was markedly attenuated by the antiadrenergic agents guanethidine or reserpine (Figs. 4.7, B and 4.8, B).[19]

The efficacy of inhaled amyl nitrite in patients with angina pectoris is related to its predominant effect on the arteriolar bed of markedly reducing systemic vascular resistance[11, 12] (Fig. 4.5). In this manner, resistance to ventricular emptying is diminished, thereby reducing both intramyocardial tension and myocardial oxygen consumption. Thus, the tendency for reflex augmentation of venous return to increase the preload and work of the ventricle is overridden by the more striking effect of inhaled amyl nitrite of reducing ventricular afterload with consequent overall reductions of intraventricular systolic pressure and volume and diminished myocardial tension and oxygen demand. Paradoxically, the possibility is suggested that, on occasion, the amyl nitrite-induced rapid and marked fall of blood pressure might actually worsen ischemia if the reduction of coronary perfusion pressure causes a decline in coronary blood flow which is relatively greater than decreased oxygen needs.

The literature concerning the cardiocirculatory actions of the nitrite compounds has been contradictory and difficult to interpret. It now appears that much of this confusion has arisen from the assumption that the actions of the nitrites and organic nitrates are similar, whether they are administered orally, intravenously, or inhaled. Thus, it is improper to conclude that the direct and reflex indirect effects of nitroglycerin given sublingually are either qualitatively or quantitatively the same as those determined from studies in which nitroglycerin is given intravenously or in which amyl nitrite is inhaled. It is concluded that each of the nitrite drugs directly relax vascular smooth muscle in all of the regional circulatory beds. When the nitrites enter the circulation slowly, such as following sublingual nitroglycerin or oral sodium nitrite, they dilate both the systemic arterial and venous beds[19],

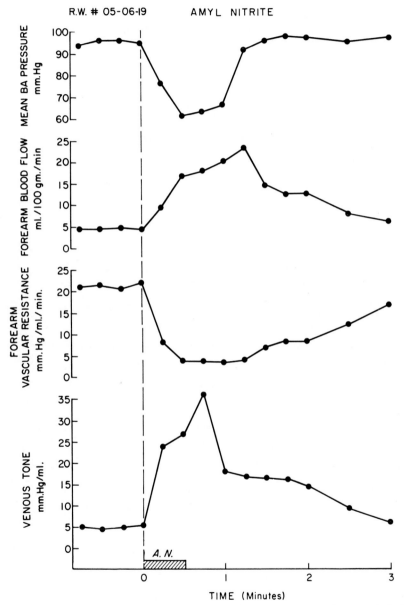

Fig. 4.6. Serial changes of forearm vascular dynamics before and after inhalation of amyl nitrite in a normal subject.

[29], [30] (Fig. 4.9). In this manner, arterial blood pressure falls slightly and central venous pressure is reduced, resulting in peripheral venous pooling and reduction in stroke volume and cardiac output.

In contrast, the rapid introduction of the nitrites into the circulation fol-

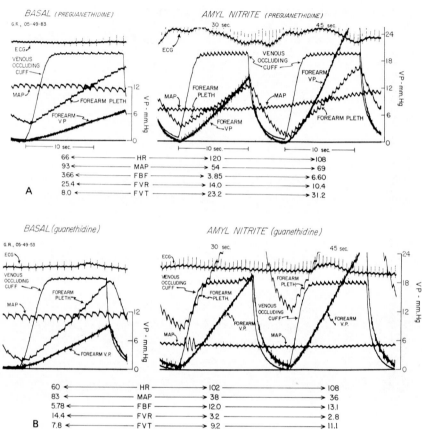

FIG. 4.7. A, two segments of the recording, obtained by the acute venous occlusion method discussed in the legend to Figure 4.2, in a normal subject before and 30 and 45 seconds after the inhalation of amyl nitrite. The tracing on the left was obtained during the control period; that on the right shows two occlusion curves recorded successively 30 and 45 seconds after the drug. For abbreviations and explanation of values below the tracing, see legend to Figure 4.2. Note that after amyl nitrite the rate of rise of pressure in the forearm vein has increased, while the rate of rise of the plethysmographic tracing has increased only slightly, indicating that profound venoconstriction had occurred. B, two segments of recordings following adrenergic blockade with guanethidine obtained in the same subject whose tracings are shown in A. Amyl nitrite increased the rate of rise of forearm circumference proportionately more than the rate of rise of venous pressure after guanethidine than before, indicating that the venoconstriction which had occurred was less than that noted before guanethidine had been given in A. (Reproduced by permission from Mason and Braunwald.[19])

lowing inhalation of amyl nitrite or the intravenous administration of nitro-glycerin[3, 19] results in profound arteriolar dilation and thereby marked fall in systemic arterial blood pressure (Fig. 4.9). This marked depressor effect leads to carotid baroreceptor stimulation and a marked reflex chronotropic

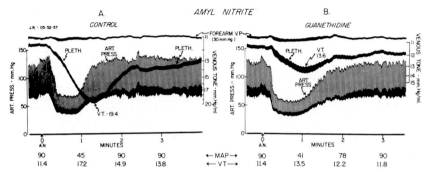

FIG. 4.8. Recordings of arterial and venous pressures and forearm circumference following amyl nitrite inhalation in a normal subject. Venous tone was determined by the same equilibration method explained in the legend to Figure 4.3. Tracing A was recorded during the control period and B after guanethidine. After adrenergic blockade (B), amyl nitrite decreased forearm volume considerably less than during the control period (A), indicating that venoconstriction was markedly diminished. For explanation of abbreviations, see legend to Figure 4.2. (Reproduced by permission from Mason and Braunwald.[19])

NITRITES

Actions on the Peripheral Circulation

	Arterial pressure	Systemic vascular resistance	Venous tone	Cardiac output
Nitroglycerin sublingual	↓	Ⓓ	Ⓟ	↓
Nitroglycerin intravenous	↓	Ⓟ	↑	↑
Amyl nitrite inhaled	↓	Ⓟ	↑	↑
Sodium nitrite oral	↓	Ⓓ	Ⓟ	↓

↑ Small increase   ↑ Large increase
↓ Small decrease   ↓ Large decrease
○ Direct action   ◎ Principal direct action

FIG. 4.9. Actions of nitrite compounds on cardiocirculatory dynamics. The effects of slowly absorbed sublingual nitroglycerin and oral sodium nitrite are contrasted to those of fast-acting inhaled amyl nitrite and intravenous nitroglycerin.

effect and some attenuation of the intense direct arteriolar dilation. Although present evidence indicates that changes in blood pressure within the physiological range in man do not produce reflex alterations in venous tone, it appears that the hyperventilation and anxiety which accompany the inhalation of amyl nitrite are largely responsible for the reflex venoconstriction.[11] The cardiac output is elevated as a consequence of the marked decline of resistance to ventricular emptying coupled with predominant reflex venoconstriction and reflex enhancement of cardiac contractility. Conversely, the decrease in blood pressure following the oral administration of nitroglycerin is less marked and is not associated with an increase in respiratory rate. Thus, reflex venoconstriction is mild or does not occur and the direct predominant action of venodilation is observed. From these observations, it appears that the principal direct action of sublingual nitroglycerin in intact man is on the veins and that of inhaled amyl nitrite on the arterial bed.

Long-acting Organic Nitrites

From the observations presented, it is evident that the therapeutic efficacy of sublingual nitroglycerin in relieving angina pectoris is dependent to a major extent on its ability to dilate the peripheral arterioles and veins, thereby reducing ventricular preload and afterload which lead to reduction of myocardial oxygen requirements. The possibility was considered that long-acting nitrites might compromise the beneficial peripheral vascular effects of nitroglycerin, if the chronic administration of long-acting nitrite compounds produces nitrite tolerance.[11, 21, 31, 32] It was found that the administration of isosorbide dinitrate for 6 weeks did not alter the sublingual nitroglycerin-induced arteriolar dilation, but it did significantly reduce the venodilator response to sublingual nitroglycerin. Thus, cross tolerance between the long-acting nitrite and nitroglycerin was demonstrated in veins, an effect which is potentially deleterious. In addition, it appears that tolerance may develop to the long-acting nitrite itself since venous tone and arterial resistance were not diminished following its chronic administration, although the possibility remains that the agent produces vasodilation initially. It is logical to postulate that chronic reduction of the loading conditions and work of the heart might reduce the frequency and intensity of angina pectoris and to speculate that the chronic administration of a long-acting vasodilator drug should affect such a decrease of ventricular loading and thereby diminish myocardial oxygen needs. In the case of the long-acting nitrite vasodilators, it appears from these studies that at least some of the potentially beneficial action of chronically reducing myocardial loading might be impaired by venodilator tolerance, an effect that also might attenuate the effectiveness of sublingual nitroglycerin.

BETA ADRENERGIC RECEPTOR-BLOCKING DRUGS

Propranolol

It is helpful both from a clinical and pharmacological viewpoint to separate the end organ receptors for the sympathetic nervous system into two functional types: alpha and beta adrenergic receptors. In the cardiovascular system, only the beta receptors are located in the myocardium, while both alpha and beta receptors are present in the peripheral vascular beds. Activation of the alpha adrenergic receptors results in arteriolar constriction, and stimulation of the beta adrenergic receptors augments cardiac contractility and heart rate and produces arteriolar dilation. Drugs that antagonize these beta adrenergic receptors have been developed only recently. The beta receptor-blocking drug now available for clinical use is propranolol, which is capable of blocking the contractile and the heart rate effects of bloodborne catecholamines and sympathetic nerve stimulation.

Propranolol is now the subject of considerable investigation for conditions in which the intensity of sympathetic drive to the heart might be excessive.[11] Since the contractility of the ventricle and the heart rate are regulated, in part, by the rate at which endogenous norepinephrine is released from sympathetic nerve endings in the heart, treatment with propranolol impairs cardiac performance during conditions such as muscular exercise in which sympathetic stimulation is one of the important adaptive mechanisms (Fig. 4.10).[33, 34] In patients with advanced cardiac disease who are critically dependent upon increased adrenergic stimulation of the heart and peripheral blood vessels for support of their failing heart, the adverse effects of propranolol on resting hemodynamics are of considerable importance.[35] Thus, propranolol may precipitate heart failure in patients with advanced cardiac disease and lead to rapid progression of hypotension and dyspnea. Indeed, the drug may actually increase the oxygen needs of the myocardium by causing ventricular dilation with resultant increases in intramyocardial tension. Also, propranolol is contraindicated in patients with serious atrioventricular conduction disturbances since the agent aggravates this condition.

One of the initial clinical applications of propranolol has been in the treatment of patients with angina pectoris.[36-41] By preventing the increase in myocardial oxygen requirements induced by stimulation of the cardiac sympathetic nerves during exertion, propranolol has proved to be of value in many patients with angina pectoris. The mechanisms by which the drug improves exercise tolerance by delaying the onset of ischemic pain in these patients depend on the effects of the agent of reducing myocardial oxygen requirements (Fig. 4.1). Most important in this regard is the capacity of propranolol to reduce heart rate and diminish the contractile state of the

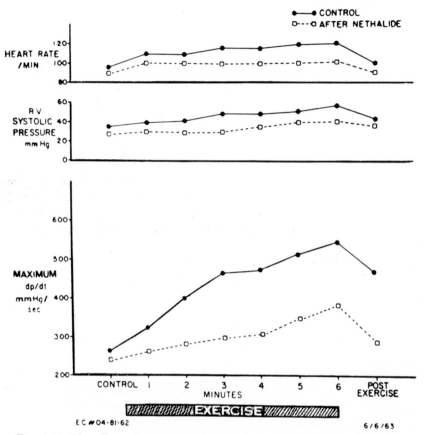

Fig. 4.10. The effect of exercise on heart rate, right ventricular (RV) systolic pressure, and maximal RV dp/dt (rate of pressure rise) during the control period (solid lines) and after beta-adrenergic blockade with the propranolol-like drug pronethalol (dotted lines). (Reproduced by permission from Harrison, D. C., Braunwald, E., Glick, G., Mason, D. T., Chidsey, C. A. and Ross, J., Jr.: Circulation 29: 84, 1964.[34])

heart. Thus, propranolol exerts its salutary clinical effects in patients whose exercise capacity is limited by angina because of an unfavorable relation between myocardial oxygen requirements and availability, while the drug is detrimental to patients whose activity is limited principally by an impairment of the pumping properties of the heart and resultant symptoms of cardiac failure. Therefore, propranolol exchanges the property of contractility for a reduction in the oxygen requirements of the heart.

The notion has arisen that drugs such as propranolol which extend exercise capacity might actually be harmful in patients with coronary disease; the contention has been that these patients might continue activity through an ischemic episode which would ordinarily produce anginal pain and serve as a warning that activity should be discontinued. However, this is not anticipated to be the case during beta blockade or treatment with nitroglycerin, since angina pectoris still occurs at the same unfavorable ratio of myocardial oxygen consumption to coronary blood flow that produced this symptom before the drug was given. What does occur is a reduction in myocardial oxygen consumption which thereby offsets the development of the unfavorable supply-demand relation in the presence of a reduced blood flow to the myocardium.[42] The development of the new beta adrenergic blocking drugs, practolol and oxprenolol, which produce effective blockade of cardiac beta receptors with apparently less direct negative inotropic action than propranolol, may represent an important advance in antianginal therapy utilizing beta-blocking drugs.[43]

Nitrites and Propranolol

The beta adrenergic receptor-blocking drug propranolol inhibits sympathetic stimulation of the heart at rest and during exercise. Thus, myocardial oxygen requirements are diminished principally by the reduction in heart rate and diminished contractility.[11, 12, 34] It is apparent that a combination of propranolol and nitroglycerin is potentially more beneficial than the use of either drug separately, since these two agents act through different mechanisms in diminishing the needs of the heart for oxygen. In addition, when used alone, the favorable dilator effects of nitroglycerin on the peripheral vessels are opposed somewhat by reflex activation of the sympathetic nervous system[19] (Fig. 4.11). Further, the extent of reduction of myocardial oxygen demands afforded by direct systemic vasodilation is opposed by the reflex chronotropic and inotropic effects of cardiac adrenergic stimulation. It is postulated that the beneficial effects of sublingual nitroglycerin of reducing myocardial oxygen requirements might even be overridden by intense baroreceptor responses in certain instances, perhaps in younger patients with angina pectoris in whom reflex activity is relatively strong. It would appear that the salutary direct vasodilator effect of nitroglycerin can be extended by its combination with propranolol. Thus, the activation of the myocardium resulting as a reflex response to the depressor action of nitroglycerin is blocked by propranolol. Recent studies have suggested a synergistic effect between isosorbide dinitrate and propranolol,[44] while other studies have not been able to demonstrate this effect.[40] The remarks outlined above refer to the use of nitroglycerin, as opposed to the long-acting nitrites, for abolishing acute ischemic pain in the presence of chronic treatment with propranolol.

CAROTID SINUS NERVE STIMULATION

The development of the technique of electrical stimulation of the carotid sinus nerves in the treatment of refractory angina pectoris represents an

NITROGLYCERIN

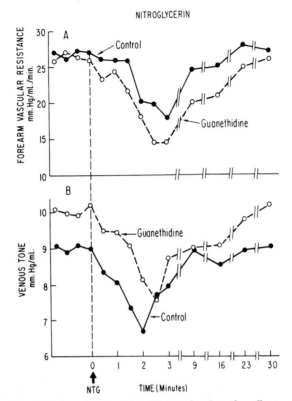

FIG. 4.11. Average values in normal subjects showing the effects of sublingual nitroglycerin (NTG) on (a) forearm vascular resistance and (b) venous tone before (solid dots and solid lines) and following intravenous administration of the antiadrenergic agent guanethidine (open circles and broken lines). The finding that adrenergic blockade accentuated the decline in arteriolar resistance produced by nitroglycerin (a) suggests that when nitroglycerin is given in the presence of a normally functioning sympathetic nervous system, the fall in resistance is partially opposed by sympathetically induced reflex arteriolar constriction.

important new approach to the management of this problem.[46, 47] This method utilizing a radio-frequency stimulator consists of surgical attachment of bipolar electrodes to both carotid sinus nerves with connection to a receiving unit beneath the skin of the anterior chest. On the surface above this receiver is fixed an induction coil which is attached to an externally placed battery-powered signal generator strapped about the patient's waist.

When the patient experiences angina pectoris or is confronted with an angina-producing situation, he may switch on the battery unit to stimulate the carotid sinus nerves. This stimulation leads to an increase in afferent impulse traffic to central autonomic centers and results in reflex diminution of adrenergic discharges to the entire cardiovascular system. Thus, arteriolar dilation is produced, myocardial contractility is diminished, and heart rate is slowed—all actions that result in a reduction of myocardial oxygen requirements. Since it is necessary to stimulate the carotid sinus nerves electrically for only a brief period until angina is relieved, this decrease in contractility persists for just a short time and does not produce cardiac decompensation in patients with advanced heart disease.

From the above observations, it is apparent that, of the major methods available for the treatment of angina pectoris, stimulation of the carotid sinus nerves is the most powerful means of reducing the requirements of the heart for oxygen (Fig. 4.1). Thus, beta adrenergic stimulation of the heart is inhibited, and thereby, negative inotropic and chronotropic effects are brought about as they are by propranolol. In addition, alpha adrenergic receptor stimulation is reduced, which brings about arteriolar dilation. Therefore, electrical stimulation of the carotid sinus nerves provides a powerful combination of indirect vasodilation and propranolol-like actions on the heart. It is of interest to postulate that the use of nitroglycerin in patients employing electrical excitation of the carotid sinus nerves would be helpful if angina were not relieved by baroreceptor stimulation, since the direct vasodilator actions of the nitrites would be additive to the indirect vasodilation produced by inhibition of the activity of the sympathetic nervous system.

Thus far the method of carotid sinus nerve stimulation has been applied in only a few patients with long-standing refractory angina; in many of these patients it has been successful.[46-48] In those in whom this method has not been useful, it would appear that the needs of the heart for oxygen cannot be reduced to the particularly low level required to relieve angina caused by severe myocardial ischemia due to very severe diminution of coronary blood flow. It should be stressed that carotid sinus nerve stimulation requires the surgical application of the electrode stimulator unit under general anesthesia, a procedure which carries with it some risk. Implantation of the pacemaker usually should be offered only to patients with severely disabling angina in whom coronary artery-saphenous vein bypass is not possible because of diffuse coronary atherosclerosis and in whom the use of nitroglycerin and propranolol has not diminished the frequency of angina pectoris.

It is of interest to point out that, in patients with coronary disease, the degree of development of collateral circulation in the heart has been demonstrated to be most dependent on the severity of regional atherosclerosis itself (Fig. 4.12).[49, 50] Thus it is postulated that, although these collateral channels appear to be of certain quantitative importance, their principal role is response to ischemia and impairment of native circulation. Also consistent with this observation quantitating collateral development solely

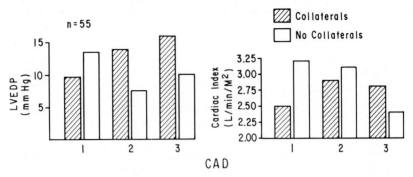

FIG. 4.12. Relation of the presence or absence of coronary collaterals to left ventricular end-diastolic pressure (LVEDP) and to cardiac index in patients with coronary atherosclerosis (CAD) with significant obstruction (greater than 75 per cent stenosis) of one, two, and three of the major coronary arteries, as determined by selective coronary cineangiography.

with the severity of coronary atherosclerosis is the finding that in patients with coronary artery disease collaterals were more extensive in those with less augmentation of coronary blood flow in response to isoproterenol;[51] and that, in anomalous origin of the left coronary artery from the pulmonary artery, the extensive network of collaterals between the right and left coronary arteries was markedly diminished on postoperative angiography several months following establishment of normal left coronary artery blood flow by saphenous vein-coronary artery bypass graft.[52] This view, which directly relates the level of coronary blood flow to the severity of occlusive disease alone, is consonant with the theme presented in this review that the antianginal action of nitrites is limited to the ability of the agents to lower myocardial oxygen demands rather than to improve the reduced coronary blood flow. Also consistent with these concepts implying that the therapeutically responsive variable in coronary disease is myocardial oxygen demand is the relief of ischemic pain by a variety of other means which also lower myocardial oxygen consumption, such as propranolol,[41, 42] carotid sinus nerve stimulation,[47] phlebotomy,[53] weight reduction, and exercise training.[54, 55] The value of maintaining plasma lipids within normal limits at present appears directed at prevention and reduction of progression of plaques rather than resolution of existing atheromas.[56] It appears that, once a patient with coronary disease develops angina pectoris, the disease itself usually worsens faster than the formation of collaterals, and perhaps any spontaneous decrease of pain might be due to necrosis of cardiac cells and thus diminished oxygen demands of the heart. From these observations, the various medical approaches in the treatment of angina are mediated by the common mechanism of lowering myocardial oxygen consumption rather than by favorably affecting the basic patho-physiological abnormality of diminished coronary blood flow.

CORONARY ARTERY-SAPHENOUS VEIN BYPASS GRAFT

It appears that the only method presently available for substantially elevating blood flow to the ischemic myocardium is coronary bypass with saphenous vein anastomosis in carefully selected patients,[42, 57] and recent data suggest that myocardial revascularization techniques to increase compromised blood flow through the development of collateral channels are largely ineffective.[8, 9] It is our current choice to carry out coronary angiography in the younger patients with active angina in their fourth, fifth, or sixth decades of life, even when this pain is relatively mild and may not necessarily be refractory to propranolol. These younger patients, in whom rehabilitation is of special importance, appear to have accelerated coronary disease most often associated with lipoprotein elevations, espe-cially the hypertriglyceridemia Type IV abnormality[60] (Fig. 4.13). Further, in our experience, the majority of these younger patients have a coronary lesion which is suitable for saphenous vein bypass: localized severe proximal obstruction (greater than 75 per cent narrowing of the luminal diameter) with relatively normal distal patency of the same vessel of at least one coronary artery. In contrast, the older patients with angina above 60 years of age usually have not had surgically amenable lesions because of the presence of diffuse coronary atherosclerosis. In these older patients, it is our current practice to reserve coronary angiography and consideration for coronary bypass surgery for those in whom angina is causing substantial disability and is unmanageable with nitroglycerin and propranolol.

Although the saphenous vein bypass graft now has been applied exten-sively in patients with angina pectoris, objective documentation of the effectiveness of this procedure has been lacking. Thus, a study was recently carried out in our laboratories to determine pre- and postoperative exercise capacity and hemodynamics with the use of the upright bicycle ergometer in patients who underwent aorta to right and/or left coronary artery-saphenous vein anastomoses.[42] The heart rate-mean systemic intraarterial pressure product was assessed as an index of myocardial oxygen consump-tion. Before surgery, intravenous propranolol delayed for about 1 to 2 minutes the onset of exercise-provoked angina, whereas myocardial oxygen consumption was not increased as examined by the heart rate-blood pres-sure product (Fig. 4.14). Strikingly, 2 to 3 months after surgery, angina disappeared and could not be provoked by exercise, which was limited only by leg fatigue. Postoperative rise in myocardial blood flow was indicated by an increase of the heart rate-blood pressure product (Fig. 4.14). In addition, preoperative electrocardiographic ischemic ST-T wave changes

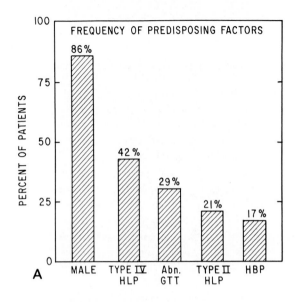

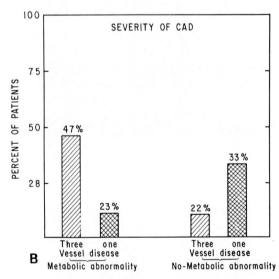

Fig. 4.13. Relation of certain factors (A) predisposing to coronary atherosclerosis and (B) to severity of coronary disease in patients with symptomatic coronary artery disease. Type II and IV refers to the specific abnormal hyperlipoprotein (HLP) pattern. GTT, abnormal elevation of glucose tolerance test; HBP, elevated systolic systemic arterial blood pressure (>150 mm. Hg). Metabolic abnormality includes Type II and IV hyperlipoproteinemia, abnormal GTT or HBP. One and three vessels refers to significant obstruction to one or three of the major coronary arteries, as defined by selective coronary cineangiography.

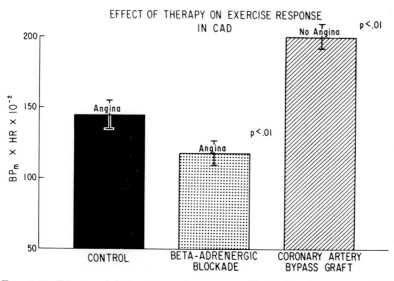

FIG. 4.14. Effects of beta-adrenergic receptor blockade with propranolol or practolol on the exercise response (heart rate (HR)-mean systemic blood pressure (BP_m) product, as an indirect measure of myocardial oxygen consumption), and of subsequent coronary artery-saphenous vein bypass graft carried out in the same patients with coronary artery disease (CAD). The values of significance refer to beta-adrenergic blockade or coronary bypass relative to the control exercise response. Patients with beta-adrenergic blockade were able to exercise for longer periods prior to angina than in the control period, while considerably greater external work was performed without producing angina following coronary bypass compared to beta-adrenergic blockade.

during exercise cleared or were improved postoperatively. These postoperative results indicate that the saphenous vein bypass technique in surgically amenable coronary artery disease increases oxygen delivery to the ischemic myocardium and is superior for relief of refractory angina in properly selected patients for surgical intervention as described above, compared to beta adrenergic blockade which acts by reducing myocardial oxygen requirements.

CONCLUSION

The fundamental action of each of the nitrite compounds is a generalized direct vasodilation. With the rapid introduction of these agents into the circulation, there is a mixture of this direct relaxing effect on vascular smooth muscle and indirect reflex vasoconstrictor actions. The relief of angina pectoris with sublingual nitroglycerin appears to be most related to direct venodilation, while with inhalation of amyl nitrite this symptom is abated by marked direct arteriolar dilation. Angina pectoris can be considered pathophysiologically to result from an unfavorable relation of myocardial oxygen requirements to coronary blood flow. In the treatment of ischemic pain, the variable factor mediating the beneficial effects of the nitrites is reduction of myocardial oxygen requirements. Moreover, the common mechanism by which all types of antianginal therapy relieve ischemic pain (except for direct coronary artery surgery itself) is reduction of oxygen needs of the heart, rather than improvement of coronary blood flow (Fig. 4.1).

The beta adrenergic receptor-blocking drug propranolol inhibits sympathetic stimulation of the heart at rest and during exercise. Thus, myocardial oxygen requirements are diminished by the reduction in heart rate and diminished contractility. As a result of this latter action, cardiac output is reduced, and thereby arterial pressure and intramyocardial tension are lowered. Electrical stimulation of the carotid sinus nerves in patients with intractable angina pectoris has provided a powerful means for the reduction of myocardial oxygen requirements. Thus, there is reflex sympathetic withdrawal throughout the cardiovascular system which leads to transient decrease in peripheral vascular resistance, systemic blood pressure, heart rate, and cardiac contractile state.

Finally, since the extent of development of coronary collateral circulation is most critically related to the severity of coronary disease itself, it appears that the responsive variable which allows improvement by both spontaneous and therapeutic means short of direct coronary surgery is reduction of myocardial oxygen consumption rather than the traditional concept of the augmentation of diminished coronary blood flow. The only effective method at present available for substantially elevating blood flow to the ischemic myocardium is the coronary bypass graft in carefully selected patients. It is our current recommendation to carry out coronary angiography for consideration of venous bypass surgery in the younger patients with angina, particularly those of less than 50 years of age, and even those with relatively mild angina, without requiring previous trial with propranolol. Surgically approachable coronary lesions are usually found by angiography in these younger patients, whereas coronary angiography is withheld until angina is disabling and refractory to nitroglycerin and propranolol in the older patients, who more often appear to have diffuse coronary atherosclerosis unamenable to bypass techniques. In any case, the coronary artery-saphenous vein anastomoses should be reserved for patients with lesions which are potentially amenable to bypass surgery: discrete, severe proximal obstruction with relatively normal distal patency of the same vessel of at least one coronary artery.

This study was supported in part by National Heart and Lung Institute Grant HE-05901.

REFERENCES

1. Wegria, R., Nickerson, J. L., Case, R. B., and Holland, J. F.: Effect of nitroglycerin on the cardiovascular system of normal persons. Amer. J. Cardiol. 10: 414–418, 1951.
2. Muller, O., and Rorvik, K.: Hemodynamic consequences of coronary heart disease: with observations during angina pain and on the effect of nitroglycerin. Brit. Heart J. 20: 302, 1958.
3. Honig, C. R., Tenney, S. M., and Gabel, P. V.: The mechanism of cardiovascular action of nitroglycerin: an example of integrated response during the unsteady state. Amer. J. Med. 29: 910, 1960.
4. Weisse, A. B., and Regan, T. J.: The current status of nitrites in the treatment of coronary artery disease. Prog. Cardiovasc. Dis. 12: 72, 1969.
5. Horwitz, D., Gorlin, R., Taylor, W. J., and Kemp, H. G.: Effects of nitroglycerin on regional myocardial blood flow in coronary artery disease. Clin. Res. 18: 312, 1970.
6. Berne, R. M.: Regulation of coronary blood flow. Physiol. Rev. 44: 1, 1964.
7. Gorlin, R., Brachfeld, N., MacLeod, C., and Bopp, P.: Effect of nitroglycerin on the coronary circulation in patients with coronary artery disease or increased left ventricular work. Circulation 19: 705, 1959.
8. Hollander, W., Madoff, I. M., and Chobanian, A. V.: Local myocardial blood flow as indicated by the disappearance of Na I^{131} from the heart muscle: studies at rest, during exercise, and following nitrite administration. J. Pharmacol. Exp. Ther. 139: 53, 1963.
9. Bernstein, L., Friesinger, G. C., Lichtlen, P. R., and Ross, R. S.: Effect of nitroglycerin on myocardial blood flow in man as measured with Xenon^{133}. Circulation 30 (Suppl. 3): 47, 1964.
10. Bing, R. J., Bennish, A., Bluemchen, G., Cohen, A., Gallagher, J. P., and Zaleski, E. J.: The determination of coronary flow equivalent with coincidence counting technic. Circulation 29: 833, 1964.
11. Mason, D. T., and Braunwald, E.: Mechanisms of action and therapeutic uses of cardiac drugs. In Fulton, W. F. M. (ed.): *Modern Trends in Pharmacology and Therapeutics*. Butterworth, pp. 112–166, 1967.
12. Mason, D. T., Spann, J. F., Jr., Zelis, R., and Amsterdam, E. A.: Physiologic approach to the treatment of angina pectoris. New Engl. J. Med. 281: 1225, 1969.
13. Maroko, P. R., Braunwald, E., Covell, J. W., and Ross, J., Jr.: Factors influencing the severity of myocardial ischemia following experimental coronary occlusion. Circulation 40 (Suppl. 3): 140, 1969.
14. Sarnoff, S. J., Braunwald, E., Welch, G. A., Jr., Case, R. B., Stainsby, W. N., and Macruz, R.: Hemodynamic determinants of oxygen consumption of heart with special reference to tension-time index. Amer. J. Physiol. 192: 148, 1958.
15. Sonnenblick, E. H., Ross, J., Jr., Covell, J. W., Kaiser, G. A., and Braunwald E.: Velocity of contraction as determinant of myocardial oxygen consumption. Amer. J. Physiol. 209: 919, 1965.
16. Covell, J. W., Braunwald, E., Ross, J., Jr., and Sonnenblick, E. H.: Studies on digitalis. XVI. Effects on myocardial oxygen consumption. J. Clin. Invest. 45: 1535, 1966.
17. Braunwald, E.: Thirteenth Bowditch lecture: the determinants of myocardial oxygen consumption. Physiologist 12: 65, 1969.
18. Brunton, T. L.: On the use of nitrite of amyl in angina pectoris. Lancet 2: 97–98, 1967.

19. Mason, D. T., and Braunwald, E.: The effects of nitroglycerin and amyl nitrite on arteriolar and venous tone in the human forearm. Circulation 32: 755, 1965.
20. Williams, J. F., Jr., Glick, G., and Braunwald, E.: Studies on cardiac dimensions in intact unanesthetized man. V. Effects of nitroglycerin. Circulation 32: 767, 1965.
21. Zelis, R., Mason, D. T., Spann, J. F., Jr., and Amsterdam, E. A.: The mechanism of action of nitroglycerin in the relief of angina pectoris: reduction of myocardial oxygen consumption by extracoronary vasodilation and its attenuation by the chronic administration of isosorbide dinitrate. Ann. Intern. Med. 72: 779, 1970.
22. Zelis, R., Amsterdam, E. A., and Mason, D. T.: Alterations in ventricular contractility produced by nitroglycerin in man. Amer. J. Cardiol. 26: 667, 1970.
23. Fam, W. M., and McGregor, M.: Effect of coronary vasodilator drugs on retrograde flow in areas of chronic myocardial ischemia. Circ. Res. 15: 355, 1964.
24. Fallen, E. L., Elliott, W. C., and Gorlin, R.: Mechanisms of angina in aortic stenosis. Circulation 36: 480, 1967.
25. Johnson, J. B., Gross, J. F., and Hole, E.: Effects of sublingual nitroglycerin on pulmonary artery pressure in patients with failure of the left ventricle. New Engl. J. Med. 257: 1114, 1957.
26. Russek, H. I., Urbach, K. F., and Zohman, B. L.: Paradoxical action of glyceryl trinitrate (nitroglycerin) in coronary patients. J. A. M. A. 158: 1017, 1955.
27. Benchimol, A., and Dimond, E. G.: The apex cardiogram in ischemic heart disease. Brit. Heart J. 24: 581, 1962.
28. Braunwald, E., Oldham, H. N., Jr., Ross, J., Jr., Linhart, J., Mason, D. T., and Fort, L.: The circulatory response of patients with idiopathic hypertrophic subaortic stenosis to nitroglycerin and to the Valsalva maneuver. Circulation 29: 422, 1964.
29. Wilkins, R. W., Haynes, F. W., and Weiss, S.: The role of the venous system in circulatory collapse induced by sodium nitrite. J. Clin. Invest. 16: 85, 1937.
30. Ablad, B., and Johnsson, G.: Comparative effects of intraarterially administered hydralazine and sodium nitrite on blood flow and volume of forearm. Acta Pharmacol. 21: 1, 1963.
31. Schelling, J. L., and Lasagna, L.: A study of cross-tolerance to circulation effects of organic nitrates. Clin. Pharmacol. Ther. 8: 256, 1967.
32. Zelis, R., and Mason, D. T.: Demonstration of nitrite tolerance: attenuation of the venodilator response to nitroglycerin by the chronic administration of isosorbide dinitrate. Circulation 40 (Suppl. 3): 221, 1969.
33. Epstein, S. E., Robinson, B. F., Kahler, R. L., and Braunwald, E.: Effects of beta-adrenergic blockade on the cardiac response to maximal and submaximal exercise in man. J. Clin. Invest. 44: 1745–1753, 1965.
34. Harrison, D. C., Braunwald, E., Glick, G., Mason, D. T., Chidsey, C. A., and Ross, J., Jr.: Effects of beta adrenergic blockade on the circulation with particular reference to observations in patients with hypertrophic subaortic stenosis. Circulation 29: 84, 1964.
35. Epstein, S. E., and Braunwald, E.: The effect of beta-adrenergic blockade on patterns of sodium excretion: studies in normal subjects and in patients with heart disease. Ann. Intern. Med. 65: 20–27, 1966.
36. Alleyne, G. A. O., Dickinson, C. J., Dornhorst, A. C., Fulton, R. M., Green, K. G., Hill, I. D., Hurst, P., Laurence, D. R., Pilkington, T., Prichard, B. N. C., Robinson, B., and Rosenheim, M. L.: Effects of pronethalol on angina pectoris. Brit. Med. J. 2: 1226–1227, 1963.

37. Gillam, P. M. S., and Prichard, B. N. C.: Propranolol in the therapy of angina pectoris. Amer. J. Cardiol. 18: 366, 1966.
38. Gillam, P. M. S., and Prichard, B. N. C.: Use of propranolol in angina pectoris. Brit. Med. J. 2: 337, 1965.
39. Grant, R. H. E., Kellam, P., Kernohan, R. J., Leonard, J. C., Nacekievill, L., and Sinclair, K.: Multicenter trial of propranolol in angina pectoris. Amer. J. Cardiol. 18: 361, 1966.
40. Srivastava, J. C., Dewar, H. A., and Newell, D. J.: Double-blind trial of propranolol in angina of effort. Brit. Med. J. 2: 724, 1964.
41. Amsterdam, E. A., Gorlin, R., and Wolfson, S.: Evaluation of long-term use of propranolol in angina pectoris. J. A. M. A. 210: 103, 1969.
42. Amsterdam, E. A., Iben, A., Hurley, E. J., Mansour, E., Hughes, J. L., Salel, A. F., Zelis, R., and Mason, D. T.: Saphenous vein bypass graft for refractory angina pectoris: physiological evidence for enhanced blood flow to the ischemic myocardium. Amer. J. Cardiol. 26: 623, 1971.
43. Amsterdam, E. A., Hughes, J. L., Mansour, E., Salel, A. F., Bonanno, J. A., Zelis, R., and Mason, D. T.: Circulatory effects of practolol: selective cardiac beta adrenergic blockade in arrhythmias and angina pectoris. Clin. Res. 19: 109, 1971.
44. Russek, H. I.: Propranolol and isosorbide dinitrate synergism in angina pectoris. Amer. J. Cardiol. 21: 44, 1968.
45. Battock, D. J., Alvarez, H., and Chidsey, C. A.: Effects of propranolol and isosorbide dinitrate on exercise performance and adrenergic activity in patients with angina pectoris. Circulation 39: 157, 1969.
46. Braunwald, E., Epstein, S. E., Glick, G., Wechsler, A. S., and Braunwald, N. S.: Relief of angina pectoris by electrical stimulation of the carotid-sinus nerves. New Engl. J. Med. 277: 1279, 1967.
47. Epstein, S. E., Beiser, G. D., Goldstein, R. E., Redwood, D., Rosing, D. R., Glick, G., Wechsler, A. S., Stampfer, M., Cohen, L. S., Reis, R. L., Braunwald, N. S., and Braunwald, E. Treatment of angina pectoris by electrical stimulation of the carotid-sinus nerves; results in 17 patients with severe angina. New Engl. J. Med. 280: 971, 1969.
48. Farrehi, C.: Stimulation of the carotid sinus nerve in treatment of angina pectoris. Amer. Heart J. 80: 759, 1970.
49. Helfant, R. H., Kemp, H. G., and Gorlin, R.: Coronary atherosclerosis, coronary collaterals, and their relation to cardiac function. Ann. Intern. Med. 73: 189, 1970.
50. Miller, R., Mason, D. T., Zelis, R., Bonnano, J. A., and Amsterdam, E. A.: Determinants of the coronary collateral circulation in man: development principally related to severity of regional atherosclerosis. Clin. Res. 19: 117, 1971.
51. Knoebel, S. B.: Correlation of arterial pathology, coronary blood flow and treadmill exercise. In Likoff, W., Segal, B. I., and Moyer, J. H. (eds.): *Hahnemann Symposium on Coronary Heart Disease*. Grune & Stratton, Inc., New York, in press.
52. Reis, R. L., Cohen, L. S., and Mason, D. T.: Direct measurement of instantaneous coronary blood flow after total correction of anomalous left coronary artery. Circulation 39 (Suppl. 1): 229, 1969.
53. Parker, J. O., Case, R. B., Fareeduddin, K., Ledwich, J. R., and Armstrong, P. W.: The influence of changes in blood volume on angina pectoris: a study of the effect of phlebotomy. Circulation 41: 593, 1970.

54. Hellerstein, H. K.: Exercise therapy in coronary disease. Bull. N. Y. Acad. Med. 44: 2, 1968.
55. Clausen, J. P., Larsen, O. A., and Trap-Jensen, J.: Physical training in the management of coronary artery disease. Circulation 40: 143, 1969.
56. Rowe, G. G., Young, W. P., and Wasserburger, R. H.: The effects of ileal bypass plus hypocholesteremic treatment on human coronary atherosclerosis. Proc. Ass. Univ. Cardiologists, February, 1970.
57. Sheldon, W. C., Sones, F. M., Jr., Shirey, E. K., Fergusson, D. J. G., Favaloro, R. G., and Effler, D. B.: Reconstructive coronary artery surgery: postoperative assessment. Circulation 39: 61, 1969.
58. Dart, C. H., Jr., Scott, S., Fish, R., and Takaro, T.: Direct blood flow studies of clinical internal thoracic (mammary) arterial implants. Circulation 41 (Suppl. 2): 64, 1969.
59. Manchester, J. H., and Gorlin, R.: Left ventricular performance after myocardial revascularization with internal mammary artery implantation. Circulation 39 (Suppl. 3): 138, 1969.
60. Salel, A. F., Amsterdam, E. A., Mason, D. T., and Zelis, R.: The importance of type IV hyperlipoproteinemia as a predisposing factor in coronary artery disease. Clin. Res. 19: 321, 1971.

5

Intractable Angina Pectoris: A Therapeutic Challenge

HENRY I. RUSSEK, M.D.

Angina pectoris may become difficult to manage or remain refractory to treatment either as the result of physiological or emotional disturbance, some additional cardiovascular problem, complicating noncoronary disease, or as a consequence of organic changes in the coronary circulation. As a first step in attempting to evaluate and treat the patient who has failed to respond to conventional modes of therapy, the physician must endeavor to determine by means of careful history and physical examination whether or not complicating noncoronary disorders are playing a major role. This will often permit him to answer the following questions:

Has resistance to usual treatment ensued from recurrent paroxysmal tachycardia or bradycardia, from hypoxia associated with congestive heart failure, or from progressive hypertension or valvular heart disease such as aortic stenosis?

Has a relatively mild angina been transformed into an intractable problem by prolonged emotional stress, anger or conflict, anemia, infection, hyperthyroidism, or obstructive prostatic hypertrophy?

In addressing himself to these questions, the physician may find that substantial improvement follows corrective measures such as antiarrhythmic therapy, digitalis, antihypertensive drugs, the resolution of emotional conflict, replacement of blood loss, antibiotics, or surgery.

INTRACTABILITY FROM ORGANIC CHANGES
IN CORONARY ARTERIES

When refractoriness to therapy cannot be explained by noncoronary conditions having an unfavorable influence on oxygen delivery and/or myocardial oxygen consumption, it must be assumed that the aggravation of symptoms has arisen from organic changes within the coronary arteries. Progressive and slow aggravation of typical angina over weeks and months reflects an increasing inadequacy of collateral channels as the main coronary arteries become narrowed and occluded. In these cases of *chronic* cardiac pain, the discomfort occurs with such frequency and with such slight provocation that it may prove not only disabling but also intolerable. The pain usually interrupts sleep many times during the night, and the relief obtained from nitroglycerin is often so brief and transient that numerous tablets must be consumed daily. A similar pattern of intractability may develop *more acutely* as a result of a more recent anatomic change characterized by partial or complete occlusion of a coronary artery without infarction or evident subendocardial necrosis. As a consequence of the sudden reduction in coronary reserve, the characteristic pattern of the anginal syndrome is altered. The episode of discomfort frequently becomes more prolonged and severe, occurring at rest and even without obvious cause. It may occur especially upon recumbency, with some degree of relief on sitting or standing. It may occur more frequently with less and less provocation so that rest or nitroglycerin or both may produce little or no relief. Although this clinical picture often denotes "impending" myocardial infarction, viability of heart muscle may be maintained by collateral circulation despite the critical level of coronary reserve. Consequently, some of the patients who escape acute infarction may gradually improve, while others remain in an intractable state similar to that observed following more gradual elimination of coronary reserve.

TREATMENT OF INTRACTABLE ANGINA PECTORIS

Nitroglycerin

At the outset, it should be recognized that one of the major causes of intractability in angina pectoris resides with the attending physician himself. Even today, almost 100 years after the introduction of nitroglycerin,[1] many patients are left completely unaware of the prophylactic value of the drug, using it only to abort an attack. Others harbor the mistaken notion that nitroglycerin may be habit-forming or harmful, or that its repeated use may lead to failure of response. These misconceptions have arisen, at least in part, from the physician's negligence, inexperience, or failure to "communicate." Frequently, I have encountered patients, referred for surgical revascularization of the myocardium allegedly for intractable angina, who had never been instructed in the proper use of nitroglycerin or long-acting nitrates for the prophylaxis of anginal episodes. Indeed, many have never received any other drug but nitroglycerin and this only for treatment of the actual attack. Consequently, as a first step in evaluating or treating the patient with refractory angina, the kind of antianginal drugs previously employed and the prior manner of their use must be carefully determined.

Long-acting Nitrates

Obviously, to obtain the full potential from any antianginal agent, it is fundamental that the drug's presumed action be permitted to coincide in time with the known pattern of occurrence of anginal episodes in the individual case.[2-9] With traditional drug administration before or after meals, a large segment of patients may be left unprotected during their most vulnerable periods, even with therapeutically active agents.[4, 5] Thus, the many patients who experience angina chiefly in the morning upon arising and the evening upon returning home from work may obtain no greater relief from a potent drug than from an inactive agent. Without carefully planned administration, a similarly negative response must be anticipated when patients with postprandial angina are given medicaments possessing delayed therapeutic effects. Inasmuch as the overwhelming majority of anginal patients seen in clinical practice present such patterns of symptomatology, lack of care in the choice of drugs and in the time of their administration may obscure valuable prophylactic activity. The effective utilization of antianginal therapy therefore requires knowledge both of the individual patient and of the drug employed.[4, 5]

When angina occurs so frequently or unpredictably that the short action of nitroglycerin cannot effectively prevent attacks without repeated administration at brief intervals, the long-acting nitrates may prove most valuable. For this purpose, none is more useful than isosorbide dinitrate (ISD), sublingually, in a 5-mg. dose, three times daily after meals and before contemplated exertion or excitement.[2-5] In contrast with the brief duration of action of nitroglycerin, a significant increase in exercise tolerance has been recorded in tests performed as early as 5 minutes and as late as $1\frac{1}{2}$ to 2 hours following sublingual administration. These observations make it clear that the drug should be administered *after* meals in order to provide the longest possible period of prophylaxis during physical exertion. Obviously, if ISD were taken *before* meals and followed by an interval of inactivity during the ingestion of food and the rest period thereafter, the subsequent duration of protection would be markedly curtailed. Inattention to such simple principles is often responsible for limited success in therapy. When angina pectoris is of appreciable frequency and severity, it has been my practice also to instruct patients to use ISD sublingually before any contemplated exertion and as often as every 1 to 2 hours during periods of physical activity. The drug may also be given orally, but by this route there is not only a 30- to 60-minute delay in the onset of action but also an attenuation of effect.[4, 5] If the oral preparation is employed, it is best administered before meals to permit time for therapeutic response at the resumption of activity following the ingestion of food.

Erythrityl tetranitrate in a sublingual dose of 5 to 15 mg. is similar to

ISD in all respects except for the more frequent occurrence of headache.[2-5] Pentaerythritol tetranitrate administered orally in a dose of 20 mg. three times daily *before* meals is a weaker long-acting nitrate, which nevertheless exerts an influence for 4 to 5 hours after a therapeutic lag of 60 to 90 minutes.[2-5] It is of particular value in patients who show hypersensitivity to the more potent nitrates.

Despite the definite value of these standard preparations for the prevention of anginal attacks, all sustained action oral formulations, whether of isosorbide dinitrate, pentaerythritol tetranitrate, or nitroglycerin, have proved uniformly ineffectual or unsatisfactory.[4, 5] It is not uncommon to recover such preparations relatively unaltered in the patient's stool. Nonetheless, American physicians unwittingly continue to prescribe these weak sustained action preparations far more frequently than the worthwhile standard preparations of the same drugs. In our experience, sustained action formulations when given in two or three times the recommended dosage at bedtime do have value for the prevention of nocturnal angina. In such instances, the small amount of nitrate slowly absorbed appears adequate to prevent coronary spasm engendered by disturbing dreams even though the same dosage has proved ineffectual for angina of effort during the waking hours.

MANAGEMENT OF INTRACTABLE ANGINA PECTORIS

It can be seen that the physician himself may be responsible for the intractability of angina both through the omission or improper use of potent preparations and the utilization of weak or useless ones.

When, however, the severity of symptoms has incapacitated the patient to a major degree despite the prudent use of potent antianginal agents, it has been accepted practice to institute a broad therapeutic regimen of coordinated measures designed primarily to correct the noncoronary factors contributing to the intractability of angina. In brief, this consists of a period of bed rest in hospital to ensure a reduction in physical activity and isolation from stressful environment, a bland, low calorie, low fat diet, abstinence from tobacco, coffee, and alcohol, and the use of sedatives, nitrates such as nitroglycerin and isosorbide dinitrate, and digitalis, if indicated. With the resolution of conflicts, adjustments in interpersonal relationships, or psychotherapy, improvement often develops and dramatic relief sometimes may ensue.

Since the benefits from this approach are in large measure or wholly attributable to the reduction in circulating catecholamines with consequent reduction of cardiac work and myocardial oxygen requirements, the same end result might be readily achieved almost immediately and without sacrifice by means of beta adrenergic receptor blockade. With the advent of propranolol[10-15] and particularly since its use in combination with isosorbide dinitrate,[16-18] bed rest and other restrictive measures are now rarely indicated. Indeed the designation "intractable angina pectoris" will be applicable to a much smaller segment of patients when propranolol-nitrate therapy is widely and effectively utilized for the treatment of severe cases.

Propranolol

Until recently, nitroglycerin and the long-acting nitrates provided the major approach to prophylaxis and treatment in angina pectoris. With the introduction of propranolol and other beta adrenergic blocking agents, a significant advance has been achieved in antianginal therapy. The versatility of cardiovascular function which allows the normal heart to adjust to varying levels of physical activity is mediated through adrenergic stimulation. Since the heart with an impoverished blood supply can ill afford the unneeded overactivity which accompanies a wide range of responses to adrenergic stimulation, beta blockade may be utilized to modify cardiac function to correspond to actual needs. Thus, by decreasing heart rate and ventricular systolic force, propranolol may reduce the myocardial oxygen requirements to a level more readily satisfied by a restricted coronary flow. In an oral dose varying from as little as 40 mg. to as much as 400 mg. per day, the drug has been found effective in alleviating angina pectoris previously refractory to conventional modes of therapy. Most patients respond to a dosage level of 40 mg. administered three or four times daily, but if this dose does not produce an attenuation of the resting heart rate to 55 to 60 beats per minute, gradual increments are made until this is achieved. The starting dose probably should be no more than 20 mg. three times daily, since absorption varies considerably among patients and a small number will respond adequately at this level.

Propranolol plus Isosorbide Dinitrate

Of far greater importance to the refractory anginal patient is the protection afforded by the synergistic interaction of propranolol and certain long-acting nitrates, notably isosorbide dinitrate administered sublingually. Our studies over the past 5 years have shown that this combination of drugs has fundamentally altered the quality of life for patients previously unresponsive to conventional modes of therapy. Thus, when these drugs were used in combination, the resultant increase in exercise tolerance was four times that observed when either drug was used alone. Strong evidence for synergism was also noted in studies of ischemic patterns observed in post-exercise electrocardiograms.

Although each drug tends to decrease the work of the heart and to prevent myocardial ischemia, it is primarily through the canceling out of adverse subsidiary effects that the two drugs appear to achieve therapeutic synergism. Propranolol, while reducing the energy requirements for cardiac contraction, also reduces coronary blood flow through vasoconstriction (or loss of vasodilation). This undesirable action, which may partially negate its benefits, is effectively blocked by the simultaneous use of an active nitrate preparation. Contrariwise, propranolol prevents the oxygen-wasting tachycardia and increased contractility induced by isosorbide dinitrate and other related compounds. These observations appear adequate to explain the fact that concurrent administration is attended by therapeutic responses which appreciably exceed the sum of those evoked when each of the two drugs is administered independently.

In a study of 100 patients maintained on combined therapy consisting of propranolol (20 to 100 mg. orally) before meals and isosorbide dinitrate (5 mg. sublingually) after meals, 85 per cent have shown not only a significant and unexpected increase in exercise tolerance but also marked improvement or complete reversal in ischemic electrocardiographic patterns induced by standard exercise. Moreover, these benefits have been consistently maintained in most patients during follow-up periods ranging from 1 to 4 years (Fig. 5.1). Patients in this study have had severe grades of angina unresponsive to conventional modes of therapy. Many have been considered poor risks for surgery because of triple coronary artery disease and diffuse involvement of the coronary system. Of the 100 patients in the series, 84 per cent are alive after 3 years; one-third have sustained myocardial infarction but more than half of these survived the attack. These results appear to indicate that the patient with severe angina pectoris or triple coronary artery disease is not necessarily in danger of immediate dissolution should revascularization surgery be delayed or omitted entirely, as some surgically oriented physicians have claimed. Only 7 per cent of patients have manifested side effects such as dyspnea or faintness, while only 4 per cent have required discontinuation of therapy.

Consideration of the time of onset and duration of action of propranolol and isosorbide dinitrate, respectively, helps to provide an optimal formula for their administration in a comined treatment program. The following facts must be borne in mind in establishing a schedule for therapy.

1. The patient's most vulnerable period is following the ingestion of food.

2. Propranolol requires 30 to 60 minutes for therapeutic effect, while ISD is active within 5 minutes.

3. Propranolol in a single dose has a duration of action of 4 to 5 hours, while ISD sublingually exerts its influence for only $1\frac{1}{2}$ to 2 hours.

In order to provide the longest period of maximal prophylaxis during physical stress, the following routine is recommended.

A. The patient is instructed to rest for at least $\frac{1}{2}$ hour after each meal whenever possible.

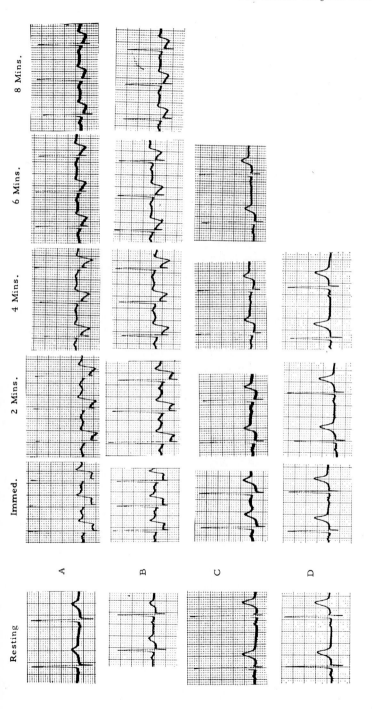

A. Placebo
B. ISD 5 mg. subling.
C. Propranolol, 40 mg.
D. ISD & Propranolol

Fig. 5.1. Electrocardiographic responses to various drugs in a patient who had been on continuous therapy with propranolol and isosorbide dinitrate (ISD) for a period of 18 months.

B. The dose of propranolol is administered before each meal, so that the drug is fully active upon the resumption of activity following the postprandial rest period.

C. Isosorbide dinitrate is taken sublingually 5 minutes before the termination of the rest period following each meal.

Given in this manner, both drugs become active at about the time that physical exertion is resumed, and no portion of the prophylactic effect is wasted during the sedentary dining period. Since ISD tapers in its effect after 1½ to 2 hours, it should be taken again between meals by those engaged in continuous activity or before any contemplated exertion by those who have no established routine of work or play. If this practice is not followed, it is evident that only the limited benefits from propranolol may be available to the patient during certain periods of activity when maximal protection may be indicated.

The schedule outlined may be modified according to need in the individual case. Thus, if angina is experienced immediately on arising in the morning, ISD is administered prior to getting out of bed. If angina is encountered during the ingestion of food, ISD is given before meals, and if nocturnal angina occurs, both propranolol and ISD are prescribed at bedtime. The basic schedule outlined previously is of course maintained with any or all of these modifications. Failure to consider the respective patterns of action of these drugs and to titrate their dosage for the individual patient has resulted not only in the denial of their synergistic activity but also in the claim that they are actually detrimental or hazardous.[19] Similar indiscriminate use of other potent drugs such as insulin, epinephrine, cortisone, or thyroxine could also have led to their unjustified condemnation.

TRANQUILIZERS AND SEDATIVES

Tranquilizers and sedatives were gaining increasing importance in the treatment of angina pectoris until the introduction of beta adrenergic blockade. Since the psychic reaction to the perception of anginal pain tends to perpetuate or augment the transient imbalance between coronary flow and myocardial requirements, it is desirable to prevent the rebound effects which are mediated by the sympathetic nervous system and catecholamine release. Among these effects are augmentation of myocardial metabolism, increase of heart rate and blood pressure, and diminution of cardiac efficiency.

Sedatives and tranquilizers, such as phenobarbital, meprobamate (Equanil, Miltown), and chlordiazepoxide (Librium), have proved valuable as adjuvant therapy in combination with "vasodilators" in the management of angina pectoris. Alcohol in moderate amounts may also be useful when employed for its tranquilizing properties, but it is not to be considered a coronary vasodilator.[20] Indeed, when anxiety states coexist, tranquilizers may be as effective as vasodilators for reducing anginal episodes. This fact may not be recognized when the physician overlooks the total patient in his zeal to treat the disease alone. Beta adrenergic receptor blockade, however, by protecting the heart from psychogenic influences, has diminished the need for tranquilizing agents.

ANTITHYROID DRUGS OR RADIOIODINE

By reducing metabolism and diminishing the work of the heart, antithyroid drugs or radioactive iodine may prevent the transient myocardial ischemia underlying the anginal syndrome. In addition to these actions, the resultant decrease in the sensitivity of the myocardium to catecholamines and possible alteration in the utilization of oxygen or in the pathways of energy release may play a significant role in clinical response. Although impressive results are occasionally observed in refractory cases of angina pectoris, the advent of beta adrenergic blockade has all but eliminated the need for consideration of induced myxedema as a therapeutic approach.

ELECTRICAL STIMULATION OF CAROTID SINUS NERVES

Surgical implantation of electrical stimulators of the carotid sinus nerve has been reported to relieve patients with incapacitating angina pectoris.[21] Activation of the stimulator allegedly terminated almost all episodes of angina in 11 of 17 patients in whom implantation was performed. Two patients experienced no benefit, while two others died from the procedure.

This high immediate mortality rate from an approach of questionable long-term value must surely be regarded as unacceptable. Moreover, inasmuch as a prerequisite for implantation was "an increase in exercise tolerance after administration of either nitroglycerin or isosorbide dinitrate," it appears more than likely that equal or better results would have been achieved from the prudent use of propranolol-nitrate therapy. If the same attention required for the repeated activation of the stimulator were given to the prophylactic and therapeutic trial of nitroglycerin or isosorbide dinitrate in conjunction with propranolol, such intervention would very likely find little or no clinical application. An occasional patient, however, may be aided by this form of therapy.

SURGICAL REVASCULARIZATION OF MYOCARDIUM

Until recently, internal mammary artery implantation into the myocardium was used extensively for the treatment of angina pectoris. While the value of such intervention in specific instances was undeniable, the dramatic results achieved in a fortunate few did not appear to justify the high price tag in morbidity and mortality for the many others. Thus, even under the most favorable circumstances, the double arterial implant was almost immediately responsible for infarction, serious complication, or death in at least one of every five patients.[22, 23] For this calculated risk, objective clinical benefit could be anticipated in less than 50 per cent of survivors, with noteworthy response in only 20 per cent. Comparable studies employing propranolol in combination with isosorbide dinitrate were attended by a much lower mortality, significantly higher incidence of benefit, and greater freedom from complications than was observed following surgical revascularization.

The relatively new surgical procedure, saphenous vein bypass from aorta to coronary artery, has been associated with the most dramatic success of all techniques utilized to date. The proper selection of patients and the careful weighing of risks should save lives and restore certain incapacitated patients to a more productive existence. Since coronary artery disease is often a diffuse and inexorable process, not all patients can be considered suitable for surgery. Unfortunately, there are no clearly defined rules by which to identify the ideal candidate for bypass surgery. Diffuse involvement of smaller branches would appear to contraindicate surgical intervention because of the likelihood of poor peripheral run-off. The desire to save myocardium should not lead us into the trap of needlessly sacrificing life. Reports of mortality undoubtedly understate the operative risk. It is well known that leading centers frequently select patients carefully and operate only upon the best surgical risks. Unaware of this selective process, other groups, encouraged by the low mortality rates reported, have been operating on almost all patients referred for evaluation. As a consequence, the mortality rate has soared in proportion to the enthusiasm that has been generated. Multiple bypass grafts may raise the operative mortality to 20 per cent or higher. Even when the outcome of surgery is apparently successful, this may be short-lived as a consequence of progression of the disease or occlusion of the venous graft. Reassessment of patients 1 to 2 years after operation has disclosed an unexplained process of profound fibroblast proliferation in the subintimal layer affecting almost a quarter of the saphenous veins used for coronary artery bypass grafts.[24] It would appear reasonable that patients should at least have the benefit of optimal medical care before surgery is considered. Unfortunately, they are still being referred often without adequate trial of medical therapy, without consideration of the relative medical and surgical risks, and in the erroneous belief that a cure is reasonably certain.

Saphenous vein bypass is undoubtedly a significant advance in the treatment of severe and refractory forms of angina pectoris. Careful study will eventually delineate the patients most likely to benefit from this procedure. Indeed, in patients with proximal coronary artery occlusion, bypass surgery may ultimately prove of prophylactic value in reducing the likelihood of myocardial infarction and in prolonging survival.

SUMMARY

Since the introduction of nitroglycerin, there have been only two major advances in the medical therapy of angina pectoris: the long-acting nitrates and propranolol. While each may be effective alone in individual patients, their combination produces striking synergistic effects constituting a major breakthrough in the management of refractory angina pectoris. In a study of 100 patients maintained on combined therapy, 85 per cent have shown not only a significant and unexpected increase in exercise tolerance but also marked improvement or complete reversal in ischemic electrocardiographic patterns induced by standard exercise. These benefits have been consistently maintained in most patients during follow-up periods ranging from 1 to 4 years. Success in therapy is dependent on careful titration of each patient to determine optimal dosage for the individual case.

The advent of beta adrenergic blockade has eliminated the need for antithyroid drugs or radioiodine for the control of intractable angina.

Electrical stimulation of the carotid sinus nerves to relieve patients with incapacitating angina pectoris is rarely necessary and is unlikely to find application in more than an occasional patient.

Surgical revascularization of the myocardium by means of saphenous vein bypass has been associated with the most dramatic success of all techniques utilized to date. Careful study will eventually delineate the patients most likely to benefit from this procedure. In the meanwhile, enthusiasm should be tempered to avoid indiscriminate surgical intervention and needless loss of life.

REFERENCES

1. Murrell, W.: Nitroglycerine as a remedy for angina pectoris. Lancet 1: 80, 113, 151, 224, 1879.
2. Russek, H. I.: The choice of a coronary vasodilator in clinical practice. G. P. 28: 84, 1963.
3. Russek, H. I.: The therapeutic role of coronary vasodilators. In *Coronary Heart Disease*. Grune & Stratton, Inc., New York, 1963, p. 332.
4. Russek, H. I.: The therapeutic role of coronary vasodilators: glyceryl trinitrate, isosorbide dinitrate, and pentaerythritol tetranitrate. Amer. J. Med. Sci. 252: 43, 1966.
5. Russek, H. I.: Antianginal drugs: current status. Cardiovasc. Clin. 1970.
6. Russek, H. I., and Howard, J. C.: Glyceryl trinitrate in angina pectoris. J. A. M. A. 189: 108, 1964.
7. Russek, H. I., Zohman, B. L., and Dorset, V. J.: Objective evaluation of coronary vasodilator drugs. Amer. J. Med. Sci. 229: 46, 1955.
8. Russek, H. I., Urbach, K. F., Doerner, A. A., and Zohman, B. L.: Choice of a coronary vasodilator drug in clinical practice. J. A. M. A. 153: 207, 1953.
9. Russek, H. I., Smith, R. H., Baum, W., Naegele, C., and Regan, F. D.: Influence of saline, papaverine, nitroglycerine and ethyl alcohol on the electrocardiographic response to standard exercise in coronary disease. Circulation 1: 700, 1950.

10. Gillam, P. M. S., and Prichard, B. N. C.: Propranolol in the therapy of angina pectoris. Amer. J. Cardiol. 18: 366, 1966.
11. Ginn, W. M., Jr., and Orgain, E. S.: Propranolol hydrochloride in the treatment of angina pectoris. J. A. M. A. 198: 1214, 1966.
12. Grant, R. H. E., *et al.*: Multicenter trial of propranolol in angina pectoris. Amer. J. Cardiol. 18: 361, 1966.
13. Hamer, J., and Sowton, E.: Effects of propranolol on exercise tolerance in angina pectoris. Amer. J. Cardiol. 18: 354, 1966.
14. Rabkin, R., Stables, D. P., Levin, N. W., and Suzman, M. M.: The prophylactic value of propranolol in angina pectoris. Amer. J. Cardiol. 18: 370, 1966.
15. Wolfson, S., *et al.*: Propranolol and angina pectoris. Amer. J. Cardiol. 18: 345, 1966.
16. Russek, H. I.: Propranolol and isosorbide dinitrate synergism in angina pectoris. Amer. J. Med. Sci. 254: 406, 1967.
17. Russek, H. I.: Propranolol and isosorbide dinitrate synergism in angina pectoris. Amer. J. Cardiol. 21: 44, 1968.
18. Russek, H. I.: New dimension in angina pectoris therapy. Geriatrics 24: 81, 1969.
19. Aronow, W. S., and Kaplan, M. A.: Propranolol combined with isosorbide dinitrate versus placebo in angina pectoris. New Engl. J. Med. 280: 847, 1969.
20. Russek, H. I., Naegele, C. F., and Regan, F. D.: Alcohol in the treatment of angina pectoris. J. A. M. A. 143: 355, 1950.
21. Epstein, S. E., *et al.*: Treatment of angina pectoris by electrical stimulation of the carotid-sinus nerves: results in 17 patients with severe angina. New Engl. J. Med. 280: 971–978, 1969.
22. Russek, H. I.: Medical vs. surgical therapy for angina pectoris. Dis. Chest 55: 269, 1969.
23. Russek, H. I.: Medical versus surgical therapy in angina pectoris. Geriatrics 25: 93–102, 1970.
24. Johnson, W. D., Auer, J. E., and Tector, A. J.: Late changes in coronary vein grafts. Paper presented at Twentieth Annual Scientific Session, American College of Cardiology, Washington, D. C., February 4, 1971.

6

Angina with Normally Patent Coronary Arteries

WILLIAM LIKOFF, M.D.

Among the determinants of coronary blood flow, the internal caliber of the arterial channels is the most important. Aortic and right atrial pressures, vascular resistance, and blood viscosity have smaller but pertinent roles.

Myocardial oxygen uptake is regulated by the size, configuration, and thickness of the ventricle and by intraventricular pressure which combine to determine systolic wall stress, by pulse rate and ejection interval which establish the duration of that stress, and by the inotropic state of the cardiac muscle fibers from which contractile force flows. Fiber shortening and the energy required for depolarization and electromechanical coupling are secondary factors.

The pathophysiological basis for angina pectoris is an unfavorable balance between coronary blood flow and myocardial oxygen uptake. In the main, it is brought about by atherosclerosis which compromises the internal caliber of the coronary vessels. Other disorders such as syphilitic occlusion of the coronary ostia, coronary embolism, dissecting aortic aneurysm, periarteritis nodosa, and thromboangiitis obliterans mimic atherosclerosis and cause angina by blocking or reducing the caliber of the coronary arteries.

Although exceptional, angina does occur when the coronary vessels are normally patent. The syndrome arises because factors other than mechanical obstruction adversely influence coronary perfusion at a time when myocardial oxygen consumption is greatly increased.

Severe aortic stenosis is a classic example. Marked elevation of intraventricular pressure increases peripheral coronary resistance, thereby diminishing coronary flow during systole. At the same time the thickened ventricular musculature, high intraventricular pressure, and prolonged ejection interval increase myocardial oxygen needs considerably.

The coronary arterial system usually is overdeveloped and widely patent in significant rheumatic aortic regurgitation. Nevertheless, angina is not

77

uncommon. The factors responsible include diminished coronary flow during diastole, resulting from abnormally depressed aortic head pressure, and increased myocardial oxygen consumption due to the size and configuration of the left ventricle.

Subjects with cardiomyopathy may suffer from angina although the coronary arteries are unobstructed. The causative mechanisms in idiopathic hypertrophic subaortic stenosis, for example, are identical with those in aortic stenosis. However, explanations are less certain in restrictive and congestive cardiomyopathies and may involve consideration of both structural and metabolic errors which impede normal cellular oxygen utilization.

Since the advent of coronary arteriography, a group of patients has been identified as having recurrent, even disabling angina although free of demonstrable obstructive coronary atherosclerosis.[1-3] The individuals comprising the group are in the main normally menstruating females without valvular or myocardial disease who are singularly free of the risk factors predisposing to atherosclerosis, especially hypertension, diabetes, and abnormal concentrations of circulating lipids.

In the majority, the presenting clinical manifestation is retrosternal discomfort brought on by physical and emotional stress. The syndrome is less typical in others but still closely resembles angina. Without exception the electrocardiogram at rest or after exercise is abnormal. The changes are limited to the RST segments and T waves and are strikingly similar to those encountered in subendocardial ischemia.

The cause of angina in these patients is not known. Abnormal hemoglobin-oxygen dissociation curves have been discovered in a number of individuals, suggesting the possibility that incomplete oxygen release is responsible.[4] Small vessel disease also has been considered as an etiological factor.[5] However, autopsy examination of three individuals did not reveal small vessel lesions.[4] Coronary arterial spasm and myocardial bridging have not been encountered consistently. The perfectly normal appearance of the arterial channels during visualization makes it unlikely that thrombotic lesions were present and recanalized.

The lack of a satisfactory explanation for angina in this particular group of patients accounts in large measure for the fact that the very existence of the clinical problem has been seriously questioned. It has been suggested that the chest pain does not resemble angina but more closely simulates the discomfort encountered in a host of inconsequential neuromuscular and psychosomatic disorders. This is not an acceptable view. Even the more atypical expressions of discomfort in these patients can hardly be confused with an anterior chest wall syndrome or the manifestations which characterize neurocirculatory asthenia. Furthermore, unmistakable electrocardiographic abnormalities do exist at rest or following exercise.

The view also has been expressed that these patients have obstructive lesions in major or lesser coronary arteries which cannot be seen because of the inherent limitations of arteriography or inadequacies in its application.[5] Admittedly, visualization underestimates vascular pathology. However, it is extremely unlikely that major obstructive lesions are mistaken for normally patent channels even by the most inexperienced hands.

At least for the present it is reasonable to conclude these are not misjudged patients but individuals who represent a distinct clinical entity. Treatment has not been particularly effective. Nitroglycerin may relieve an attack of acute discomfort as readily as it controls the pain caused by coronary vascular disease. However, long-acting nitrates are notoriously ineffective. Beta blockade has been helpful but not consistently so.

Even though an imbalance between coronary perfusion and the metabolic needs of the myocardium does develop when the internal caliber of the coronary arteries is not compromised, the occasions and clinical examples are limited. In no way do they appreciably modify the basic axiom that angina pectoris is a clinical syndrome usually arising as a result of obstructive coronary artery disease.

REFERENCES

1. Likoff, W., Segal, B. L., and Kasparian, H.: Paradox of normal selective coronary arteriograms in patients considered to have unmistakable coronary heart disease. New Engl. J. Med. 276: 1063, 1967.
2. Gorlin, R.: Anginal pain without atherosclerosis. J. A. M. A. 201: 27, 1967.
3. Dwyer, E. M., Jr., Winener, L., and Cox, W.: Angina and normal coronary arteriogram. Amer. J. Cardiol. 23: 639, 1969.
4. Eliot, R. S., and Bratt, G.: The paradox of myocardial ischemia and necrosis in young women with normal coronary arteriograms: relation to abnormal hemoglobin-oxygen dissociation. Amer. J. Cardiol. 23: 633, 1969.
5. James, T. N.: Angina without coronary disease. Circulation 62: 109, 1970.

7

Diagnosis and Treatment of Cardiomyopathy

GEORGE E. BURCH, M.D. AND T. D. GILES, M.D.

The continuing difficulty with the clinical and pathological classification of heart muscle disease was emphasized again recently.[1, 2] Nevertheless, the patient with a large dilated heart and congestive heart failure is a common problem which demands an accurate and early diagnosis and proper treatment. Therefore, this presentation is concerned with practical clinical aspects of the cardiomyopathies. Because of limited space, only the cardiomyopathies most commonly encountered in the United States are considered.

GENERAL CONSIDERATIONS

Cardiomyopathy literally means pathology of heart muscle. Myocardial pathology exists because of, and in association with, numerous disease states (Table 7.1), many of which have no specific treatment. This is of clinical importance because, until specific therapy is available for each etiological type of heart muscle disease, broad general principles of clinical management must be applied to the cardiomyopathies.

Regardless of etiology, patients with cardiomyopathy have in common many clinical manifestations.[3-5] For example, these patients complain of weakness, fatigue, dyspnea on exertion, palpitation, orthopnea, paroxysmal nocturnal dyspnea, peripheral edema, and the many other manifestations of congestive heart failure. Palpitation, pleuritic chest pain, syncope, cough, and hemoptysis, often indicative of pulmonary embolism, are also frequent complaints. The clinical manifestations of systemic and pulmonary emboli are protean.

Because so little is known concerning the possible causes of cardiomyopathy, meticulous history-taking is always essential, not only for the sake of patient management but also for the advancement of knowledge concerning the disease process. There are particular areas in history-taking

80

Table 7.1. *Types of cardiomyopathy*

I. Primary heart muscle disease
  A. Familial cardiomyopathy
    1. with ventricular outflow tract obstruction
    2. without ventricular outflow tract obstruction
  B. Nonfamilial idiopathic cardiomyopathy
    1. with ventricular outflow tract obstruction
    2. without ventricular outflow tract obstruction
  C. Endomyocardial fibrosis
II. Secondary heart muscle disease
  A. Infectious cardiomyopathy
    1. viral
    2. bacterial
    3. rickettsial
    4. protozoal
    5. metazoal
  B. Alcoholic cardiomyopathy
  C. Postpartal cardiomyopathy
  D. Metabolic cardiomyopathy
    1. hyperthyroidism
    2. hypothyroidism
    3. amyloidosis
      a. secondary
      b. primary
      c. primary cardiac
    4. glycogen storage disease
      a. Pompe's disease
      b. Forbe's disease
    5. nutritional deficiency
      a. thiamine deficiency (beriberi)
      b. protein deficiency
      c. avitaminosis
  E. Allergy-related cardiomyopathy
    1. post-vaccinal
    2. serum sickness
    3. urticaria
  F. Toxic cardiomyopathy
    1. drugs (emetine, arsenic, isoproterenol)
    2. anesthetic gases
    3. poisons
    4. foods
    5. heavy metals (cobalt, cadmium, etc.)
  G. Cardiomyopathy associated with systemic disease of unknown etiology
    1. rheumatoid arthritis
    2. autoimmune disease
  H. Infiltrative cardiomyopathy
    1. carcinomatosis (lung, thyroid)
    2. leukemia
    3. hemochromatosis
    4. sarcoidosis

Table 7.1.—*Continued*

I. Cardiomyopathy due to physical agents
  1. nonpenetrating chest injury
  2. heat sickness
  3. ionizing radiation
  4. electric shock
  5. solar radiation
J. Cardiomyopathy associated with neuromuscular disorders
  1. progressive muscular dystrophy
    a. Duchenne dystrophy
    b. limb-girdle (Erb)
    c. fascioscapulohumeral (Landouzy-Déjérine)
K. Primary tumor of the myocardium
L. Senile cardiomyopathy
M. Ischemic cardiomyopathy

which often give clinicians difficulty. For example, a history of precordial pain, angina, or myocardial infarction may often be difficult to obtain.[6] Likewise, much patience and effort may be required to evaluate the role of hypertension in a particular patient with cardiomyopathy. In the latter instance, records of blood pressure from previous examinations, *e.g.*, pre-employment, insurance, or military, are often invaluable.

Many patients with cardiomyopathy may be said to have pre-existing "rheumatic" heart disease. Such patients must be carefully questioned since rheumatic heart disease has not been clearly defined. Indeed, the accepted criteria change every decade.[7]

Many toxic agents are often not appreciated as etiological factors capable of producing myocardial damage. Regardless of how remote the possible role of such agents may be, these agents must be carefully considered. Industrial solvents, patent medicines, insecticides, drugs, alcohol, and other chemicals can injure the myocardium. Past infections which may elude the unsuspecting clinician, such as forgotten colds, so-called viral infections, or upper respiratory tract infections, are important clues to the cause of myocardial disease. Since malnutrition alone can produce cardiomyopathy as well as complicate other types of heart muscle disease, a meticuluous dietary history should always be obtained. Unfortunately, a history of malnutrition is often difficult to obtain because challenging the dietary adequacy of some people places them in a position of defending their pride. Furthermore, people often do not remember what they eat. Thus, much perseverance and effort are required to obtain a fairly reliable history of dietary habits.

A history of the intake of alcoholic beverages is extremely important since alcohol, alone or in association with malnutrition, infection, and other conditioning factors, may produce cardiomyopathy. The relationship of alcoholic intake and malnutrition to the production of cardiomyopathy is similar to their relationship to the production of liver disease.

The general appearance of the patient with advanced cardiomyopathy and dilated heart is that of a person with right and left ventricular congestive heart failure. On physical examination, patients with cardiomyopathy[3-5] are usually found to have a narrow pulse pressure resulting from an elevated arterial diastolic blood pressure, often to 110 mm. Hg or more, in association with a relatively low systolic pressure. Restoration and maintenance of normal arterial blood pressure following successful treatment of the congestive heart failure is a common occurrence in cardiomyopathies and is a good sign of improvement. A wide pulse pressure should alert the physician to suspect a specific cause for the cardiomyopathy, such as thyrotoxicosis, or to search for an associated circulatory disturbance, such as aortic insufficiency. A weak peripheral arterial pulse and jugular venous distention, often with a large *v* wave secondary to tricuspid insufficiency, are frequent physical findings. Careful examination of the ocular fundi and peripheral blood vessels provides important information concerning hypertensive and arteriosclerotic processes.

The apex beat of the heart is usually displaced laterally and inferiorly, and a left ventricular heave may be seen and palpated—findings indicative of left ventricular enlargement. A left parasternal lift is usually also present, indicating enlargement of the right ventricle. On auscultation, the heart sounds at the apex may be of poor quality and somewhat muffled in intensity. A protodiastolic gallop rhythm is usually present, at times appreciated by palpation as well as by auscultation. An atrial gallop is a frequent auscultatory finding, and the clinician may palpate an associated double apical impulse. When the cardiac rate is sufficiently rapid, summation gallops, *i.e.*, superimposition of protodiastolic and atrial gallop sounds, may be heard. The second heart sound at the pulmonic area may have a loud pulmonic component and may at times exhibit paradoxical splitting.

Apical systolic murmurs, often pansystolic, are common in cardiomyopathy and are probably related in large part to papillary muscle dysfunction.[8, 9] The murmur is due to one or both of the following factors which result in papillary muscle dysfunction: (1) as the ventricles dilate, their walls and attached papillary muscles are displaced centrifugally, thus holding the valve leaflets partially open during systole, and/or (2) disease of the papillary muscles themselves is present which interferes with their contraction, resulting in impairment of valve closure, as discussed previously.[9] Generally, when heart failure improves, especially when there is reduction in the size of the left ventricle, the murmur of papillary muscle dysfunction decreases in intensity and changes in quality, whereas the opposite may be true in acquired, organic disease of the mitral valve. Occasionally, the murmur of papillary muscle dysfunction may have an ejection quality, and amyl nitrite may be useful in the differential diagnosis involving subaortic hypertrophic stenosis by causing the murmur of papillary muscle dysfunction to become less audible and the obstructive murmur to become louder.

Of course, various types of cardiomyopathy may occur in association with any type of valvular heart disease. Cardiomyopathy should be considered by the clinician when a patient's signs and symptoms are out of proportion to those expected for the valve disease alone.

Roentgenograms of the chest reveal generalized cardiomegaly and evidence of pulmonary vascular congestion. The presence of a significant pericardial effusion may be excluded by carboangiography, echocardiography, or radioisotope scans. We have found carboangiography most reliable and least expensive.[10]

The electrocardiogram (ECG) and vectorcardiogram are abnormal in all patients with cardiomyopathy and congestive heart failure (Fig. 7.1). The electrocardiographic changes associated with the different types of cardiomyopathy are discussed below.

Cardiac catheterization in patients with cardiomyopathy adds little if any clinically useful information, is usually unnecessary, and can be dangerous. In fact, over-reliance on cardiac catheterization procedures in a noncritical fashion may even mislead the physician. A low cardiac output, elevation of the mean right atrial and right ventricular diastolic pressures, and normal or slightly elevated pulmonary artery and capillary wedge pressures are found when expected from the clinical data.[3] In fact, pulmonary capillary wedge pressure is almost always elevated. The left ventricular

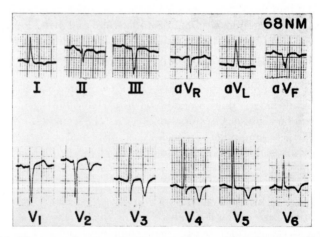

Fig. 7.1. Electrocardiogram of a 68-year-old man with ischemic cardiomyopathy. The ECG shows evidence of diffuse myocardial disease found frequently in patients with all types of cardiomyopathy.

end diastolic pressure is elevated as well as the left atrial pressure, as would be expected, in patients who manifest left ventricular congestive heart failure clinically. Left atrial pressure usually exceeds right atrial pressure by more than 10 mm. Hg in those patients. The capable cardiologist, after a thorough clinical evaluation, can usually establish the diagnosis in any patient with cardiomyopathy and can understand the pathological physiology involved. Only when another diagnosis is suspected clinically should extensive diagnostic procedures be performed. For example, when subaortic hypertrophic stenosis is suspected, left heart catheterization is useful.

The clinical course of patients with cardiomyopathy varies with the etiology, extent of the damage to the myocardium, and duration of the illness and treatment. Recurrent small pulmonary emboli are a common complicating feature of all types of cardiomyopathies and often originate from the heart.

SPECIFIC TYPES OF CARDIOMYOPATHY

The grouping of cardiomyopathy into **primary,** *i.e.*, when the heart is the only diseased organ, and **secondary,** *i.e.*, when the heart is involved as part of a systemic illness or illness elsewhere, is purely arbitrary (Table 7.1). Whether a cardiomyopathy is diagnosed as primary or secondary often depends on how thorough the clinician has been in taking the history and in performing the physical examination. The history is usually the most important part of the work-up in establishing etiological factors.

Idiopathic cardiomyopathy, as in any idiopathic disease, simply refers to the cardiomyopathy for which the etiology remains unknown. In the presence of a strong family history, the disease may be termed **familial,** but care must be taken not to interpret this as meaning genetically inherited. Environmental factors such as crowded living areas, poor nutrition, common infectious agents in a family environment, and the like may all be responsible for familial as well as sporadic cardiomyopathy.

Since any systemic illness may damage the myocardium to varying degrees, it should be expected that in some people it may ultimately produce sufficient myocardial damage to result in myocardial insufficiency with manifestations of congestive heart failure. It should also be remembered that many of the cardiomyopathies may be due to interrelated factors, *e.g.*, alcohol, viral infections, and coronary artery disease, rather than one pathogenic process alone.

Alcoholic cardiomyopathy[11-19] is fairly common in the United States. Unfortunately, sufficiently accurate data are not available to determine its exact incidence. A history of excessive alcohol intake is of paramount importance in the diagnosis of alcoholic cardiomyopathy. Although there may be some disagreement concerning the definition of the word "excessive" with respect to alcoholic intake, most patients with this disease consume large quantities of alcoholic beverages. Patients intentionally or unintentionally underestimate considerably their consumption of alcohol unless carefully questioned. Any type of alcoholic beverage apparently can damage the myocardium if imbibed in sufficiently large quantities, but it is quite likely that some people are more sensitive to the cardiotoxic effects of alcohol than others. Daily large consumption of alcohol seems to be more important in the pathogenesis of alcoholic cardiomyopathy than infrequent episodes of acute intoxication.

Although some patients with alcoholic cardiomyopathy are malnourished, the majority of them appear well fed. A stereotyped concept of the patient with alcoholic cardiomyopathy as a "skid row bum" will cause the clinician frequently to miss the diagnosis. The bulk of experimental evidence suggests that alcohol alone may cause cardiomyopathy.[19]

In contrast to ischemic cardiomyopathy, which affects the older age group, the usual age of patients with alcoholic cardiomyopathy is 30 to 50 years. However, alcoholic cardiomyopathy may occur in any age group provided that large quantities of alcohol are consumed.

Palpitation and the insidious onset of dyspnea are early symptoms characteristic of this group of patients. Premature contractions and other arrhythmias may occur early. In fact, in a patient found to have atrial fibrillation with no obvious cause, cardiomyopathy, including alcoholic, should be strongly considered. The changes in the T waves of the electrocardiogram (alcoholic T waves)[12] discussed below may also be manifestations of early myocardial damage. Recognizing these early electrocardiographic changes and correlating them with the use of alcohol are extremely important since, with proper advice, advanced cardiomyopathy can be prevented. The symptoms of congestive heart failure usually develop so insidiously that the patient and even his physician fail to recognize the disease until it is far advanced. However, occasionally congestive heart failure has a fairly explosive onset.

Findings on physical examination are described above. The clinican should try to distinguish between the rapid, hyperkinetic circulation associated with predominantly right-sided congestive heart failure seen in beriberi and low cardiac output with predominantly left-sided congestive heart failure of alcoholic cardiomyopathy. However, both types of heart disease are eventually associated with biventricular failure. If, after careful examination of the patient, the question of whether or not thiamine deficiency exists is still unresolved, a therapeutic trial of thiamine is advisable.

Occasionally, one may find clinical and laboratory evidence of severe hepatic disease, but it is unusual to find alcoholic cirrhosis associated with alcoholic cardiomyopathy and congestive heart failure.

The ECG of patients with alcoholic cardiomyopathy may often show characteristic T wave changes early in the course of the disease, as mentioned above.[12] The T waves associated with alcoholism are of several types. Spinous T waves are tall ones with a needle-like point at the apex. Low T waves with a cleft in the summit are referred to as cloven (Fig. 7.2). Dimpled T waves are characterized by a shallow, narrow, dimple-like interruption of an otherwise isoelectric S-U interval. Uncomplicated alcoholic T wave changes are often associated with a short Q-T interval. Of course, continued myocardial degeneration, as well as certain therapeutic measures, will modify these T waves and tend to prolong the Q-T interval. Arrhythmias, particularly atrial fibrillation, are common and may also be one of the earliest manifestations of the disease. The QRS complexes may show left ventricular hypertrophy in the early stages of the disease, but the voltage usually decreases as the disease progresses. In the final stages, the QRS complexes are abnormally low, slurred, and characteristic of those associated with diffuse myocardial disease.

If alcoholic cardiomyopathy is treated early and properly, the prognosis is good, provided, of course, that the patient abstains completely from alcoholic beverages and follows the general regimen for large dilated hearts discussed below. If the patient continues to drink alcohol and does

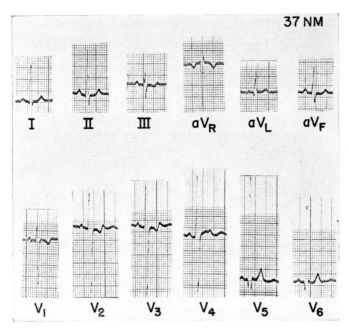

Fig. 7.2. Electrocardiogram of a 37-year-old man with alcoholic cardiomyopathy, showing cloven T wave in V_4 and peaked or spinous T waves in V_5 and V_6.

not follow the therapeutic regimen, progressive cardiac decompensation and death follow.

Viral cardiomyopathy is common. Many viruses and other infectious agents are capable of causing heart disease.[20-24] However, since a great deal of experimental and clinical experience has been accumulated for the Coxsackie group of the picornaviruses,[25-27] these viruses may serve as a prototype for some other viral infections of the heart. Although the original association of Coxsackie infection with heart disease was found in infants, it is now known to occur frequently in adults.[26] The usual clinical history is one of a biphasic illness beginning with malaise, loss of appetite, nausea, and abdominal discomfort, often described as a flu-like illness by the patient. After an asymptomatic period of several days, fever, myalgia, weakness, and chest pain develop. It is important that the physician realize that this asymptomatic period exists or he may fail to associate the cardiac disease with the previously fairly benign respiratory illness. In fact, this type of biphasic clinical response to this viral infection is characteristic of many viral diseases.[28] Outbreaks of Coxsackie infection simplify the etiological diagnosis. The presence of aseptic meningitis, pleurodynia, and encephalitis, which are frequently seen with Coxsackie infections, suggests the etiological viral agent to the physician. Most of the viral diseases responsible for viral cardiomyopathy go unnoticed.

On physical examination, the degree of cardiac decompensation will vary with the severity of the disease. The ECG reveals a decrease in amplitude or inversion of the T waves, reflecting in various ways the diffuse myocardial disease. Low voltage, widened and slurred QRS complexes, and widespread S-T segment and T wave changes may be seen. The P-R interval may be prolonged, or more severe A-V nodal and/or bundle branch block may be present.

The hemogram may be normal or there may be a slight leukocytosis. The serum glutamic oxalacetic transaminase (SGOT) is usually normal. When the diagnosis of acute viral heart disease is suspected, an attempt should be made to establish the agent responsible. Isolation of the virus from the feces, pharyngeal washings, effusions, etc. should be attempted. Acute and convalescent sera should be obtained in search of elevations in type-specific neutralizing antibodies and/or complement fixation antibodies. In autopsied patients, an effort to clarify the etiology and extent of the cardiac damage should be made by careful microscopic examination, immunofluorescent studies for viral antigen, and electron microscopy.

Occasionally, patients with chronic alcoholism will present with a history similar to that just described for acute viral heart disease. In such patients it is possible that alcohol simply acts as a conditioning factor for the viral infection. Other possible conditioning factors for viral infections of the myocardium include malnutrition, pregnancy, bacterial infections, and toxic and other agents. It should be remembered that acute viral myocardial infection may complicate any chronic cardiomyopathy and produce sudden deterioration of a patient's clinical state.

The role of viruses in the production of chronic cardiomyopathy has not been fully understood. However, the possibility exists that viruses may play an important etiological role in many of the clinical syndromes associated with chronic cardiomyopathy.[4, 22, 27,29]

Postpartal cardiomyopathy[30-32] probably occurs one or two times per 1,000 term births. The diagnosis of postpartal cardiomyopathy should be restricted to women who develop signs and symptoms of heart disease between the 2nd and 20th weeks following delivery and in whom the presence of a normal cardiovascular system can be documented during gestation. There should also be an inability to establish another accepted etiology for the heart disease.[31] It should be remembered that a pregnant woman may acquire any disease that a nonpregnant woman can acquire. Meticulous examination of previous and current clinical records, previous X-rays, and the patient's clinical course should be obtained to exclude chronic hypertension, chronic renal disease, or toxemia of pregnancy. A history of malnutrition is often obtained from women whose illnesses meet the criteria for postpartal cardiomyopathy, and thus malnutrition may be an important contributing factor. Another possible etiological agent in the production of postpartal heart disease is a viral infection. Coxsackie viral infections have been found to be responsible for heart disease in some patients whose illnesses fulfilled the criteria for postpartal heart disease.[33]

Physical examination of patients with postpartal cardiomyopathy reveals the usual signs associated with the other cardiomyopathies. With proper treatment, the prognosis for the patient with postpartal heart disease is good, but the illness may recur with subsequent pregnancies.

Ischemic cardiomyopathy is of considerable importance but is traditionally excluded by most clinicians from the heart muscle diseases. Nevertheless, ischemia of the myocardium secondary to coronary artery disease is the most common cause of cardiomyopathy in the United States.[34, 35] Patients with ischemic cardiomyopathy are clinically indistinguishable from patients with any other type of cardiomyopathy except for a history of angina pectoris and/or myocardial infarction and other manifestations of coronary artery disease with myocardial ischemia. Occasionally, a history of angina or myocardial infarction may be extremely difficult to obtain.[6, 34, 35] Nevertheless, the diagnosis of ischemic heart disease is not difficult to make. Patients with this type of cardiomyopathy have an extremely grave prognosis once the heart is large and associated with congestive heart failure.

Other types of cardiomyopathy make up an almost endless list.[1, 2, 4] Table 7.1 is a partial list of factors that may cause cardiomyopathy. In many types of cardiomyopathy, the diagnosis is facilitated by the general clinical picture. For example, in thyrotoxicosis, the fine skin, tremor, weight loss, eyelid lag, weakness, etc. make the diagnosis of thyrotoxic cardiopathy apparent. Likewise, collagen diseases are usually suspected from specific, extracardiac clinical manifestations. It should be remembered that almost any infectious organism, toxin, drug, or other agent may produce myocardial damage. Thus, a history of exposure to toxins, drugs, chemicals, cosmetics, heavy metals, physical stress, etc., regardless of how remote, should be considered and recorded in the study of patients with cardiomyopathy. A classic example of the benefit of careful history taking and clinical investigation was the finding of cobalt cardiomyopathy in beer drinkers in Quebec.[36, 37]

TREATMENT

General Principles

Regardless of etiology, patients with cardiomyopathy associated with congestive heart failure have a common problem, *i.e.*, a large, dilated, flabby, and failing heart. When the myocardium is normal, a slight amount of ventricular dilation provides a useful cardiac compensatory mechanism, as indicated by the Frank-Starling principle. However, when ventricular dilation occurs in association with cardiomyopathy, an increased load is imposed upon the myocardium, as previously discussed.[38] Because of the small amount of blood ejected during ventricular systole, the radius of the dilated ventricle is changed little and, therefore, cardiac work must increase greatly throughout systole,[39] whereas in the normal sized heart the load progressively decreases throughout systole. Ventricular dilation also disrupts spatial orientation of the myocardium with a loss of mechanical advantage of the myocardium and papillary muscles. These factors, and the associated papillary muscle diseases, are responsible for dysfunction and mitral regurgitation.[8, 9]

Thus, decreasing the size of the heart must be one of the major objectives in the treatment of patients with cardiomyopathy. To accomplish this objective, the diseased heart must be "unloaded" as much as possible. One might reasonably expect to accomplish the unloading by decreasing systemic blood pressure, reducing heart rate, decreasing cardiac output and stroke volume, reducing the vigor or rate of contraction and, in general, reducing the metabolic demands on the heart. Virtually all of the requirements for unloading the heart are accomplished to some extent by prolonged bed rest.[40-42] For this reason, bed rest for periods of 6 months to 1 year or longer is the therapeutic foundation for patients with cardiomyopathy (Fig. 7.3). For several months the patient is allowed only to feed himself and to use a bedside commode. If objective improvement occurs,

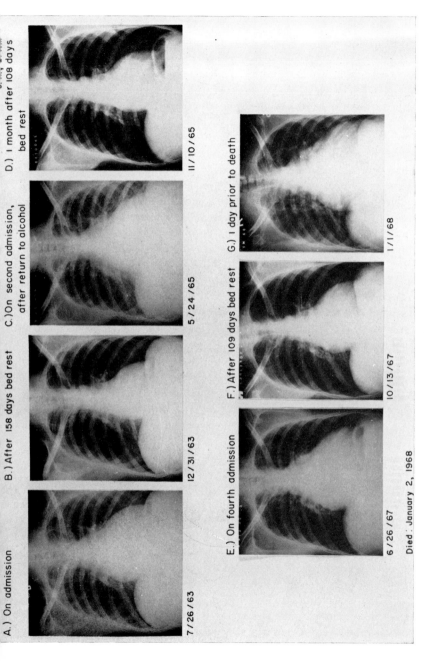

A.) On admission

B.) After 158 days bed rest

C.) On second admission, after return to alcohol

D.) 1 month after 108 days bed rest

7/26/63

12/31/63

5/24/65

11/10/65

E.) On fourth admission

F.) After 109 days bed rest

G.) 1 day prior to death

6/26/67

10/13/67

1/1/68

Died: January 2, 1968

FIG. 7.3. Serial teleoroentgenograms of a 51-year-old man with alcoholic cardiomyopathy, illustrating the therapeutic value of prolonged bed rest and abstinence from alcohol. The reduction in cardiac size during three periods of bed rest is evident from the teleoroentgenograms.

such as a decrease in the size of the heart, the patient is then allowed some light occupational therapy in bed. This form of treatment should be carried out in a facility where temperature and humidity can be controlled by air-conditioning, which further unloads the heart during hot and humid weather. Extreme variations in temperature, especially hot and humid atmosphere, have deleterious effects on the heart.[43]

Obviously, the usual therapeutic procedures for congestive heart failure are employed in the treatment of patients with cardiomyopathy. Because most patients with cardiomyopathy are extremely sensitive to digitalis, they should be given this drug very carefully. Failure to use digitalis cautiously may produce serious and even fatal cardiac rhythm disturbances.

The need for proper (not excessive) restriction of dietary sodium and the use of diuretics vary with each patient. Mercurial diuretics, which are only slightly, if at all, kaliuretic, should be used rather than the kaliuretic oral diuretics. A low concentration of potassium in the myocardial intra- and extracellular fluids, as well as hypokalemia, predisposes to digitalis intoxication with resultant serious cardiac arrhythmias. The low potassium concentration may also produce injury to the myocardial cells.

Anticoagulants may be useful in preventing venous thrombi and embolization in patients with congestive heart failure who are consigned to bed rest for long periods of time, especially if these problems existed prior to bed rest therapy. Other general therapeutic measures which may be started in hospital are institution of good dietary habits with the proper types of food in proper quantities, cessation of smoking and of the use of caffeine and alcoholic beverages, and development of good personal health habits. Sedatives and other drugs and supportive agents should be used only as indicated.

Specific Therapy

Patients with **alcoholic cardiomyopathy** must maintain strict abstinence from alcoholic beverages and receive a well-balanced diet and supplemental vitamins. The initial response to therapy is good even in patients with associated congestive heart failure. For example, of 37 patients with alcoholic cardiomyopathy who were treated with bed rest, 57 per cent had a return of heart size to normal and another 30 per cent had significant reduction in heart size. The long-term prognosis also seems good in patients who are treated early and properly. The most common causes for therapeutic failure are delay in diagnosis, unwillingness to accept prolonged bed rest therapy, continual consumption of alcohol, poor nutrition, and excessive physical activity.[44]

Patients with acute **viral myocarditis** should be kept at bed rest until all signs and symptoms of the disease have abated in an effort to prevent chronic cardiomyopathy. The importance of bed rest is particularly emphasized for patients with mild viral myocarditis because physicians often tend to ambulate such patients too soon. The need for bed rest is supported by experimental studies which have shown fatigue and exercise to have deleterious effects on viral diseases.[45, 46] Patients with severe viral myocarditis and residual cardiomegaly should be treated with prolonged bed rest to rest the heart.

Steroids may be used in patients with life-threatening or severe, progressive viral myocardial disease. Although some theoretic danger exists in their use early in the treatment of viral diseases,[47, 48] steroids have been found to be useful on occasion.[49] Digitalis, if required, should be used very cautiously in patients with viral myocarditis in order to prevent the occurrence of serious arrhythmias.

Although the decision must be individualized, patients with **postpartal cardiomyopathy** probably should have no other pregnancies. Subsequent pregnancies result in a worsening of the disease process. Proper nutrition is extremely important in such patients.

Patients with **ischemic cardiomyopathy** must have therapy directed toward the coronary artery disease, the details of which are beyond the scope of this discussion.

The management of the cardiomyopathies is too complex and extensive to present in complete detail. All patients with cardiomyopathy, regardless of cause, should avoid exposure to viral and other infections. Immunization against influenza and other viral illnesses should be recommended for all patients with cardiomyopathy. Sustained systemic hypertension must be controlled for satisfactory therapeutic response, whether it is the primary cause of the heart disease or an associated factor. It is evident that cardiomyopathy secondary to curable diseases, *e.g.*, hyperthyroidism, hypothyroidism, anemia, malnutrition, toxic agents, etc., is reversible and can be cured if the disease is recognized early and the etiological factor promptly removed.

This study was supported by Grants from the National Heart Institute of the U. S. Public Health Service (HE-06769), the Rudolph Matas Memorial Fund for the Kate Prewitt Hess Laboratory, and the Rowell A. Billups Fund for Research in Heart Disease.

REFERENCES

1. Hudson, R. E. B.: The cardiomyopathies: order from chaos. Amer. J. Cardiol. 25: 70, 1970.
2. Mattingly, T. W.: Diseases of the myocardium (cardiomyopathies): the viewpoint of a clinical cardiologist. Amer. J. Cardiol. 25: 79, 1970.
3. Burch, G. E., and DePasquale, N. P.: *Heart Muscle Disease* (monograph). Disease-a-Month, Year Book Medical Publishers, Chicago, May 1968.
4. Mattingly, T. W.: Clinical features and diagnosis of primary myocardial disease. Mod. Concepts Cardiovasc. Dis. 30: 677, 686, 1961.

5. Fowler, N. O., and Gueron, M.: Primary myocardial disease. Circulation 32: 830, 1965.

6. Raferty, E. B., Banks, D. C., and Oram, S.: Occlusive disease of the coronary arteries presenting as primary congestive cardiomyopathy. Lancet 2: 1147, 1969.

7. Burch, G. E., Giles, T. D., and Colcolough, H. L.: Pathogenesis of "rheumatic" heart disease: critique and theory. Amer. Heart J. 80: 556, 1970.

8. Burch, G. E., DePasquale, N. P., and Phillips, J. H.: Clinical manifestations of papillary muscle dysfunction. Arch. Intern. Med. 112: 112, 1963.

9. Burch, G. E., DePasquale, N. P., and Phillips, J. H.: The syndrome of papillary muscle dysfunction. Amer. Heart J. 75: 399, 1968.

10. Burch, G. E., and Phillips, J. H.: Methods in the diagnostic differentiation of myocardial dilatation from pericardial effusion. Amer. Heart J. 64: 266, 1962.

11. Eliaser, M., Jr., and Giansiracusa, F. J.: The heart and alcohol. Calif. Med. 84: 234, 1956.

12. Evans, W.: The electrocardiogram of alcoholic cardiomyopathy. Brit. Heart J. 21: 445, 1959.

13. Brigden, W.: Uncommon myocardial diseases. The non-coronary cardiomyopathies. Lancet 2: 1243, 1957.

14. Burch, G. E., and Walsh, J. J.: Cardiac insufficiency in chronic alcoholism. Amer. J. Cardiol. 6: 864, 1960.

15. Evans, W.: Alcoholic cardiomyopathy. Amer. Heart J. 61: 556, 1961.

16. Ferrans, V. J.: Alcoholic cardiomyopathy. Amer. J. Med. Sci. 252: 89, 1966.

17. Burch, G. E., and DePasquale, N. P.: Alcoholic cardiomyopathy. Cardiologia 52: 48, 1968.

18. Burch, G. E., and DePasquale, N. P.: Alcoholic cardiomyopathy. Amer. J. Cardiol. 23: 723, 1969.

19. Burch, G. E., and Giles, T. D.: Alcoholic cardiomyopathy: concept of the disease and its treatment (editorial). Amer. J. Med., 50: 141, 1971.

20. Lyon, E.: *Virus Diseases and the Cardiovascular System.* Grune & Stratton, Inc., New York, 1956.

21. Weinstein, L.: Cardiovascular manifestations in some of the common infectious diseases. Mod. Concepts Cardiovasc. Dis. 23: 229, 1954.

22. Silber, E. N.: Respiratory viruses and heart disease. Ann. Intern. Med. 48: 228, 1958.

23. Woodward, T. E., McCrumb, F. R., Jr., Carey, T. N., and Togo, Y.: Viral and rickettsial causes of cardiac disease, including the Coxsackie virus etiology of pericarditis and myocarditis. Ann. Intern. Med. 53: 1130, 1960.

24. Pankey, G. A.: Effect of viruses on the cardiovascular system. Amer. J. Med. Sci. 250: 103, 1965.

25. Burch, G. E., and DePasquale, N. P.: Viral myocarditis. In Wolstenholme, G. E. W., and O'Connor, M. (eds.): *Ciba Foundation Symposium on the Cardiomyopathies.* London, J. & A. Churchill, Ltd., 1964, p. 376.

26. Smith, W. G.: Coxsackie heart disease in adults. Amer. Heart J. 73: 439, 1967.

27. Grist, N. R., and Bell, E. J.: Coxsackie viruses and the heart. Amer. Heart J. 77: 295, 1969.

28. Habel, K.: The nature of viruses and viral illness. Med. Clin. N. Amer. 43: 1275, 1959.

29. Christian, H. A.: Clinically, the myocardium. Arch. Intern. Med. 86: 491, 1950.

30. Hull, E., and Hafkesbring, E.: Toxic postpartal heart. New Orleans Med. Surg. J. 89: 550, 1937.

31. Walsh, J. J., Burch, G. E., Black, W. C., Ferrans, V. J., and Hibbs, R. G.: Idio-

pathic myocardiopathy of the puerperium (postpartal heart disease). Circulation 22: 19, 1965.

32. Stuart, K. L.: Peripartal cardiomyopathy. Cardiologia 52: 44, 1968.
33. Sainani, G. S., Krompotic, E., and Slodki, S. J.: Adult heart disease due to the Coxsackie virus B infection. Medicine 47: 133, 1968.
34. Burch, G. E., Giles, T. D., and Colcolough, H. L.: Ischemic cardiomyopathy. Amer. Heart J. 79: 291, 1970.
35. Burch, G. E., and Giles, T. D.: Ischemic cardiomyopathy (to be published).
36. Parker, J. S. M., and Carson, S. B.: Tissue cobalt content in "beer drinkers'" myocardiopathy. J. Lab. Clin. Med. 71: 893, 1968.
37. Wiberg, G. S., Munro, I. C., and Morrison, A. B.: Effect of cobalt ions on myocardial metabolism. Can. J. Biochem. 45: 1219, 1967.
38. Burch, G. E., Ray, C. T., and Cronvich, J. A.: The George Fahr Lecture: Certain mechanical pecularities of the human cardiac pump in normal and diseased states. Circulation 5: 504, 1952.
39. Burch, G. E.: Theoretic considerations of time course of pressure developed and volume ejected by normal and dilated left ventricle during systole. Amer. Heart J. 50: 352, 1955.
40. Burch, G. E., and Walsh, J. J.: Cardiac enlargement due to myocardial degeneration of unknown cause. Preliminary report on effect of prolonged bed rest. J. A. M. A. 172: 207, 1960.
41. Burch, G. E., Walsh, J. J., Ferrans, V. J., and Hibbs, R. G.: Prolonged bed rest in the treatment of the dilated heart. Circulation 22: 852, 1965.
42. Burch, G. E., and DePasquale, N. P.: On resting the human heart. Amer. Heart J. 41: 422, 1966.
43. Burch, G. E., and DePasquale, N. P.: *Hot Climates, Man and His Heart.* Charles C Thomas, Publisher, Springfield, Ill., 1962.
44. McDonald, C. D., Burch, G. E., and Walsh, J. J.: Alcoholic cardiomyopathy managed with prolonged bed rest. Ann. Intern. Med. 74: 681, 1971.
45. Tiller, J. G., Elson, S. H., Ihaka, J. A., Abelmann, W. H., Lener, A. M., and Finland, M.: Effects of exercise on Coxsackie A-9 myocarditis in adult mice. Proc. Soc. Exp. Biol. Med. 177: 777, 1964.
46. Rosenbaum, H. E., and Harford, C. G.: Effect of fatigue on susceptibility of mice to poliomyelitis. Proc. Soc. Exp. Biol. Med. 83: 678, 1953.
47. Kilbourne, E. D., Wilson, C. B., and Perrier, D.: The induction of gross myocardial lesions by a Coxsackie (pleurodynia) virus and cortisone. J. Clin. Invest. 35: 362, 1956.
48. Kilbourne, E. D., Smart, K. M., and Pokoy, B. A.: Inhibition by cortisone of the synthesis and action of interferon. Nature 190: 650, 1961.
49. Voight, G. C.: Steroid therapy in viral myocarditis. Amer. Heart J. 75: 575, 1968.

8

Pulmonary Thromboembolism

HAROLD M. LOWE, M.D.

In this presentation, the diagnostic aspects of pulmonary embolism are emphasized, and a high index of suspicion is encouraged regarding the possibility of this very common complication of injury, surgery, or illness requiring bed rest. Even when not by itself fatal, pulmonary embolism often seriously complicates other illnesses. Although the difficulties in the diagnosis justify inclusion of this subject in this panel, a substantial factor resides in the observer's cerebral cortex and its connections with auditory, visual, and tactile stimuli.

The incidence of pulmonary emboli has been and is difficult to estimate. Most reported studies of incidence are based on autopsy series, and the incidence is therefore grossly underestimated. The death rate is more accurately known, obviously, and accounts for about 3 to 5 per cent of all hospital deaths. Suffice it to say that the magnitude of the problem is substantial, and the more often pulmonary embolism is suspected and diligently investigated, the more often it is found and successfully treated.

One problem in suspecting and making this diagnosis is the extremely variable clinical picture. It used to be said that syphilis was the "great imposter" and perhaps, with the current moral climate, this may yet be said again. At the present time, pulmonary thromboembolism, of all disease entities, appears to be best qualified for this title.

Let us begin by considering the various clinical manifestations. Perhaps it is more meaningful to relate briefly some case experiences which illustrate the extremes of clinical findings. The first clinical example is that of a 78-year-old woman with attacks of syncope thought to be due to transient cerebral ischemia on the basis of extracranial carotid artery narrowing, and with a persistent low grade fever up to 100.6°F. The cerebral arteriograms were equivocal, and the surgeon requested consultation at this point. On examination, the patient had signs of slightly increased right heart pressure with evidence of mild biventricular failure and bilateral, indurated, tender, deep calf veins with definite palpable clots. Cultures of urine, blood, throat, and sputum were negative. The chest film was not helpful, and the lung scan was interpreted as negative. The electrocardiogram (ECG) taken during an episode of further temperature increase showed rotation of the axis to the right and clockwise, with T wave inversion in V_2 and V_3. No disturbances of rhythm were ever demonstrated. The patient was anticoagulated, first with subcutaneous heparin, later switching to oral drugs, and the heart failure was treated, with the disappearance of all symptoms and signs.

A second patient is a 52-year-old man who suffered a compound fracture of the tibia and avulsion of the skin and subcutaneous tissue of the heel when riding his son's motorcycle. Appropriate immediate surgical treatment was performed, and he did well for 12 days. He then developed a spiking fever, pain in the calf of the uninjured leg, and increased pain with dorsiflexion of that foot.

The symptoms were not mentioned to his physician. Mild shortness of breath followed, again not admitted. He was started on antibiotics after blood and urine cultures were obtained. No abnormal findings indicative of infection were present at the time of changing the cast. He then had an episode of rather severe shortness of breath with marked apprehension, depression, and anxiety. The calf of the leg not in a cast was noted to be swollen and tender, the lungs were clear, there was hyperpnea, tachypnea, and accentuation of P_2 with a RV-S_3, and a 20 mm. Hg paradoxical pulse was present. An inspiratory pulmonic systolic murmur was heard in the right lateral chest but not in the pulmonic area or left chest. The ECG showed changes consistent with acute right ventricular strain. Chest X-ray was reported negative, but actually the entire right lung field was relatively avascular. The diagnosis seemed obvious, but a lung scan was done in order to convince his personal physician, who doubted the diagnosis. The scan showed virtual absence of blood flow to the right lung. Rapid improvement occurred with heparin anticoagulation, but 15 days later he suffered another embolus while adequately anticoagulated. A vena caval ligation was then performed, anticoagulants were reinstituted 12 hours later, and complete recovery followed. The lung scan, which had become normal 1 week after the first scan, again showed evidence of emboli to the right lung at the time of the second major embolus.

There are several points of importance illustrated by these two cases. First, and deserving of the greatest emphasis, is the fact that, in order to diagnose and effectively treat pulmonary embolism, one must be willing to accept relatively subtle findings (as in the first case) as indicative that the problem under discussion is present. There is no single sign, symptom, or test which is unequivocally diagnostic, with the possible exception of pulmonary angiograms. Second, the size of the embolus and degree of pulmonary vascular occlusion do not always correlate with the clinical manifestations. A large and major embolus may produce only mild dyspnea and tachycardia, whereas a small embolus may result in a sufficiently marked decrease in cardiac output to produce shock.

The second case illustrates a degree of disparity in the clinical picture related to the extent of pulmonary vascular occlusion. At the time the lung scan was done, the patient was only mildly tachypneic and in no distress. The third point that needs to be stressed is the often considerable difficulty in convincing the referring physician that the patient has had an embolus. Surgeons in particular are reluctant to believe that such a complication could occur in one of their patients, especially if the scan and X-rays are negative. Further, the site of origin of the clot often becomes apparent only after an embolus has occurred, or it is ignored by patient and physician prior to the acute event.

The following list of symptoms and signs which may occur is offered to further illustrate the variable expression and the necessity of a high index of suspicion. These are given in approximate order of frequency.

Dyspnea, apprehension and anxiety, cough, attacks of asthma, syncope, chest pain (pleuritic or anginal), and hiccoughs. Hemoptysis often accompanies pulmonary infarction. Signs which may be present are tachypnea, tachycardia, fever, tenderness of leg or pelvic veins, increased P_2, RV-S_3, RV-S_4, distended neck veins, cyanosis, hypotension, paradoxical pulse, pulmonary systolic murmur increased with inspiration and often heard only unilaterally, supraventricular arrhythmias, or evidence of shock with right heart failure. Often the sudden drop in cardiac output may precipitate and, in the patient with marginal cerebral or myocardial blood supply, may present as an acute myocardial infarction or stroke. Acute abdominal disease may initially be a primary consideration as a result of diaphragmatic irritation and referred pain.

DIAGNOSIS

The symptoms listed above are familiar and are obviously nonspecific. Most observers have been impressed with the degree of anxiety and apprehension which, with tachypnea, may occur in the absence of chest pain or dyspnea and be misinterpreted as the hyperventilation syndrome. Low grade or recurrent spiking fever may also be the only apparent manifestation of pulmonary emboli.

The physical examination will be most rewarding and revealing to the skillful examiner. There are two diagnostic aspects to the physical examination: first, determination of the presence of right heart overload, often transient, and second, the localization of the source of the emboli. The most frequent evidence of the former are: (1) increased amplitude of P_2, (2) distended neck veins, (3) paradoxical pulse, and (4) RV-S_3. Since about 80 per cent of pulmonary emboli originate in the leg veins, a careful examination will reveal palpable tender indurated veins in the calf between the heads of the gastrocnemius, tenderness over the popliteal or femoral veins, or in the sural plexus of the sole of the foot. Edema of greater magnitude on the right compared to the left is usually related to proximal venous obstruction. A thigh blood pressure cuff inflated to 40 mm. Hg may produce pain in the area of phlebothrombosis distal to the cuff, but Homan's sign is unreliable if negative and does not rule out the presence of deep venous clots. A pelvic and rectal examination should be performed; this is of greatest importance if the legs are negative.

Of the simpler, noninvasive diagnostic procedures, the ECG is the most sensitive (although often temporary), particularly if there are previous tracings for comparison. Most frequently, there is rightward and anterior rotation of the mean QRS and P vectors, ST depression and T wave inversion in V_1 and V_2, or transient RBBB, or the pattern of inferior myocardial infarction. The latter tends to occur where there has been a previous horizontal or left axis.

It is to be emphasized that neither a negative chest X-ray or lung scan rules out the diagnosis of pulmonary embolus. Atelectasis is probably the most common X-ray finding resulting from a pulmonary embolus. Only if there is infarction does the typical wedge or triangular shaped peripheral lesion appear and then only in about 50 per cent of cases of infarction. On close inspection, a relatively bloodless area involving a lobar distribution or an entire lung field may be present. False-negative lung scans may result from atelectasis of the involved area, masking by the diaphragms, or in instances of small areas of involvement.

False-positive scans are also a problem in patients with pre-existing lung disease or with congestive failure. This problem can be largely eliminated by doing sequential radioactive gas **ventilation** scans and I^{131} macroalbumin **perfusion** scans. In chronic lung disease, the ventilatory abnormalities are usually associated with perfusion abnormalities in the same location. If there is a disparity, especially if the perfusion abnormality without ventilatory abnormality is present in the lower lobes, then the clinician can be more certain of the diagnosis.

Pulmonary angiography is the most definitive examination but also the most formidable in the critically ill patient. Proper interpretation and performance of this examination require considerable skill and experience.

So far there has been little presented that could be categorized as belonging in the "New Frontiers" title of this program. What is hoped is that an awareness of present capabilities and the often sadly neglected art of physical examination will result in earlier and more effective treatment and, more importantly, prevention of phlebothrombosis, thrombophlebitis, and pulmonary embolism.

There are two New Frontier techniques which are expected to be of great value in diagnosis and therapy of thromboembolic disease. One is a radioisotope technique using I^{125}-labeled fibrinogen and scanning of both legs. A localized accumulation indicates deposition of the labeled fibrinogen, therefore clotting.

The second procedure is more sensitive to the presence of thrombotic and/or fibrinolytic activity but does not aid in localization. This is plasma fibrinogen chromatography which demonstrates deviations from the normal molecular weight pattern of fibrinogen. There are increased high molecular weight derivatives with thrombosis, and with fibrinolysis a preponderance of lower molecular weight derivatives is seen. When both thrombosis and fibrinolysis are going on, there is a mixed pattern of high and low molecular fractions. Present studies suggest that this test may be the first really objective guide to anticoagulant and thrombolytic therapy.

TREATMENT

The ideal treatment of pulmonary embolism is prevention. The routine use of elastic stockings in hospitalized patients was shown nearly 20 years ago to reduce the incidence of fatal pulmonary embolism by at least half. Early ambulation, leg exercises, and daily examination of the legs will prevent or permit effective anticoagulant treatment of thrombotic leg vein problems before serious complications can develop. Since the site of origin of thrombi is usually in the legs (70 to 90 per cent), the measures mentioned above are of demonstrated effectiveness in the vast majority of patients.

Anticoagulation with heparin as the preferred agent should be instituted immediately when the diagnosis of thrombotic venous disease and/or pulmonary embolism is suspected, unless there are absolute contraindications. Fibrinolytic therapy may become the treatment of choice, but at present it is limited by availability of urokinase. Anticoagulation prevents propagation of the thrombus and in most instances recurrence of pulmonary embolism. If a pulmonary embolus occurs while the patient is adequately anticoagulated, vena caval ligation should be performed, provided that massive re-embolization has not occurred. In the latter instance, pulmonary embolectomy may be lifesaving. Unfortunately, about half of individuals with massive embolism die within 1 hour of the acute event. In a retrospective study of 101 patients at the Cleveland Clinic who died of major pulmonary embolism, only six would have been considered for pulmonary embolectomy, primarily because of the time factor. Cooley and Beall were successful in so treating five of 11 patients with massive pulmonary embolization. They state that patients who require vasopressors after embolization will probably not live long enough for lytic changes to clear the pulmonary arterial tree, but those who survive the acute event, are not in shock, and have half or less of the total pulmonary circulation occluded, will usually not have a fatal outcome. The operation should therefore be reserved for those who would probably not survive without it.

In acute ileofemoral venous occlusion, thrombectomy under local anesthesia is probably an improvement over conservative therapy. It is important to achieve meticulous hemostasis so that immediate heparin therapy can be instituted. In some instances, inferior vena caval ligation immediately prior to thrombectomy may be prudent.

Inferior vena caval ligation in the patient with massive embolism who requires vaspopressor therapy is unwise and usually fatal since it produces a sudden drop in the necessarily high right ventricular filling pressure and it may result in a pronounced sudden decrease in cardiac output. A second point of caution is the necessity for ligation of the left ovarian vein in association with inferior vena caval ligation in female patients.

The assumption in the foregoing discussion is that the source of emboli is in the venous system distal to the renal veins. It should be remembered that about 12 per cent of patients who die following an acute myocardial infarction have mural thrombi in the right ventricle, and that embolization is not rare from indwelling subclavian catheters or hemodialysis shunts.

The rewards in diagnosis and treatment of venous thromboembolism and in the prevention of morbidity and death are readily available. The requirements are simple. A physician, not just a doctor, is all that is needed.

9

Management of Dissecting Aneurysm of the Aorta

JAMES R. MALM, M.D.

Acute dissecting aneurysm is the most common acute catastrophe that befalls the aorta, and the thoracic aortic aneurysm is almost twice as prevalent as the abdominal variety. Although this condition is associated with a high mortality rate of 80 per cent within 1 month from the onset of symptoms, only 20 per cent succumb within the first 24 hours. The mechanism of death is the continued dissection with ultimate rupture produced by the continued cardiac impulse and pulsatile blood pressure acting upon the intimal tear.[1] The rationale for therapy by the drug-induced hypotensive regimen is to lower the blood pressure and thereby reduce the pulse width or driving pressure against the site of the aortic dissection.[2] Patients suspected of having acute dissecting aneurysms of the aorta should be placed in an intensive care unit. Other cardiopulmonary catastrophies such as acute myocardial infarction must be ruled out by appropriate studies. The electrocardiogram and blood pressure should be monitored and a Foley catheter inserted to record urinary output. The aim of therapy is to reduce the systolic blood pressure to 100 to 120 mm. Hg whenever possible. The level of consciousness and the urinary output are valuable guides to the appropriate blood pressure level. Although a systolic pressure level of 100 to 120 mm. Hg is preferred, the regimen can be modified as the patient's condition dictates, provided that an hourly urinary output of 25 to 30 ml. is maintained. In order to lower the blood pressure acutely, trimethaphan (Arfonad), 1 to 2 mg. per ml., is administered as an intravenous drip; or reserpine, up to 1 mg. intravenously every 3 to 4 hours, is employed. The blood pressure response to these drugs is rapid and can be profound if not carefully regulated. As a rule, when the blood pressure is lowered, the chest or back pain or both are greatly relieved. The relief of pain is an important clinical guide to the efficacy of the drug in arresting the "dissecting hematoma." It is important to begin both guanethedine (25 to 50 mg.) twice a day by mouth and either propranolol or Diuril simultaneously with the intravenous medication so that sufficient blood levels of these drugs may be obtained in 48 hours to allow discontinuance of the intravenous drugs. As the patient's clinical status stabilizes and the intravenous drug is discontinued, he can be transferred out of the intensive care unit for progressive ambulation and final regulation of drugs. At some time during the hospital stay, an aortogram should be done to establish the diagnosis and to locate the site and extent of the dissection. Serial chest radiographs are important in following the size of the aneurysm and discovering localized saccular aneurysms that may develop in about 15 per cent of patients with aneurysms in the chronic follow-up phase.[3] Utilization of this regimen in a large series of patients in the acute situation has been associated with a reduction in mortality rate to 10 to 12 per cent, when compared to a 25 to 40 per cent risk for immediate surgery in all patients. Major surgical intervention, that is, the use of cardiopulmonary bypass, is indicated, however, in the acute situation when there is leaking of the aneurysm, severe aortic valve insufficiency, occlusion of major branches of the aorta, or inability to maintain lowered blood pressure with the drug regimen. After successful surgical therapy for dissecting aneurysm, it is important to maintain these patients, as well as those treated only with drugs, on an appropriate drug regimen for the rest of their lives.

REFERENCES

1. Prokop, E. K., Palmer, R. F., and Wheat, M. W.: Hydrodynamic forces in dissecting aneurysms. Circulation (Suppl. 6), 158, 1968.
2. Wheat, M. W., and Palmer, R. F.: Dissecting aneurysms of the aorta. Present status of drug versus surgical therapy. Progr. Cardiovasc. Dis. 11: 198, 1968.
3. Wheat, M. W., Harris, P. D., Malm, J. R., Kaiser, G. A., Bowman, F. O., and Palmer, R. F.: Acute dissecting aneurysms of the aorta—treatment and results in 64 patients. J. Thorac. Cardiovasc. Surg. 58: 344, 1969.

10

Today's Concept of Adequate Therapy for Essential Hypertension

JOHN H. MOYER, III, M.D.

In setting up a therapeutic program for the treatment of hypertension, the primary emphasis is oriented to regulating the blood pressure so as to maintain it within approximately normal limits. Although it cannot always be done readily, this at least is the objective. If it can be achieved, the prognosis should be greatly improved. In fact, if the blood pressure is treated early enough, before atherosclerosis and vascular damage have occurred, the prognosis should be equal to that of a normotensive person of the same age and sex.

This presentation is divided into four parts: (1) pharmacodynamics and the rationale of antihypertensive therapy; (2) the specific drug regimen in the treatment of hypertension; (3) the effect of antihypertensive therapy; and (4) some special problems related to the treatment of hypertension.

PHARMACODYNAMICS AND DYNAMICS OF HYPERTENSION

Role of Autonomic Nervous System in Regulation of Blood Pressure

Figure 10.1 is a diagrammatic representation of the physiology and pharmacology of the autonomic nervous system, specifically as it relates to blood pressure regulation and cardiovascular hemodynamic control. The final regulatory mechanism responsible for the elevation of blood pressure in essential hypertension rests at the neuroeffector site of the blood vessel. When this area is stimulated and the arteriole constricts, the blood pressure increases. It is quite likely that the hereditary component of the hypertensive syndrome is carried as a defect in function at this site.

The preganglionic neurons of the sympathetic nervous system, which innervates the blood vessels, are located in the spinal cord and receive impulses originating in the brain, particularly from the vasoregulatory area of the medulla. After the axon of the preganglionic neuron leaves the spinal

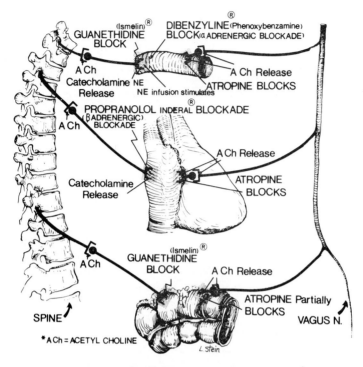

α & β ADRENERGIC BLOCKADE

FIG. 10.1. Sympathetic and parasympathetic innervation of blood, vessel, heart, and gut. Parasympathetic innervation (shown here proceeding from the vagus nerve) in cholinergic; impulses are transmitted by release of acetylcholine (ACh). Sympathetic innervation, from the thoracolumbar ganglia, is mostly adrenergic; impulses are transmitted by release of catecholamines (epinephrine and norepinephrine). Receptors at the neuroeffector sites are of two types, alpha and beta. Those in the blood vessel are of the alpha type; those in the heart are of the beta type. Drugs that block the action of catecholamines at the neuroeffector sites by occupying the receptors are known as adrenergic blocking agents, alpha or beta according to the type of receptor they occupy. Phenoxybenzamine is an example of the former; propranolol, of the latter. The alpha adrenergic blockers prevent vasoconstriction in response to either endogenous or administered catecholamines, and the beta adrenergic blockers prevent catecholamine stimulation of the heart.

canal, it forms a synapse at the sympathetic ganglia with the postganglionic neuron, which goes to the blood vessel and innervates the vasoconstrictor fibers of the vessel wall. At this point (*i.e.*, the neuroeffector site), norepinephrine and epinephrine are released, producing vasoconstriction through their action on receptors at the neuroeffector site. These receptors are known as alpha receptors. Thus, drugs used to depress the release of catecholamines (epinephrine and norepinephrine) at the level of the blood vessel are alpha depressants. A blocking agent that blocks the vasoconstrictor impulses at the blood vessel itself is an alpha blocking agent; a typical agent of this kind is phenoxybenzamine (Dibenzyline).

Concurrently, the sympathetic nervous system also innervates the heart. When the sympathetic nerves to the heart are stimulated, the response is quite similar to that produced by administration of epinephrine. The primary type of receptor found at the neuroeffector sites in the heart is known as a beta receptor. Drugs that block the ability of epinephrine and norepinephrine to stimulate the myocardial fibers, such as propranolol (Inderal), are beta blockers. Thus the alpha blocking agents are primarily effective in reducing the response to sympathetic stimuli in the blood vessel, and the beta blockers are primarily responsible for reducing the response to sympathetic stimuli in the heart (Fig. 10.1).

In addition to the heart and blood vessels, the sympathetic nerves, together with the parasympathetic nerves, also innervate numerous other tissues, such as the gastrointestinal tract. In the gastrointestinal tract, the motor component is carried in the parasympathetic system, so that when this is stimulated the gut constricts and peristalsis increases. Here, sympathetic stimulation is inhibitory rather than stimulant as in the case of the blood vessel. Thus, we have a balance and counterbalance throughout the various tissue beds and particularly in the cardiovascular system, which is of primary interest here. The parasympathetic nervous system releases acetylcholine, which has an inhibitory or vasodilator effect on the blood vessel, as well as on the myocardium and its rate of constriction.

Certain drugs used to lower blood pressure, such as guanethidine and reserpine, depress the release of catecholamines at the neuroeffector site of the blood vessel. They do not block the effect of administered norepinephrine circulating in the blood but only the release of "sympathins" at the blood vessel level. Therefore when the blood pressure is reduced with a drug such as guanethidine, it should be kept in mind that the patient will still respond to infused norepinephrine. This is particularly important if overdosage occurs and if the blood pressure falls excessively during a surgical procedure, since the pressure can readily be raised with infused norepinephrine. Under the circumstances, the blood vessel is more sensitive and responsive to infused norepinephrine than it is in the normotensive patient who has not received drugs. Consequently, excessive hypotension that might occur, as for example in the patient who has received antihypertensive drugs and is undergoing an operation, can be quickly reversed with vasopressor agents.

Pharmacology of Autonomic Drugs

Figure 10.2 represents the pharmacodynamics of blood pressure reduction by sympathetic depression or blocking effect produced by different

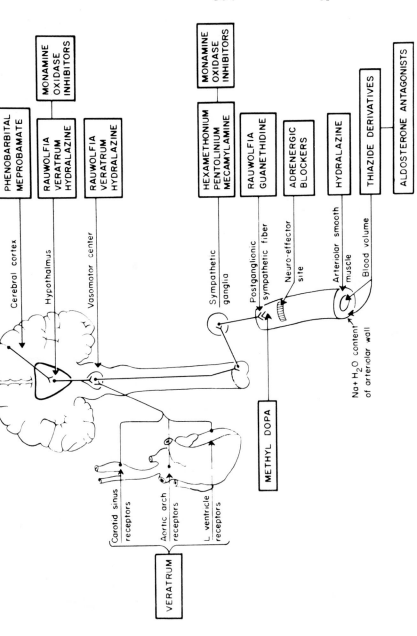

FIG. 10.2. Anatomic sites of action of various drugs that decrease blood pressure. Several of these exert hypotensive effects through action at more than one site. (Reprinted from Moyer, J. H., and Brest, A. N.: Changing outlook for the patient with hypertension. Amer. J. Cardiol. 17: 673, 1966.)

types of drugs in separate areas of the sympathetic nervous system. The predominant effect of sympathetic stimulation to the blood vessels and heart is motor; therefore, when sympathetic blocking agents are used, the blood pressure is reduced and the strength of cardiac contraction is slightly reduced, as is the pulse rate when increased by overactivity of the sympathetic nervous system. By far the most potent antihypertensive action is exhibited by drugs which block either the release of norepinephrine at the neuroeffector site or the transfer of the sympathetic impulse at the sympathetic ganglia. The difference in suitability for clinical use between drugs of the first type and those which block at the ganglia is attributable to the fact that no drug is yet available that blocks at the sympathetic ganglia and not at the parasympathetic ganglia. Therefore, when a ganglionic blocking agent is given, it blocks both sympathetic and parasympathetic motor impulses, resulting in a series of significant side effects resulting from the parasympathetic blockade, such as decreased peristalsis (even to the point of ileus), eye manifestations (*e.g.*, blurred vision), salivation, sweating, and other undesirable effects. On the other hand, a drug like guanethidine, which simply depresses the release of norepinephrine, only blocks the sympathetic component of the autonomic nervous system. As a result, we do not get the side effects of parasympathetic blockade.

As discussed later, it is important to remember that these drugs are quite potent and the patient response is extremely variable. Some patients will require much larger dosages than others in order to achieve the same result. Therefore dose titration is the cornerstone of proper therapeutic management of patients receiving antihypertensive drugs of this variety. Probably the simplest aspect of therapy but the most overlooked requirement of proper management is this simple principle: proper dose titration so that each patient receives exactly that dose which is no less and no more than the amount required to control the blood pressure at a level of 150/90 mm. Hg (or less) without producing excessive hypotension.

SPECIFIC DRUG REGIMEN IN TREATMENT OF HYPERTENSION

General Principles of Therapy

The usual approach to antihypertensive drug therapy is to give the diuretic first and evaluate the response to the diuretic before starting other (sympathetic depressant) drugs, unless blood pressure regulation within a matter of days to weeks is quite urgent. The diuretic is then continued, following which, after about 1 month's delay, the sympathetic depressant drugs are started. The reason for this is discussed later. The dosage of the diuretic would be: chlorothiazide, 500 mg. b.i.d. or its equivalent in other thiazide diuretics; or chlorthalidone (Hygroton), 50 mg. daily; or, in some instances, the shorter acting, potent drugs such as furosemide or ethacrynic acid in comparable doses.

In minimal to moderately severe hypertension, methyldopa is then tried, starting with 250 mg. and increasing by 250 mg. each week until the blood pressure is reduced below 150/100 mm. Hg. If the blood pressure cannot be adequately controlled with a maximal dose of 2000 mg. of methyldopa per day, then guanethidine (Ismelin) might be required if it is thought that a more potent and effective antihypertensive agent is needed. The approach to guanethidine is to start with a dose of 12.5 mg. given each morning, while continuing the diuretic and methyldopa. The dose of guanethidine should then be increased each week by 12.5 mg. daily until the blood pressure taken with the patient standing is regulated below 150/100 mm. Hg (Fig. 10.3). It is usually not advisable to give a larger dose of guanethidine than 300 mg. daily because of the side effects. When doses larger than this are required, it is better to investigate the possibility of alternate therapeutic approaches for that particular patient.

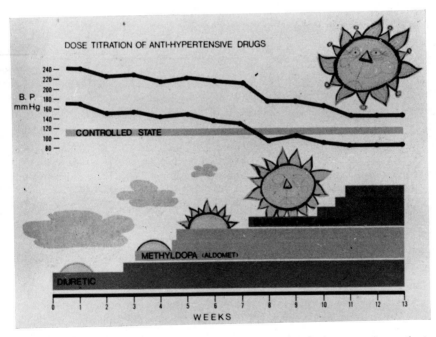

Fig. 10.3. Before treatment, the outlook is gloomy for the hypertensive patient. As optimal control of the blood pressure is gradually achieved by individual dose titration of, first, a diuretic and then antihypertensive agents of increasing potency, the outlook becomes progressively brighter, with the blood pressure finally stabilized at normotensive levels as the successful result of painstaking therapeutic trial.

In treating patients whose diastolic pressure before therapy is more than 120 mm. Hg, there is frequently little reason for trying the intermediate drug methyldopa; rather, treatment should be started directly with guanethidine as described above, increasing it until the blood pressure is adequately regulated in the standing position. In these patients, when the orthostatic effect is excessive, the dosage of guanethidine may be decreased somewhat and methyldopa administered as a third drug in order to get the maximal antihypertensive effect with the minimal orthostatic effect.

For the patient with minimal to moderately severe hypertension who has been given methyldopa plus guanethidine, it is usually good to back-titrate the dose of methyldopa after about 6 months to see whether any antihypertensive effect is lost. Usually in these patients the component of blood pressure reduction attributable to methyldopa is not very great, and it is frequently easier to maintain the patient on a two-drug regimen by gradually reducing the dose of methyldopa and finally withdrawing it completely, perhaps then increasing the dose of guanethidine by a small amount until the blood pressure is adequately regulated.

Use of Diuretics in Antihypertensive Therapy

The reason for giving the diuretic before the sympathetic depressant and continuing it while the sympathetic depressant drug is being titrated is well exemplified in Figure 10.4. The diuretic enhances the antihypertensive effect of the sympathetic depressant at a smaller dose and, in addition, prevents the development of tolerance. Therefore, if the drugs are given in reverse order, the blood pressure may drop excessively when the diuretic is started.

When methyldopa (Aldomet) is given, tolerance occurs in well over 50 per cent of the patients, and probably in almost 90 per cent of patients within 1 year if diuretics are not given concurrently. Therefore methyldopa should never—or rarely—be given alone but rather should always be given concurrently with a diuretic, if only for this reason. The decrease in the incidence of side effects is also significant, since the dosage of methyldopa and/or guanethidine can be reduced by 40 or 50 per cent, as contrasted with the dosage requirement of these drugs for equivalent effect when given alone.

The choice of a diuretic is not made, in general, solely on the basis of antihypertensive potency, since all of the drugs are about equally potent. Table 10.1 shows the results of a comparative study of different diuretics administered under similar circumstances; it is readily evident that these diuretics differ very little in effectiveness. However, the choice of a diuretic may depend on other considerations. For example, it is usually not wise to give ethacrynic acid or furosemide when a thiazide or chlorthalidone is available. Ethacrynic acid and furosemide, because of their potency, are more likely to

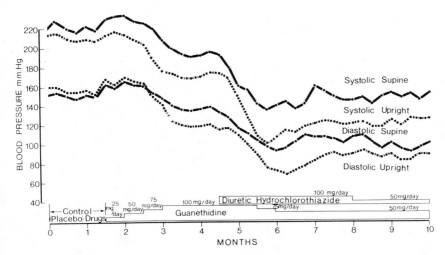

FIG. 10.4. Blood pressure response when diuretic is given to a patient partially blocked with guanethidine (Ismelin). In a patient whose pretreatment blood pressure was 215/160 mm. Hg (upright), partial control was eventually achieved with 100 mg. of guanethidine daily, and the blood pressure was fairly well stabilized at about 170/120 mm. Hg. With the addition of a thiazide diuretic, the patient became normotensive and remained so even after the dosage of both drugs had been gradually reduced to one-half the maximal dosage given to achieve this result initially. (Preferably, however, the diuretic should be given first and other antihypertensive agents added later.)

produce hypokalemia or a total body sodium deficiency state (reflected as hyponatremia) than are the other diuretics. The very reason for not using these drugs in the routine treatment of hypertension is the same reason why they are such important drugs in the overall management of other conditions: *i.e.*, their potency and the fact that they continue to produce natriuresis, kaliuresis, and diuresis even in the presence of electrolyte aberrations when the thiazides and mercurials are no longer effective. Therefore these agents, because of their continued activity, will aggravate electrolyte loss and create a much greater electrolyte abnormality before they lose their effectiveness and ability to act as diuretic (natriuretic) and kaliuretic agents.

It is worth pointing out, however, that skin reactions and other idiosyncratic or side reactions are frequently not observed with ethacrynic acid or furosemide in patients who may have such reactions when given thiazides, and vice versa. Therefore, should a patient have a skin reaction while taking a thiazide, it is worth a trial of ethacrynic acid or furosemide, since the antihypertensive effect is equally potent and it is unlikely that the latter drugs will exhibit this side effect.

Table 10.1. *Comparison of blood pressure response to various diuretics given orally to patients with hypertension*

Drug	Dose	Response		Normotensive	
		supine	upright	supine	upright
	mg./day	%		%	
Chlorothiazide	1000	36	46	18	24
Hydrochlorothiazide	100	39	39	20	22
Chlorthalidone	200	40	50	17	27
Ethacrynic acid	150–400	53	53	7	20

Prevention of Hypokalemia

Finally, we should emphasize that, in treating the patient who becomes hypokalemic, it is worthwhile to administer spironolactone (Aldactone) or triamterene (Dyrenium), which will block off the potassium loss and, at the same time, slightly enhance the natriuretic effect. For patients who tend to lose large amounts of potassium, this is certainly preferable to giving larger amounts of potassium in the diet each day. Once a patient is in a hypokalemic state, it is virtually impossible to continue the diuretic and correct the hypokalemia, since under these circumstances a dosage of 250 or 300 mEq of potassium daily may be required over an extended period in order to correct the deficiency. Therefore a dose of 50 mg. a day of spironolactone is an effective way of blocking loss of potassium sufficient to cause hypokalemia.

After the patient is stabilized on the anti-aldosterone agent, the intake of potassium must be adjusted so as to maintain a normal plasma potassium level. This can be done with K-Lyte or, if the deficiency state is not too severe, by administration of potassium through the use of orange juice and other fruit juices. Potassium triplex and various mixtures of potassium salts are also quite effective, but the incidence of nausea is relatively high after continued use. In my experience, nausea occurs less often with K-Lyte than with the liquid mixtures of potassium salts.

In patients with severe heart failure and renal damage especially, it is very important to monitor the blood level of potassium when giving added potassium in the diet, until the patient is well stabilized. On occasion the level of potassium can rise rapidly in these patients when large amounts are present in the diet and spironolactone or triamterene is given concurrently.

Stabilization of Sympathomimetic Activity

Finally, relative to drug administration, I should like to conclude by again emphasizing the importance of adjusting the dosage of potent sympathomimetic drugs for each individual patient. Basically, the patient's general condition must be stabilized insofar as possible so as to minimize the peaks and valleys in the day-to-day blood pressure. It should be kept in mind that sympathomimetic blocking drugs are used at a fixed dose, and that the degree of blockade is relatively fixed. Therefore it is important that the sympathomimetic activity be stable so as to minimize variation in blood pressure from day to day, thus standardizing the dose requirement. This allows the dosage to be adjusted properly for each patient, a procedure frequently referred to as sympathomimetic blocking agent dose titration.

Figure 10.5 is an example of a patient who experienced strong sympathomimetic response to environmental stimuli. This was a trial lawyer who became quite tense during legal procedures in court. It can be seen that his blood pressure rose rather precipitously. When the stimulus was removed by his preparing the brief and having his partner do the trial work in court, the blood pressure smoothed out and was well regulated with a lower dose of a sympathomimetic blocking agent. Thus, the drug must be adjusted and tailored to the patient's day-to-day activity. The greater the patient's stability, no matter how severely the blood pressure is elevated, the easier it will be to find the dose regimen which just fits that particular patient, with his various idiosyncrasies and hourly variations in blood pressure each day.

EFFECT OF BLOOD PRESSURE REGULATION ON VASCULAR DETERIORATION AND CLINICAL MANIFESTATIONS OF HYPERTENSION

Effect of Treatment on Renal Function

Blood pressure control effectively arrests disease of the small arterioles, particularly as seen in the kidney glomeruli. In the patient with malignant hypertension, renal damage—manifested by glomerular deterioration and fibrinoid changes in the nephron—progresses very rapidly. It can be completely arrested by blood pressure control if the hypertension is treated vigorously and early enough, before renal excretory failure has developed. In the average patient with malignant hypertension (*i.e.*, the patient with retinopathy, severe blood pressure elevation, and renal damage) the renal excretory function deteriorates by about 5 to 10 per cent per month. Thus, the patient will lose 25 to 50 per cent of his renal excretory function in 6 months. When the function drops below 40 to 50 per cent, the blood urea nitrogen is elevated, and that usually ensues rather rapidly, especially if the blood pressure is not lowered. This vascular deterioration can be controlled by blood pressure regulation.

Associated Atherosclerosis

On the other hand, the patient with milder disease, or even one who has severe disease associated with atherosclerosis, is a different problem. Athero-

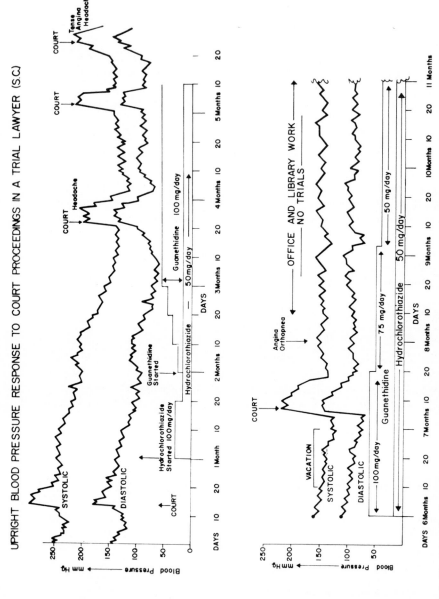

Fig. 10.5. Upright blood pressure response to court proceedings in a trial lawyer (S. C.). The blood pressure of a lawyer, normally well controlled with a combination of a thiazide diuretic and guanethidine, consistently rose to severely hypertensive levels whenever his work required his presence in court. After he restricted himself to preparing the cases and arranged to have a partner handle the trial work in

sclerosis occurs not only in the patient with hypertension but in the normo-tensive patient as well; in fact, it causes occlusive lesions (*i.e.*, thrombosis) in the normotensive state in patients who have never had hypertension. Hypertension merely accelerates the development of the atherosclerosis and makes it more likely that thrombosis, or even rupture of the vessel, will occur during sudden increases in the blood pressure. This component of the pathophysiology and clinical manifestations can be removed by blood pressure regulation. However, the hypertension is only a complication of this diphasic disease, and even though that component of the morbidity and mortality due to blood pressure elevation is removed by controlling the blood pressure, the basic atherosclerotic disease progresses.

Until atherosclerosis as such can be better treated, it is not likely that we will significantly alter the prognosis, the morbidity, and the mortality in these patients. Furthermore, atherosclerotic disease is a multicentric disease, as seen in Figure 10.6. In this patient renal arterial occlusive disease was noted, and as can be seen, there was clear-cut evidence of associated carotid occlusive disease. When occlusive disease of the renal artery is diagnosed, more than 50 per cent of the patients are found to have multicentric disease of the renal artery, either multicentric areas in the same artery or lesions on the opposite side. Furthermore, 75 or 80 per cent of these patients have as-sociated coronary artery disease as evidenced by changes in the electro-

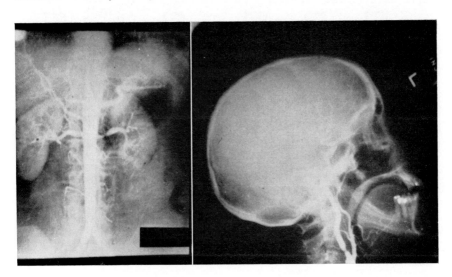

Fig. 10.6. In this patient with stenosis of a renal artery, as seen in the renal arteriogram on the left, carotid arteriogram (shown at the right) demonstrated stenosis of the right common carotid artery as well. This is not unusual, since athero-sclerosis is a multicentric disease and may cause vascular obstruction in widely separated locations. (The renal, cerebral, and cardiac vessels are most vulnerable.)

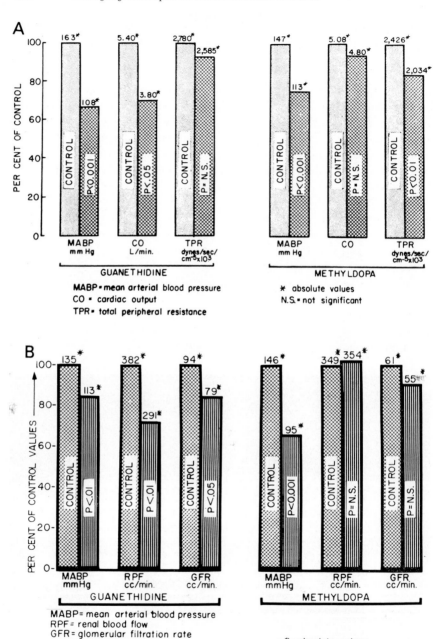

Fig. 10.7. A, cardiovascular hemodynamic response to intravenous guanethidine compared with response to intravenous methyldopa (supine). Guanethidine reduces the blood pressure slightly more than a comparable dose of methyldopa but does so

cardiogram, and 25 per cent have associated carotid disease, again emphasizing the multicentric character of this disease. Again, hypertension is
merely an aggravating complication and not the basic determinant of prognosis and morbidity.

SOME SPECIAL PROBLEMS RELATED TO THE TREATMENT OF HYPERTENSION

Finally, I should like to emphasize the problem of renal damage, especially in the presence of malignant hypertension: *i.e.*, in the patient with
papilledema and blood pressure elevation and secondary renal damage to
the glomeruli. In these patients, the blood pressure elevation is directly
related to the glomerular damage and fibrinoid changes in the nephrons.
The sooner treatment is instituted, the better for the patient. However, in
some patients, the blood urea nitrogen is elevated and evidence of excretory
failure has already occurred before the patient is brought under therapy.
When this occurs, the therapist is on the horns of a dilemma. If he does not
reduce the blood pressure and control it adequately, the disease progresses
with the usual fibrinoid and associated pathological changes in the kidney.
On the other hand, when the blood pressure is reduced, there is an additional
reduction in filtration rate on a hemodynamic basis. This only aggravates
the renal excretory failure.

The only approach to this problem is to gingerly reduce the blood pressure
as far as can be tolerated hemodynamically by the patient. Best results are
achieved through the use of parenteral methyldopa. When this drug is administered, it maintains cardiac output, thus permitting the maintenance of
renal blood flow so that there is less reduction in glomerular filtration rate
than is observed with the other antihypertensive agents for an equivalent
reduction in blood pressure. This is evident from the hemodynamic studies
shown in Figure 10.7. As soon as the blood pressure has been reduced for 10
days to 2 weeks and the renal hemodynamics have become adjusted, then
the parenteral methyldopa is gradually withdrawn and the usual oral antihypertensive measures are instituted, consisting of a diuretic and more potent drugs, such as guanethidine.

---

largely by reducing cardiac output rather than peripheral resistance, whereas methyldopa significantly reduces peripheral resistance and causes only a slight decrease in
cardiac output. B, comparison of the effects of intravenous guanethidine and the
effects of intravenous methyldopa on renal function. The difference in action between
guanethidine and methyldopa is reflected in their effects on renal function. By maintaining cardiac output at nearly normal levels and decreasing peripheral resistance,
methyldopa maintains renal blood flow, and glomerular filtration rate is reduced very
little. By contrast, the reduction in cardiac output caused by guanethidine substantially decreases renal blood flow and, consequently, glomerular filtration rate.
(Reprinted from Moyer, J. H., and Brest, A. N.: Amer. J. Cardiol. 17: 673, 1966.)

After the blood urea nitrogen is elevated, however, the prognosis is much poorer, even with adequate blood pressure regulation. However, the only way to offer the patient any future at all is to try to control the blood pressure to the maximal degree that he can tolerate, following the blood urea nitrogen carefully.

Renal function is also reflected in mortality. As Figure 10.8 shows, mortality in untreated malignant hypertension is 100 per cent within 5 years. In the treated patient, on the other hand, the 5-year mortality is reduced to 25 per cent, a considerable improvement. If the blood pressure is treated early enough, before renal damage is significant, then the mortality is reduced even more markedly. However, it is of some significance that the patient has then been converted to a candidate for intermittent hypertension and, after a period of years, atherosclerosis will rear its head. Referring to Table 10.2, it can be seen that, of those patients who died in the first 2 years, a significant number died of renal failure caused by progression of the renal damage, indicating that therapy had not been instituted early enough. Of the patients who died after 2 years, however, all died of a complication of atherosclerosis such as thrombosis of the coronary vessels or of a cerebral vessel, or from another complication related primarily to the atherosclerosis. Here the hypertension was merely a complicating phenomenon and not the direct cause of progressive renal disease, as is seen in the kidneys in untreated malignant hypertension.

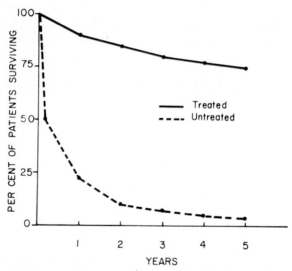

Fɪɢ. 10.8. Course of malignant hypertension. Patients with malignant hypertension whose blood pressure is effectively controlled have a good prognosis: 75 per cent survive for more than 5 years after treatment is started. Untreated patients, on the other hand, have a 5-year mortality rate of nearly 100 per cent.

Table 10.2. *Cause of death in 12 of 48 patients treated for malignant hypertension*

Year	Renal	CVA*	Coronary
1st	2	1	
2nd	1	1	1
3rd		2	
4th		1	2
5th			1
Total	3	5	4

Mortality after 5 years due to hypertension: 25%
Unrelated cause of death: 3 patients

* Cerebrovascular accident.

SUMMARY AND CONCLUSIONS

1. The control of blood pressure is quite possible if one pays strict attention to pharmacodynamics of the drugs, the proper selection of a drug, and some basic principles related to drug administration, particularly the autonomic drugs. Obviously the most important consideration is that of proper dose titration of sympathetic depressant drugs.

2. Diuretics are cornerstones of antihypertensive therapy for several reasons. They not only have some antihypertensive properties in their own right, but in addition they prevent the development of tolerance to other drugs such as methyldopa. They also decrease the dose requirement of the more potent antihypertensive drugs, thereby decreasing side effects due to the latter agents.

3. In the patient whose blood pressure is not so severely elevated, atherosclerosis and fluctuating blood pressure may become the predominant determinant of morbidity and mortality. Under these circumstances, the hypertension is merely a complicating phenomenon, and controlling the blood pressure only removes that component of the morbidity and mortality determinant related to blood pressure elevation; it does not affect the basic morbidity and mortality related to the atherosclerotic disease. In these patients the primary problem is that of occlusive lesions—*i.e.*, thrombosis, not rupture—of the diseased, atherosclerotic vessel.

4. If treated early enough, the small vessel disease of malignant hypertension can be completely arrested. However, atherosclerotic disease later becomes manifest, and then becomes the primary disease even in well-controlled patients. Eventually many of these patients will die of atherosclerotic disease even if the blood pressure is regulated at the normotensive level.

5. Again, it cannot be sufficiently emphasized that, in the therapeutic

management of hypertension, probably the most important simple consideration, yet the most frequently overlooked, is that of appropriate dose titration, in which the dose of the sympathetic depressant drug is adjusted exactly to the requirement of the patient for blood pressure regulation.

This study was supported by the Mary Bailey Institute for Heart Research.

11

Pulmonary Heart Disease: Highlights of Etiology, Diagnosis, and Treatment

HAROLD M. LOWE, M.D.

GENERAL CONSIDERATIONS

This discussion focuses on the basic pathophysiological concepts which characterize the clinical syndrome of cor pulmonale and points out how this information may be used as a basis for diagnosis and therapy.

It is appropriate at the outset to offer a definition of the subject. Cor pulmonale is the clinical syndrome of right heart failure occurring as a result of a primary disease process affecting the pulmonary parenchyma, pulmonary vessels, or chest bellows function. No other well-defined clinical syndrome has such a vast array of various disease processes which may produce this clinical picture. Table 11.1 is an admittedly incomplete list of some of the primary disease processes which may produce cor pulmonale. They are grouped according to their major pathophysiological effects on the respiratory apparatus. Despite this wide variety of disease processes, there is a factor common to all which produces cor pulmonale. The final common pathway is pulmonary vascular obstruction sufficient to cause pulmonary hypertension (Fig. 11.1).

Anatomic fixed pulmonary vascular obstruction is rarely the most important factor in producing pulmonary hypertension. The capacitance reserve of the pulmonary vessels is so large that it is possible to experimentally reduce the pulmonary vascular tree to 15 per cent of normal without affecting cardiac output or resting pulmonary pressures. Increased pulmonary flow without increased resistance is also very unlikely to produce right heart failure. Therefore we shall concentrate on reversible causes of increased pulmonary vascular resistance, namely hypoxemia and acidosis, or a combination of the two. Figure 11.2 illustrates the mechanisms by which hypoxemia and acidosis may be produced. Either acidosis or hypoxemia alone may cause pulmonary hypertension. The combination of the two is additive in the degree of elevation of pulmonary pressures.

The pathophysiological mechanisms resulting in significant degrees of hypoxemia and respiratory acidosis fall into the following general categories:

Table 11.1. *Etiological classification of cor pulmonale*

I. Pulmonary parenchymal and tracheo-
bronchial diseases
  A. Obstructive airway disease
    1. Emphysema
      a. panlobular
      b. centrilobular
      c. bullous
      d. postpneumonectomy
    2. Asthma
    3. Chronic bronchitis
  B. Restrictive pulmonary disease
    1. Infective agents
      a. Tuberculosis
      b. Fungal infections
        (1) actinomycosis
        (2) blastomycosis
        (3) coccidioidomycosis
        (4) histoplasmosis
      c. Bacterial
        (1) recurrent pneumonia
        (2) bronchiectasis
    2. Fibrocystic disease
    3. Carcinoma
    4. Unknown or uncertain etiology
      a. scleroderma
      b. Hamman-Rich syndrome
      c. idiopathic fibrosis
    5. Due to irritants and destructive
      agents
      a. berylliosis
      b. silicosis
      c. various noxious gases
    6. Pleural calcification

II. Diseases affecting the chest bellows
function
  A. Neurological disorders
    1. Poliomyelitis
    2. Amyotrophic lateral sclerosis
    3. Multiple sclerosis
    4. Depression of respiratory
      center
      a. encephalitis
      b. bulbar polio
      c. primary
  B. Musculoskeletal
    1. kyphoscoliosis
    2. rheumatoid spondylitis
    3. thoracoplasty
    4. muscular dystrophy
    5 dermatomyositis
III. Lesions of the pulmonary vascula-
ture
  A. Primary pulmonary hyperten-
sion
  B. Pulmonary emboli
    1. acute
    2. chronic, recurrent, multiple,
      small
  C. Schistosomiasis
  D. Carcinoid syndrome
  E. Pulmonary arteriovenous fistu-
lae
  F. Sickle cell anemia
  G. Pulmonary venous sclerosis

I ↑ Pulmonary <u>flow</u> with resistance unchanged

II ↑ Pulmonary vascular <u>resistance</u>
    independent of flow

    A. Anatomic-fixed pulmonary vascular obstruction

    B. Functional-potentially reversible

III   Combined ↑ flow and resistance

FIG. 11.1. Mechanisms of pulmonary hypertension.

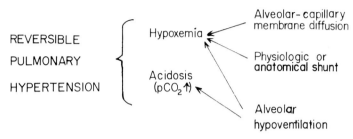

FIG. 11.2. Pathological aspects of reversible pulmonary hypertension.

(1) alveolar hypoventilation, (2) pulmonary vascular obstruction, (3) anatomic or physiological shunts, (4) disturbed gas diffusion across the alveolar capillary membranes, and (5) abnormal structure or function of the thoracic cage bellows action. It should be obvious by this time that a logical approach to treatment of cor pulmonale demands that the major effort be directed at the primary lung disorder, and that only in this way can therapy be effective.

The incidence of chronic respiratory disease continues to rise and, since emphysema and chronic bronchitis are by far the most common causes of cor pulmonale, the reported incidence of cor pulmonale is highest where climate, air pollution, and occupational factors influence their occurrence. Compared to all forms of heart disease, pulmonary heart disease varies from 3.3 per cent in Buenos Aires, Argentina to 25 per cent in Sheffield, England.

It is hoped that no one is tired of hearing about air pollution and ecological problems, since our responsibility is evident. Chronic respiratory disease and air pollution are obviously related and are a prime example, certainly in weight of numbers, of an ecological problem demanding a solution. That the emphasis in medicine must shift from *quantity* of life to *quality* has already been pointed out, unfortunately from outside the medical profession more often than from within. This brief editorial seems appropriate because the individual with cor pulmonale so often has advanced and irreversible changes, and the prognosis is so dismal. Roughly 25 per cent die with their first attack of overt failure, and another 25 per cent within 2 years. Even if death does not occur, the majority are disabled in their most productive years.

Nevertheless there is often a great deal that can be done, particularly for the acutely ill patient. Since the treatment of the basic pathological process depends on definition of the process, it is obvious that we cannot consider all or even a few of the various disease states listed in Table 11.1. Therefore it may be useful to consider some specific aspects of the treatment of acute respiratory failure in patients with chronic lung disease of the emphysema-bronchitis type, in whom right heart failure is inevitably present.

ACUTE RESPIRATORY FAILURE

Keeping in mind the fact that hypoxemia, acidosis, and pulmonary hypertension are the common denominators of cor pulmonale, effective therapy must accomplish correction or partial correction of these problems by concentrating on improvement of ventilation.

Acute respiratory failure superimposed on chronic lung disease most frequently occurs as a result of acute lower respiratory infection, though injudicious use of sedatives, narcotics, and anesthesia may also frequently precipitate the problem.

Diagnosis

The patient in acute respiratory failure is not difficult to recognize clinically. He may be obtunded, comatose, semicomatose, or acutely agitated and nearly unmanageable. The patient who is less severely ill may state that he is afraid to go to sleep, or it may be noted that he becomes quite drowsy or unresponsive while receiving oxygen or intermittent positive pressure breathing (IPPB) treatment. The usual signs of cor pulmonale are present: cyanosis, tachycardia, distended neck veins, enlarged liver, and peripheral edema. If the respiratory noise does not completely obscure the heart sounds, a ventricular gallop over the xyphoid or in the epigastrium is heard. Tachypnea with poor air exchange is evident. The patient may complain of anterior substernal chest pain. Ineffective cough without purulent sputum is common, even though infection is present. A variety of cardiac arrhythmias unrelated to digitalis may be noted. Sinus tachycardia or other supraventricular tachycardias are the rule, and ventricular arrhythmias are rare. The latter usually indicate the presence of underlying heart disease or digitalis toxicity.

Treatment

Effective therapy demands, first of all, correction of the ventilatory problem, and secondarily, treatment of the heart failure. One must have the capability of obtaining accurate and frequent arterial blood gas determinations. The sample must be drawn anaerobically in a heparinized syringe. A bubble as small as 0.1 ml. will change the pH and pCO_2 significantly. The higher the actual pCO_2 the greater the error, producing falsely low values. In the range of an actual pCO_2 of 60 to 70, a bubble error can be demonstrated to be as high as 10 mm. Hg. Since the changes in the blood gases dictate initial treatment and alterations in therapy, it is essential that an accurate and consistent technique be followed. In the patient who requires frequent arterial gas analysis, it is useful to insert an indwelling arterial catheter with a heparin lock.

Other laboratory studies of immediate pertinence include blood count, urinalysis, posterior-anterior and lateral chest film, electrocardiogram, sputum culture, serum electrolytes, and blood urea nitrogen.

Primary therapeutic problems requiring immediate attention are as follows in approximate order of priority: (1) airway obstruction, (2) hypoxemia, (3) hypercapnea and respiratory acidosis, (4) infection, (5) right ventricular failure, (6) metabolic alkalosis and acidosis, and (7) dehydration.

1. *Airway Obstruction*

Bronchospasm and accumulated secretions are the two major reversible causes of airway obstruction which can be treated effectively. Intravenous aminophylline and aerosol bronchodilators (isoproterenol, racemic epinephrine) are standards of bronchodilator therapy. Aerosol-administered drugs are not effective, however, if the tracheobronchial tree is filled with secretions so that the drugs cannot reach the desired site of action.

In the patient with ineffective cough, tracheal or transtracheal intubation, irrigation and suction are necessary and tracheostomy may be the only satisfactory solution. In the comatose or semicomatose patient, immediate tracheostomy and insertion of a cuffed tube are essential. Emergency bronchoscopy with suction under direct vision and with lavage may at times be even more effective as the initial measure. The double cuffed large bore Portex tracheostomy tube has been the most satisfactory, in our experience, for two very important reasons. Alternate cuff inflation permits uninterrupted mechanically assisted or controlled ventilation, and the large bore connector avoids an artificial increase in airway resistance to flow. Tubes with small diameter external connections interfere with effective air exchange, particularly when pressure-cycled respirators are used.

There are a few other problems with respirator therapy which have not been emphasized in the literature and which, when not recognized, may unnecessarily reduce the effectiveness of or may defeat therapeutic efforts.

Pressure-cycled respirators without flow control are worthless in effecting adequate air exchange in the patient who requires assisted or controlled ventilation. The high airway resistance cycles the respirator before any effective input of air is accomplished.

The flow and pressure settings should always be adjusted to the individual patient's need. The physician should adjust the settings himself and not rely on either a routine or recommended set of flow and pressure settings, nor should he rely on the oxygen therapist. In the conscious patient, there is considerable variation in requirements for flow and pressure to really assist ventilation rather than having the patient fight the machine.

It has been observed that there is a consistent inconsistency in the percentage of O_2 delivered on the dilute (or supposedly 40 per cent) O_2 setting of pressure-cycled respirators as well as the percentage of O_2 setting of volume respirators. The delivered supposedly 40 per cent has gas mixtures varying from 20 per cent O_2 to 80 per cent O_2. High O_2 enrichment in excess of requirements may be particularly undesirable.

More than an occasional patient with acute respiratory failure has extremely high airway resistance requiring very high inflation pressures for adequate ventilation. For these patients, a volume respirator must be used. These patients also require constant close monitoring of blood pressure, since the pressure needed for ventilation may restrict or shut off venous return. There often is a narrow margin to accomplish adequate ventilation and to avoid the circulatory problem.

2. *Hypoxemia*

Correction of hypoxemia to a PO_2 of at least 50 mm. Hg is the minimal objective and is accomplished by relief of airway obstruction, by assisted ventilation to improve alveolar ventilation, and by increasing inspired O_2 concentration sufficiently but cautiously. In the conscious and cooperative patient, one can accurately deliver known concentrations of oxygen using a Venturi type mask which permits accurate stepwise increments of O_2 enrichment without over-oxygenation. For many years the dangers of uncontrolled oxygen administration have been emphasized as the cause of a further decrease in alveolar ventilation and development of CO_2 narcosis. The toxicity of 100 per cent oxygen and the resulting pathological changes in the alveoli have been more recently reported.[1-3] Furthermore, it has been pointed out by McNichol and Campbell that extreme respiratory acidosis is probably always iatrogenic.[4] The pCO_2 cannot exceed 80 mm. Hg, nor can the pH be below 7.19 while the patient is breathing room air. Any further reduction in alveolar ventilation would result in death from hypoxia.

Despite the well-recognized hazards of O_2 therapy, the patient with acute respiratory failure must have an increase in the level of inspired O_2 to achieve a normal arterial PO_2. The only way in which one can give enough, but not too much, is to have an accurate knowledge of how much is being given and to assess accurately its effect on the blood gases. The necessary additional oxygen can be given at low flow rates and/or controlled concentrations with frequent blood gas determinations as the guideline.

High fever superimposed on hypoxemia may frequently result in irreversible brain damage and should be controlled by whatever means are necessary.

3. *Hypercapnea and Respiratory Acidosis*

Hypercapnea and respiratory acidosis are essentially a direct reflection of the degree of alveolar hypoventilation. Those measures already discussed are the major features of treatment of these problems. Two items deserve mention here in addition to the previously described means of improving

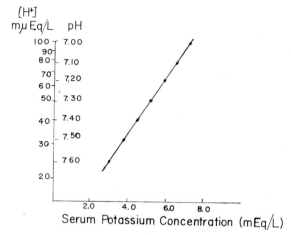

Fig. 11.3. Effect of change in acid-base status on serum potassium concentration.

alveolar ventilation. First, the acidosis may be severe enough to require treatment before much has been accomplished in the way of increasing alveolar ventilation. A pH below 7.20 or one which remains below 7.25 should probably be treated with judicious amounts of sodium bicarbonate. It is the consensus of opinion that the organic buffers are less effective than sodium bicarbonate. Second, the changes in serum potassium associated with changes in pH deserve re-emphasis (Fig. 11.3). Rapid correction of acidosis may precipitously lower the serum potassium and cause digitalis toxicity. Previous diuretic therapy and malnutrition may have already reduced body potassium stores, thus magnifying the problem.

4. *Infection*

Since lower respiratory infection is the most common precipitant of acute respiratory failure, adequate material for culture is essential and should represent the bacterial flora of the lower respiratory tract. In the absence of an effective cough, tracheal suction or even bronchoscopy may be necessary.

The patient with a non-hospital-acquired infection may be treated, while awaiting results of the cultures, with tetracycline or ampicillin. A hospital-acquired infection is usually a resistant staph or more often *Escherichia coli*, *Pseudomonas*, or *Proteus*. In the case of the last three organisms, therapy with nebulized aerosol antibiotics such as gentamycin may at times be more effective than parenteral administration.

5. *Right Heart Failure*

Since the primary cause of right heart failure in cor pulmonale is pulmonary hypertension as a result of increased pulmonary vascular resistance, and since this is in turn due to hypoxemia and acidosis, the single most important aspect of treatment of the heart failure is relief of hypoxemia and acidosis. Digitalis is indicated, as in the presence of any congestive heart failure, along with salt restriction, bed rest, and aminophylline. Diuretics are useful but should be used cautiously, and phlebotomy may be more effective, particularly in the presence of a marked increase in red cell mass. There is no longer any argument among authorities as to the use of digitalis in cor pulmonale. The failing right ventricle needs glycoside support; the problem lies in determining the optimal clinical effect. Use of the resting pulse rate, in the absence of atrial fibrillation, in any type of heart failure as an index of digitalis therapy is generally unsatisfactory, but in cor pulmonale it may lead to serious overdosage. The tachycardia which is almost invariably present should be viewed as a compensatory mechanism to maintain cardiac output. The controversy over whether left ventricular failure is commonly present in cor pulmonale appears to have been resolved in the negative; however, it is well to remember that an occasional patient with left ventricular decompensation may present as having primary pulmonary disease, with associated right heart failure.

6. *Metabolic Alkalosis and Acidosis*

Provided that renal function is adequate, potassium chloride supplementation is usually advisable, particularly in the presence of metabolic alkalosis with low serum potassium and while respiratory acidosis is being corrected.

7. *Dehydration*

Correction of water deficit is usually necessary and often neglected. Decreasing the viscosity of sputum and blood are valuable and often necessary adjuncts in therapy. Adequate humidification of inspired gas is essential.

In summary, this presentation has attempted to offer current pathophysiological concepts upon which rational treatment of cor pulmonale can be based. It has been one clinician's approach to a clinical problem. Specific observations have been offered in regard to problems in treatment, particularly of the patient in acute respiratory failure. After effective therapy, it is frequently most gratifying to see your patient walk out of the hospital, often in better health than in the months preceding his acute episode. The clinical syndrome of acute respiratory failure does not imply terminal irreversible lung disease.

REFERENCES

1. Nash, G., Blennerhassett, J. B., and Pontoppidan, H.: Pulmonary lesions associated with oxygen therapy and artificial ventilation. New Eng. J. Med. 276: 368, 1967.

2. Soloway, H. B., Castillo, Y., and Martin, A. M.: Adult hyaline membrane disease: Relationship to oxygen therapy. Ann. Surg. 168: 937–945, 1968.
3. Barter, R. A., Frulay-Jones, L. R., and Walters, M.: Pulmonary hyaline membrane: Sites of formation in adult lungs after assisted respiration and inhalation of oxygen. J. Path. Bact. 95: 481–488, 1968.
4. McNichol, M. W., and Campbell, E. J. M.: Severity of respiratory failure. Arterial blood-gases in untreated patients. Lancet 1: 336, 1965.

12

Recent Advances in the Understanding of Congestive Heart Failure

DEAN T. MASON, M.D., ROBERT ZELIS, M.D.,
EZRA A. AMSTERDAM, M.D., AND
RASHID A. MASSUMI, M.D.

Congestive heart failure is the pathological condition in which severely abnormal cardiac performance is responsible for the inability of the heart to deliver blood at a rate commensurate with the basal metabolic requirements of the organs throughout the body. Intensive investigation in the past few years has provided important new information concerning the physiological derangements and certain biochemical abnormalities comprising the heart failure state. Considered in this chapter are recent advances in the elucidation of disturbed cardiac function, alterations of hemodynamics and myocardial mechanics, cardiocirculatory compensatory mechanisms, and underlying derangements of myocardial ultrastructure and metabolism which have provided an improved comprehension of clinical heart failure. In this review, the concept is developed that the fundamental physiological abnormality in congestive heart failure resides in depression of myocardial contractility in disorders characterized by ventricular pressure or volume overloading, as well as in cardiac abnormalities due to primary defects of contractility.

PRINCIPAL DETERMINANTS OF CARDIAC FUNCTION AND ASSESSMENT OF CONTRACTILITY

The principal determinants of stroke volume, cardiac output, and other variables of ventricular performance are now acknowledged to be the loading conditions of the ventricle (preload: left ventricular end diastolic volume and pressure; afterload: aortic impedence and systemic arterial resistance), contractile state, heart rate and, in certain types of heart disease, the synergy or temporal sequence of ventricular contraction.[1] Interplay among these five major determinants of cardiac function governs ventricular pump performance (cardiac output) and related hemodynamic variables and the mechanics of ventricular contraction (force, velocity, and length characteristics).

In the clinical assessment of cardiac function, the determinant which requires a precise assessment that is most difficult to obtain is the contractile state of the myocardium. Two general approaches are available for the evaluation of contractility in the intact heart.[1] (1) The traditional hemodynamic methods utilize measurements of blood pressure and flow, usually within the framework of the Frank-Starling ventricular function principle, which provide qualitative information concerning directional alterations of inotropic state. (2) More recently it has become possible to evaluate the mechanics of myocardial contraction by study of the force-velocity-length relations which allow quantitative assessment of the determinants of cardiac function, including the numerical analysis of contractile state. In this discussion, the terms cardiac performance and ventricular function are used in a general sense to refer to all five of the principal determinants of pump and muscle function and not necessarily to the specific determinant of contractile state itself.

Within the approach of myocardial mechanics, two general lines of development have taken place: (1) analysis of the properties of the isovolumic phase of ventricular contraction and (2) study of the characteristics of ventricular ejection. The precise determination of isovolumic mechanics has offered quantitative methods for the evaluation of contractility, usually in terms of maximal contractile elemental velocity (V_{max}) by employing high fidelity recordings of intraventricular pressure and corresponding rate of pressure rise (dp/dt).[1-4] These isovolumic methods are suitable for serial intrapatient studies and for interpatient studies. Further, these isovolumic techniques can usually be carried out without difficulty, since only non-artifactual ventricular pressure recordings are necessary. The new method of determining instantaneous contractile element velocity (VCE) and isovolumic pressure-velocity curves, which allow extrapolation of V_{max} solely from instantaneous high fidelity intraventricular pressure and dp/dt, has provided a practical, sensitive, and valid means of quantifying left ventricular contractility without influence of preload or afterload from beat to beat in individual patients and in specific comparison of basal inotropic state among different patients.[3]

Study of the mechanics of ventricular ejection usually requires complex angiographic analysis for the determination of fiber shortening rate (VCF) in order to obtain a single VCE point on the force-velocity curve.[5] These techniques based on ventricular ejection mechanics are often not suitable for serial study, do not afford measurement of V_{max}, and are influenced by ventricular loading. However, these methods provide estimation of contractility between patients and obviate potential problems of mitral regurgitation and different series elastic properties in evaluation of inotropic state.

ALTERATIONS OF HEMODYNAMICS AND MYOCARDIAL MECHANICS

The performance of the failing heart has recently been defined in terms of hemodynamics and the mechanics of ventricular contraction. Patients with overt congestive heart failure have marked elevation of ventricular end diastolic pressure and reduced cardiac output at rest (Fig. 12.1); thus they experience dyspnea and fatigue with rest or with ordinary activity and exhibit pulmonary and systemic edema.[1, 6] In contrast, patients with heart disease without circulatory decompensation manifest shortness of breath only with more than ordinary activity, generally have moderate elevations of ventricular end diastolic, pulmonary, and systemic venous pressures, and demonstrate normal cardiac output at rest (Fig. 12.1), although elevation of cardiac output during exercise is compromised.[1, 6]

In normal subjects, when venous return to the heart is briefly diminished by inflation of a catheter-tip balloon in the inferior vena cava, small reductions of ventricular filling pressure result in large reductions in stroke volume, thereby describing a steep ascending limb of the function curve.[7] However, patients with ventricular failure demonstrate little change in their reduced stroke volume with large decreases in elevated end diastolic pressure.[7] When resistance to left ventricular ejection is increased by the arteriolar constricting action of angiotensin in normal subjects, marked rises in stroke volume occur with small increments of end diastolic pressure.[8] In contrast, small or no alteration in stroke volume is observed with large elevations of ventricular filling pressure in the diseased left ventricle.[8] Thus, the failing ventricle in patients operates on a lowered and flattened function

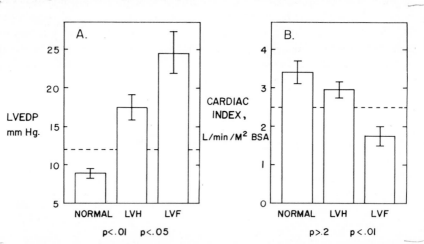

FIG. 12.1. Average values (± standard error of the mean (SEM)) of left ventricular end diastolic pressure (LVEDP) in A, and of the cardiac index in B, in three groups of patients studied. LVH, left ventricular hypertrophy; LVF, left ventricular failure; BSA, body surface area.. (Reproduced by permission from Mason, D. T., *et al.*[6])

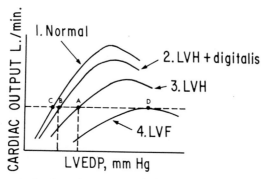

Fig. 12.2. Ventricular function curves relating cardiac output to left ventricular end diastolic pressure (LVEDP) in the normal heart: (1), left ventricular hypertrophy (LVH) with (2) and without (3) digitalis, and left ventricular failure (LVF) (4). Points C, B, A, and D on these curves indicate the level of LVEDP necessary to achieve normal resting cardiac output (horizontal broken line).

curve and exhibits a depressed response to changes in preload (Fig. 12.2). The dysfunctioning left ventricle in man does not usually operate for long periods of time on the descending limb of the Frank-Starling curve. Since the apex and ascending and descending limbs of the depressed ventricular function curve are not clearly distinct, it is often difficult clinically to ascertain precisely the point on the curve at which the failing ventricle is operating.

The examination of ventricular performance within the Frank-Starling framework during muscular exercise has demonstrated impaired ability of the human failing ventricle to shift its function curve to a more elevated and steeper position in response to the positive inotropic influence of increased adrenergic activity.[9] In contrast to normal subjects who exhibit large increases in stroke volume and decreases or slight increases in ventricular end diastolic pressure during exercise, patients with heart failure respond with little change or reduction in stroke volume and large elevations of filling pressure.[9] Thus, in patients with depressed ventricular function, the failing ventricle is less capable of increasing its diminished contractile state in response to sympathetic stimulation accompanying exercise.

Although the measurement of ventricular end diastolic pressure and cardiac output provides useful information concerning cardiac function, it is now quite clear that these variables do not always afford accurate assessment of ventricular contractility since they are influenced by changes in loading imposed on the heart by valvular lesions, pericardial disease, cardiac shunts, and peripheral circulatory dynamics. Thus, in the study of cardiac function by pump characteristics alone, it is difficult to differentiate between the principal determinants of ventricular performance as to which one or a combination of these factors is primarily responsible for the inability of the failing heart to eject an adequate stroke volume. The recent development of techniques and concepts for the analysis of the performance of the intact human myocardium in terms of the mechanics of contraction allows separation of the effects of preload and afterload from the inotropic state of heart muscle.

Thus, very recently it has been possible to document the observation that the contractile state is reduced in the failing human left ventricle.[6] Myocardial contractility is reduced both in patients with primary and in those with secondary ventricular hypertrophy even before the onset of failure; reduction in inotropic state is greater in cardiomyopathies than in long-standing ventricular hemodynamic overloading.[10] It appears that, in the presence of heart disease with ventricular hypertrophy without decompensation, the increased preload or Frank-Starling mechanism and ventricular hypertrophy maintain cardiac output at normal levels, despite the presence of diminished contractility. The initial series of observations which allowed these conclusions concerning the quantification of contractility in patients with heart disease with and without decompensation is based on clinical studies of the force-velocity properties of the intact ventricle.[6] Thus, the maximal velocity of contractile element shortening (V_{max}) was reduced in hypertrophy without failure and more severely diminished in heart failure (Fig. 12.3). The same conclusions were possible when instantaneous contractile element velocity (VCE) and V_{max} were calculated utilizing total or developed isovolumic pressure. Also, contractility has been shown to be diminished in the primarily and secondarily hypertrophied left ventricle in patients before the onset of failure, by the finding in these individuals that there was depression of the ratio of dp/dt at the common isovolumic pressure of 50 mm. Hg divided by the ventricular end diastolic volume index.[6]

In addition, other findings are consistent with these observations that the inotropic state is reduced in the failing left ventricle in patients. Thus, the maximal rate of left ventricular pressure rise (dp/dt) is lower in patients with left ventricular failure compared to normal subjects,[6] and the mean systolic ejection rate of the failing left ventricle is reduced at rest and during exercise,[11] as is the mean rate of circumferential fiber shortening.[12] In patients with ventricular disease, the extent and velocity of shortening of circumferential myocardial fibers is reduced at levels of wall tension comparable to those in normal subjects.[5] In normal subjects, maximal tension occurs soon after the onset of ejection and then diminishes rapidly to levels lower than at the onset of ejection; while in patients with left ventricular disease the development of peak tension is delayed, as is its decline throughout the ejection phase to tensions higher than at the onset of this period.[5] In normal subjects, concerning the instantaneous relation between developed tension and fiber shortening rate during ejection, velocity attains high levels during the rapid rise of tension and is sustained as tension falls. In

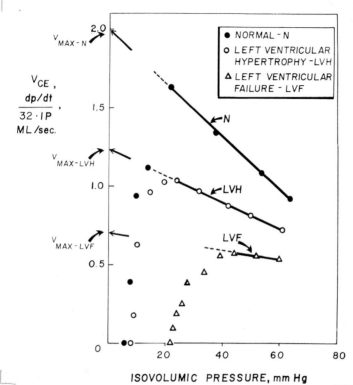

Fig. 12.3. Representative comparison of the pressure-velocity relation during isovolumic contraction of the left ventricle in a normal patient, a patient with left ventricular hypertrophy in the absence of failure, and a patient with left ventricular failure. The diagonal broken lines indicate extrapolation of the isovolumic segment to V_{max} at zero load, shown by the arrows. Instantaneous VCE and V_{max} are expressed in muscle lengths per second (ML/sec.) as the relation $(dp/dt)/(32 \times IP)$ where IP = instantaneous isovolumetric left ventricular pressure. (Reproduced by permission from Mason, D.T., *et al.*[6])

contrast, in patients with left ventricular disease, the velocity of fiber shortening declines as tension decreases during ejection.[5] At the point of maximal developed tension during ejection, the fiber shortening rate (VCF) is equal to instantaneous VCE, since the velocity of the series elastic element (VSE) is zero. At peak tension the velocity of contraction is reduced in patients with heart failure, despite the increase in left ventricular end diastolic volume.[5] In patients with aortic valvular insufficiency, VCE at peak tension has been observed not to be depressed until the onset of clinical and hemodynamic evidence of left ventricular decompensation, suggesting that cardiac failure in these patients occurred as a consequence of impairment of ventricular contractility and not entirely as the result of chronic hemodynamic overloading alone.[13]

From these observations in patients, as well as those in animals with experimentally induced heart failure,[14, 15] it appears that congestive heart failure is a relatively late manifestation of the severely depressed heart, and substantial losses of ventricular function precede detectable abnormalities of hemodynamic performance. There appears to be a spectrum of decreasing ventricular function between left ventricular hypertrophy without failure and left ventricular hypertrophy with failure. In hypertrophy without failure (Class I of the functional classification of the New York Heart Association), the absolute increase in total muscle mass with or without elevated ventricular end diastolic pressure maintains cardiac output at rest, although during strenuous exertion the cardiac output does not increase to a normal extent with increased rise of end diastolic pressure. In compensated heart failure, the basal cardiac output is maintained at a normal level as a result of increased end diastolic pressure, and pulmonary and systemic venous congestion occurs with excessive elevations of end diastolic pressure with marked exercise (Class II) or mild activity (Class III). In hypertrophy with overt congestive heart failure and decompensation (Class IV), despite the striking increase in ventricular end diastolic pressure and muscle mass, cardiac output falls in the basal state as a result of the markedly reduced level of contractility.

COMPENSATORY MECHANISMS

When an excessive pressure or volume load is imposed upon the heart, three major adaptive mechanisms are available for the direct support of myocardial function that provide a limited amount of cardiac reserve and offset the development of overt congestive heart failure. Thus, the force of contraction can be improved by (1) ventricular dilation attributable to the Frank-Starling principle, (2) increase in the number of contractile units by the development of ventricular hypertrophy, and (3) augmentation of activity of the sympathetic nervous system to enhance depressed cardiac contractility.

The Frank-Starling mechanism is immediately available to aid the ventricle in the maintenance of cardiac output in the presence of an increased hemodynamic overload or primary depression of the contractile state. Not only does the increase in end diastolic volume of the ventricle permit more forceful contraction, but also the increase in ventricular size permits a greater stroke volume to be ejected with less extent of shortening of the circumferential myocardial fibers. On the other hand, the efficiency of the Frank-Starling mechanism is somewhat encroached upon in the heart failure state, since the function curve of the abnormally performing ventricle is less steep and the point of end diastolic pressure at which maximal cardiac output can be delivered is delayed (Fig. 12.2).

The development of ventricular hypertrophy provides a second compensatory mechanism available to the heart when its load is excessive or the contractile state is impaired. An increase in contractile element mass occurred within 2 days in the right ventricle of cats in which pulmonic stenosis was produced[14]; left ventricular mass rapidly increased in guinea pigs after constriction of the ascending aorta[16]; and protein synthesis was accelerated within 1 day in the secondarily hypertrophied rat heart.[17] In this process of hypertrophy, perhaps the level of intramyocardial tension serves as the mechanical-biochemical transducer or coupling mechanism responsible for increased protein synthesis in secondary hypertrophy, and an abnormality of this transducer might be responsible for primary hypertrophy. It is of nterest that positive inotropic support provided by digitalis is capable of reducing the degree of ventricular hypertrophy resulting from a chronic pressure overload.[18] Since the three principal hemodynamic-related determinants of myocardial oxygen requirements are: (1) intramyocardial systolic tension, (2) heart rate, and (3) contractility, digitalis may reduce the elevated myocardial oxygen requirements in heart failure by the drug's predominantly indirect action in this condition of decreasing heart size and tension, despite the positive inotropic effect of the glycoside.[19]

In a recent clinical study carried out in our laboratories, the inotropic state and compensatory mechanisms were compared in primary myocardial disease and in ventricular hypertrophy secondary to chronic hemodynamic overloading.[10] The possibility was considered that quantitative differences in contractility and utilization of reserve mechanisms might exist between the primarily and secondarily hypertrophied ventricles. The results of this investigation are shown in Figure 12.4 in which the contractile state and

COMPENSATORY MECHANISMS FOR MAINTAINING NORMAL CARDIAC OUTPUT IN PRIMARY AND SECONDARY LVH

	V_{MAX}	LVEDV	LVH
MYOCARDIOPATHY (primary LV inotropic defect)	↓↓	↑	↑
AORTIC STENOSIS (primary LV pressure overload)	↓	0	↑↑
MITRAL REGURGITATION (primary LV volume overload)	↓	↑	↑

Fig. 12.4. Compensatory mechanisms for maintaining normal cardiac output in primary and secondary left ventricular hypertrophy (LVH). V_{max}, maximal contractile element velocity (contractile state); LVEDV, left ventricular end diastolic volume (preload).

compensatory mechanisms for the maintenance of cardiac output are compared in these groups of patients. In aortic stenosis, the major physiological abnormality is the primary excessive afterload opposing ventricular ejection, in response to which the compensatory mechanism of ventricular hypertrophy appears to be the principal reserve mechanism supporting cardiac output. Although the contractile state of this hypertrophied muscle appears to be diminished, as shown by studies discussed above, cardiac output is maintained in chronic pressure overloading of the ventricle by development of more contractile units without increasing end diastolic volume.

In contrast, in patients with cardiomyopathies, the basic physiological derangement is reduction of the inotropic state, and cardiac output is maintained by the operation of the compensatory mechanisms of both ventricular hypertrophy and increased end diastolic volume (Fig. 12.4). In these patients, normal cardiac output and ventricular compensation are achieved, despite more severe depression of the contractile state compared to aortic stenosis, since the ventricle is not operating against a mechanical abnormality opposing ventricular ejection. In primary myocardial disease, cardiac output falls and decompensation occurs when the contractile state becomes further depressed, despite greater employment of the hypertrophy and Frank-Starling mechanisms. In aortic stenosis, congestive heart failure occurs with decrease of the basal cardiac index when the contractile state is further depressed by the chronic adverse effect of the pressure overload on the myocardium, despite further hypertrophy and, late in decompensation, the development of ventricular dilation. In compensated chronic volume overloading of the ventricle, it appears that both hypertrophy and dilation maintain cardiac output despite diminished contractility, and heart failure occurs with further reduction of contractility but at a higher level than in cardiomyopathies (Fig. 12.4). Thus, the basal cardiac index is unable to be maintained when the contractile state falls below a certain critical level in both primary and secondary ventricular hypertrophy, with this critical level being lower in primary myocardial disease compared to secondary ventricular hypertrophy.

From these data, the concept is formulated that the fundamental abnormality in congestive heart failure is depressed contractility, and that basal cardiac output can be achieved by use of reserve mechanisms until the level of the contractile state becomes depressed below a critical level. Thus, congestive heart failure is defined as the inability of the heart to maintain basal cardiac output. The compensatory mechanisms and the extent to which they are utilized differ in primary and secondary ventricular hypertrophy, and the level of contractile state below which normal cardiac output cannot be maintained appears to be lower in cardiomyopathies than in chronic pressure and volume overloading of the ventricle.

The failing heart is dependent in part on the support mechanism provided by the adrenergic nervous system in which the endogenous neurotransmitter, norepinephrine, increases myocardial contractility and the frequency of contraction through stimulation of the beta adrenergic receptors in the myocardium. Thus, increased sympathetic activity is immediately available to the stressed ventricle, and there now is abundant clinical and experimental evidence indicating that overall adrenergic activity in the body is augmented in congestive heart failure.[20] Paradoxically, there is reduction in the concentration and content of norepinephrine in the failing myocardium (Fig. 12.5) as a result of defects in the synthesis and uptake and binding of the catecholamine by cardiac sympathetic nerves, while net turnover of norepinephrine in the failing heart is normal.[16, 21, 22] Depletion of norepinephrine occurs in both ventricles, regardless of which ventricle develops hypertrophy or failure in response to a hemodynamic burden.[14, 16] The intrinsic defect of cardiac contractility in the failing heart is not the direct consequence of depletion of myocardial norepinephrine, since the contractile state is normal in catecholamine-depleted muscle from the surgically denervated normal heart.[23] However, the reduced myocardial norepinephrine has important functional consequences since stimulation of the sympathetic nerves to the heart results in abnormally small increments in heart rate and myocardial contractile force[24] and thus impairs availability of the

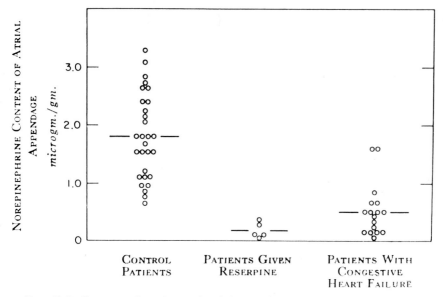

Fig. 12.5. Concentration of norepinephrine in the atrial appendages excised at operation in 29 control patients who had not been in congestive heart failure, in five patients who had been treated with reserpine, and in 17 patients who had been in congestive heart failure. (Reproduced by permission from Chidsey, C. A., *et al.*[21])

sympathetic compensatory mechanism to augment depressed contractile performance in the failing heart. On the other hand, it appears that beta receptors in the failing heart are intact and perhaps even supersensitive to circulating catecholamines.[14] Thus the increased level of blood-borne catecholamines from the peripheral vasculature may be important in restoring, in part, the adrenergic supporting mechanism to the failing heart.[25] It is apparent that beta adrenergic receptor-blocking drugs must be administered with caution to patients with reduced cardiac function, since their use might precipitate or intensify heart failure.

An important principle developed in this review is that the primary objective of compensatory mechanisms in clinical heart failure is to maintain the basal cardiac output at a normal level. Thus, the first symptoms accompanying cardiac dysfunction are related to unfavorable side effects necessarily resulting from the action of these reserve mechanisms in performance of their compensatory role, and the late symptoms in heart failure are due to low cardiac output which is the last hemodynamic variable to become abnormal when myocardial function is reduced. The deleterious symptoms accompanying the compensatory mechanisms for maintaining resting cardiac output limit the extent to which they can be employed. Therefore, when the increased work load and depression of myocardial contractility exceed the reserve of these compensatory mechanisms, the heart is unable to maintain normal cardiac output (decompensated congestive heart failure). In compensated congestive heart failure, pulmonary and systemic venous congestion results from increased use of the Frank-Starling principle prior to reduction of cardiac output.

From these observations, the clinical manifestations of advancing heart failure develop initially (Class II) with dyspnea on exertion (early use of the Frank-Starling mechanism), fatigue with more than ordinary activity (reduced response of cardiac output with exercise as a result of diminished cardiac contractility), exertional angina pectoris (ventricular hypertrophy with consequent increase in myocardial oxygen demands), and excessive tachycardia and sweating with exercise (augmented sympathetic discharge). The clinical picture worsens (Class III) with dyspnea, fatigue, angina, tachycardia, and sweating with ordinary activity (further depression of contractility with increased use of compensatory mechanisms). Finally, these symptoms become very severe and occur even at rest (Class IV) with the addition of weakness, cachexia, mental confusion, oliguria, and hypotension (due to reduced basal cardiac output and poor organ perfusion despite maximal use of compensatory mechanisms). It is recognized that there may be considerable overlap between the relations of altered hemodynamics and clinical features. Thus, when diuretic treatment decreases congestive symptoms and concurrently reduces the use of the Frank-Starling mechanism by causing the ventricle to operate at a lower point on the ascending limb of its function curve, a Class III patient may be converted to one with Class II symptoms with reduced cardiac output at rest. Further, it is realized that these functional classifications of patients comprise a continuum rather than discrete categories. In Class II (congestion with moderate activity) and in Class III (congestion with mild activity), heart failure is compensated (normal basal cardiac output), and in Class IV (congestion at rest) decompensation occurs (low basal cardiac output). It is evident from these considerations of the correlation of clinical signs and symptoms with pathophysiological mechanisms that the traditional clinical classification of heart failure is principally based upon deleterious expressions of the activity of compensatory mechanisms and is not directly founded on the fundamental abnormality of cardiac function (contractile state) in the heart failure state and/or on the fundamental hemodynamic variable (cardiac output), the maintenance of which is responsible for the congestive symptoms.

In addition to the cardiac compensatory mechanisms in heart failure, adjustments in the peripheral circulation are important in the support of depressed cardiac performance and maintenance of regional blood flow. Thus, arteriolar and venous constriction is characteristic of human congestive heart failure.[26, 27] The increase in total systemic vascular resistance maintains organ perfusion pressure in the face of a low cardiac output. This arteriolar constriction in heart failure is produced mainly by increased sympathetic nervous activity and by a stiffness component in the arteriolar wall (Fig. 12.6).[28, 29] In contrast to the failing myocardium, there are increased labile stores of norepinephrine in the arteriolar beds of skeletal muscle in patients with heart failure (Fig. 12.7).[30] The altered mechanical properties of the arterioles in heart failure result from increased sodium and water content in the vessel itself,[31, 32] and they are responsible in part for the decreased arteriolar dilator capacity which has recently been demonstrated in these patients;[28] the increased tissue pressure in heart failure which offers increased resistance to flow through the capillary bed arises similarly.[33]

With the failure of the heart as a pump, there is a decrease in blood flow to most regions of the body. However, since the uniform reduction of flow to all areas might result in a critical decline of tissue oxygen tension in some organs, in severe heart failure this reduction of flow is not uniform and redistribution of flow occurs (Fig. 12.8).[34, 35] Blood flow to an organ is determined by the ratio of the driving pressure (difference between the arterial and venous pressures) to the resistance to flow offered by the vessels. This resistance governing regional blood flow is determined by interplay between sympathetic activity and local production of vasodilator metabolites. The mechanism by which redistribution of blood flow is accomplished is thought to be the augmentation of local flow in response to the accumulation of vasodilator metabolites, while blood flow to other areas is reduced reflexly in

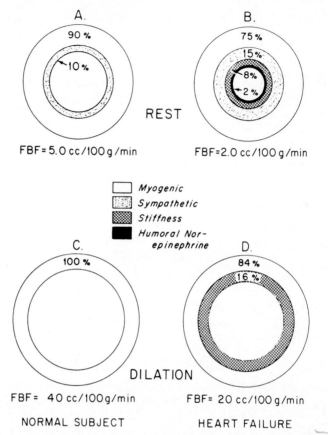

Fig. 12.6. Diagram represents the components of vascular resistance in the arterioles of the forearm at rest (A and B) and during maximal vasodilation (C and D) in a normal patient (A and C) and in a patient with heart failure (B and D). Components are expressed as percentage of radius of arteriolar lumen; the value is estimated from changes in blood flow induced by certain interventions and based on the Poiseuille relationship which indicates that flow varies directly as the fourth power of the inner radius of the vessel. FBF, forearm blood flow. (Reproduced by permission from Mason, D. T., and Zelis, R.[27])

order to maintain arterial pressure. Thus, reflex sympathetic discharge occurs in most of the regional circulations but, in the organs with high metabolic requirements relative to blood flow, this action is overridden by locally produced vasodilator influences.

Although it has been appreciated for many years that the venous system participates actively in alterations of venous return to the heart, recent evidence suggests that the capacitance beds play somewhat less of a responsive role in the regulation of circulatory function. Thus, the sympathetic nervous

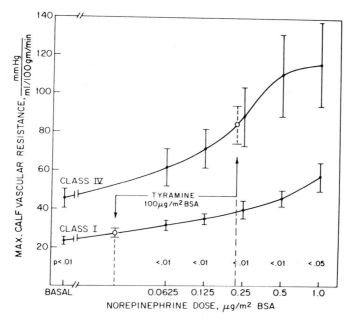

Fig. 12.7. Norepinephrine dose-response curves, in patients without heart failure (Class I) and patients with heart failure (Class IV). The average peak values of vascular resistance (± SEM) elicited by intra-arterial injections of graded doses of norepinephrine are shown. The probability values indicate the significance of the difference of the responses between the two groups. The mean maximal resistance in response to tyramine (open circles and vertical broken lines) is positioned on the appropriate curve, providing an expression of the tyramine response in terms of "norepinephrine-equivalent dose." (Reproduced by permission from Kramer, R. S. *et al.*[30])

system does not appear to innervate the veins in skeletal muscle,[36] and moderate stimulation of the carotid baroreceptors does not produce venoconstriction in the skin.[37] Nevertheless, the overall capacitance bed is relatively indistensible in heart failure and thereby affords another peripheral circulatory mechanism for aid of the failing heart. This reduced compliance of the venous system appears to result in part from increased stiffness of the venous wall similar to that in the arteriolar bed in congestive heart failure.[38] Thus, the increased venous tone characteristic of congestive heart failure, produced by the augmented adrenergic activity and a vascular stiffness factor, is accompanied by a shift of blood in the systemic venous reservoir toward the central circulation, which augments venous return to the heart and assists in utilization of the Frank-Starling mechanism to maintain cardiac output by elevating ventricular diastolic filling.

In addition, renal mechanisms contribute actively to the altered hemodynamics comprising the heart failure state by the influence of the kidneys

REGIONAL DISTRIBUTION OF BLOOD FLOW

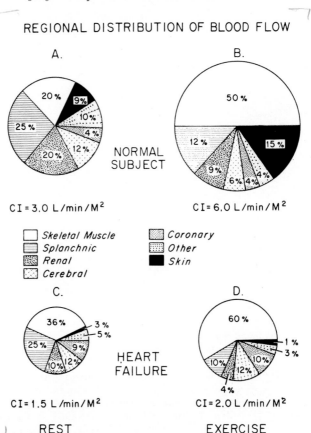

FIG. 12.8. Regional distribution of blood flow at rest and during exercise in normal subjects and in patients with heart failure. CI, cardiac index. (Reproduced by permission from Mason, D. T.[34])

on total blood volume through their action on salt and water balance. When renal blood flow is reduced, which may occur prior to reduction of cardiac output because of increased adrenergic activity and redistribution of total blood flow, the kidneys retain sodium and water, which increases intravascular volume, thereby enhancing ventricular filling and use of the Frank-Starling mechanism for control of cardiac output. Early in heart failure, blood flow to the kidney is reduced to a greater extent than reduction of glomerular filtration rate. Thereby the filtration fraction is increased and the reabsorption of sodium rises in the proximal convoluted tubules. With more advanced heart failure, the renin-angiotensin-aldosterone system is activated, and inappropriate increased secretion of antidiuretic hormone occurs as well, thus leading to enhanced sodium and water reabsorption in the distal tubules. Unlike normal subjects who exhibit diuresis with adrenergic blockade,[39] in the patient with congestive heart failure, any tendency for an antiadrenergic effect to enhance sodium excretion is overcome by worsening of the depressed cardiocirculatory state, which produces further retention of sodium and water.[40]

ABNORMALITIES OF MYOCARDIAL ULTRASTRUCTURE AND METABOLISM

The sarcomere is the basic contractile unit within the myocardium and, in cardiac dilation, there is increase in sarcomere length accompanying the greater use of the Frank-Starling preload mechanism.[41] Thus, there is a direct relationship between sarcomere length and myocardial length throughout the ascending limb of the ventricular function curve. In severe cardiac dysfunction resulting from primary myocardial weakness or mechanical overloading, ventricular dilation often occurs beyond the size that would be anticipated from increased sarcomere length at the peak of the ventricular function curve or at the apex of the length-tension curve of the myocardium. Present evidence indicates that, in extreme clinical cardiac dilation, the sarcomeres do not become overstretched, but slippage occurs among the myofibrils.[42]

Considerable attention has been devoted to research for a specific biochemical abnormality responsible for the altered performance of the failing myocardium. In the consideration of possible abnormalities of myocardial energy supply and utilization, it is useful to consider substrate availability, energy production, energy storage, and energy utilization and conversion, and the process of excitation-contraction coupling. Concerning substrate availability, recent investigations have demonstrated a subcellular lesion that appears to prevent the full utilization of fatty acid by the failing myocardium.[43] In the heart, metabolism of fatty acids requires a carnitine-dependent system that allows the entrance of fatty acids into the mitochondria for beta oxidation. In the experimental failing heart, this carnitine-dependent system is depressed to one-half of normal. However, it is not thought that this abnormality is causally related to the basic abnormality of performance of the failing heart.

In the consideration of energy utilization, in the cardiac mitochondria the energy from substrate oxidation is converted into terminal bond energy of creatine phosphate and adenosine triphosphate (ATP). This process of oxidative phosphorylation has been studied in experimental animals and man, and the more recent data indicate that it is not impaired in heart failure.[44] Concerning energy storage, the terminal bond energy resulting from oxidative phosphorylation is stored in the myocardium in the form of creatine phosphate which serves as a reservoir to maintain ATP, the more immediate source of chemical energy for heart muscle. The energy stores of creatine phosphate are depressed in the chronically failing heart of experimental animals.[45] Since this suppression of high energy phosphate stores can be experimentally dissociated from depression of contractility, depression of energy stores is not thought to be the primary cause of the failing myocardium.

In the area of energy utilization and conversion, there have been no conclusive demonstrations of alterations of the physical properties of the contractile proteins in failing heart muscle. The experimental failing heart has not been thought to be inefficient in the conversion of chemical energy to mechanical work,[46] although there have been conflicting reports in this regard.[47] On the other hand, the activity of myofibrillar ATPase, which splits the terminal phosphate bond off ATP and thereby liberates energy for the contractile process, is severely depressed in the failing heart and thereby may reduce the rate of energy released.[48]

The process of excitation-contraction coupling occurs at the level of the sarcoplasmic reticulum surrounding each myofibril. Since the release of calcium ions from the sarcoplasmic reticulum into the vicinity of the contractile proteins is of fundamental importance in cardiac muscle contraction, a metabolic defect in this area has been proposed as a possible basic mechanism in the failing myocardium. Thus, it is possible that a fundamental subcellular abnormality responsible for myocardial failure is related to an inadequate release of calcium from the sarcoplasmic reticulum or a related defect of the contractile apparatus, which could result in an abnormality of excitation-contraction coupling and a weak contraction. Fragments of sarcoplasmic reticulum isolated from spontaneous failing heart-lung preparations have demonstrated depressed calcium uptake and a parallel depression in ATPase activity.[49] Harigaya and Schwartz have demonstrated a diminution in calcium binding in fragments of sarcoplasmic reticulum obtained from diseased hearts of patients undergoing heart transplantation.[50] Abnormalities in microsomal calcium transport have been reported in the hamster with myocardial dystrophy.[51] It is now recognized that the role of calcium is complex in the excitation-contraction process. Not only is calcium released from sarcoplasmic reticulum into the area of the myofibrils important, but also it appears that calcium transferred across the cell membrane may be important in excitation. The process of myocardial relaxation is thought to involve the recapture of calcium back into the sarcoplasmic reticulum and perhaps also the movement of calcium across the cell membrane into the extracellular space.

Adenyl cyclase is thought to be present in cardiac microsomal preparations believed to represent sarcoplasmic reticulum. Production of cyclic adenosine 3′,5′-monophosphate (AMP) through adenyl cyclase activation has been suggested to augment calcium accumulation in cardiac microsomes, which in turn may be related to positive inotropic actions produced by beta receptor stimulation.[52] Adenyl cyclase activity itself does not appear to be changed by chronic heart failure,[52] although there is lack of stimulation of this enzyme by glucagon in the failing heart.[53] There is debate as to whether there is an altered capacity of norepinephrine to enhance adenyl cyclase activity in the failing myocardium.[52, 54] The possibility has been suggested that a cyclic AMP-dependent protein kinase might be responisble for phosphorylation of protein components of sarcoplasmic reticulum and of myofibrillar proteins responsible for the regulation of contraction and relaxation[55]; the possibility of an abnormality in this area in heart failure is currently under investigation.

Protein synthesis is essential to the process of compensatory hypertrophy which results from mechanical systolic overloading of the ventricle. In the experimental animal, excessive systolic overloading of the ventricle consistently leads to an activation of protein synthesis. Thus, constriction of the aorta in the guinea pig[16] or constriction of the pulmonary artery in the cat[14] quickly leads to ventricular hypertrophy of the ventricle under stress. Increased amino acid incorporation into protein occurs as early as 3 hours after an elevated pressure load, and the weight of the ventricle doubles in 2 days and triples within 1 month.[14, 16, 17] As discussed previously, there is evidence that this increased contractile mass is characterized by diminished inotropic state per unit of muscle. However, the increased number of contractile units aids in the maintenance of ventricular compensation. The intriguing sequence of events coupling mechanical work, tension, and dilation of the ventricles to the process of protein synthesis has not been fully elucidated. There is activation of all stages of protein synthesis with cardiac hypertrophy: desoxyribonucleic acid (DNA), ribonucleic acid (RNA), and transcription of new proteins.[56-59] This increased activity is particularly associated with earlier stages of hypertrophy which precede congestive heart failure. The diminution of these processes in congestive heart failure suggests that they might contribute to the heart failure state but do not appear to be causative in this regard. Thus, protein synthesis is stimulated very early in the course of cardiac hypertrophy and remains elevated during stress and, with prolonged severe hemodynamic overloading, the production of protein is diminished.

Therefore, evidence to date suggests that changes in protein synthesis, alterations in energy metabolism, and disturbances of myocardial catecholamine metabolism all may ultimately contribute to the process of heart failure, but these mechanisms probably are not the primary metabolic defect responsible for the heart failure state. In this regard, it is more likely that the principal causative role of heart failure resides in a defect or group of abnormalities in the excitation-contraction process.

CONCLUSIONS

The derangements of hemodynamics and myocardial mechanics characteristic of the congestive heart failure state have been defined precisely in patients. Thus, the basal stroke volume is decreased, despite marked elevations of left ventricular end diastolic pressure, and the force-velocity properties are reduced in the decompensated failing human ventricle in idiopathic cardiomyopathies and in chronic pressure or volume overloading. From these data in patients and observations in experimental heart failure, the concept is developed that, of the determinants of ventricular function, the fundamental abnormality in human congestive heart failure is depressed cardiac contractility. There is lesser extent of reduced contractile state with normal basal cardiac output and moderate rise in end diastolic pressure in compensated ventricular hypertrophy before the onset of overt congestive heart failure. Thus, a spectrum of decreasing inotropic state is demonstrated between ventricular hypertrophy without failure and hypertrophy with failure.

When an excessive pressure or volume load or a primary defect in contractility is imposed upon the heart, there are three principal cardiac compensatory mechanisms available for the direct support of myocardial performance and the fundamental goal of maintaining normal cardiac output at rest: (1) Frank-Starling principle, (2) ventricular hypertrophy, and (3) sympathetic nervous system. Symptoms necessarily accompany the action of each of these reserve mechanisms in their primary role of maintaining basal cardiac output, and these symptoms limit the extent to which these compensatory mechanisms can be employed. It is pointed out that the traditional functional classification of heart failure is principally coupled to the results of secondary factors (compensatory mechanisms) and not directly to the fundamental abnormality of hemodynamics (cardiac output) and ventricular function (contractility) characteristic of heart failure.

Concerning disorders of myocardial metabolism, recent investigations indicate that changes in protein synthesis, alterations in energy metabolism, and abnormalities of myocardial catecholamine metabolism all may ultimately contribute to the process of heart failure. However, these mechanisms probably do not represent the primary metabolic defects responsible for the heart failure state. At the present time, on a biochemical basis, it appears that the primary causative role of heart failure is the result of disturbances in the process of excitation-contraction coupling.

REFERENCES

1. Mason, D. T., Spann, J. F., Jr., Zelis, R., and Amsterdam, E. A.: Alterations of hemodynamics and myocardial mechanics in patients with congestive heart

failure: pathophysiologic mechanisms and assessment of cardiac function and ventricular contractility. Prog. Cardiovasc. Dis. 12: 507, 1970.

2. Mason, D. T.: Usefulness and limitations of the rate of rise of intraventricular pressure (dp/dt) in the evaluation of myocardial contractility in man. Amer. J. Cardiol. 23: 516, 1969.

3. Mason, D. T., Spann, J. F., Jr., and Zelis, R.: Quantification of the contractile state of the intact human heart: maximum velocity of contractile element shortening determined from the instantaneous relation between the rate of pressure rise and pressure in the ventricle during isovolumic systole. Amer. J. Cardiol. 26: 248, 1970.

4. Mason, D. T., Braunwald, E., Covell, J. W., Sonnenblick, E. H., and Ross, J., Jr.: Assessment of cardiac contractility: the relation between the rate of pressure rise and ventricular pressure during isovolumic systole. Circulation 44: 47, 1971.

5. Gault, J. H., Ross, J., Jr., and Braunwald, E.: Contractile state of the left ventricle in man: instantaneous tension-velocity-length relations in patients with and without disease of the left ventricular myocardium. Circ. Res. 22: 451, 1968.

6. Mason, D. T., Spann, J. F., Jr., Zelis, R., and Amsterdam, E. A.: Comparison of the contractile state of the normal, hypertrophied, and failing heart in man. In Alpert, N. R. (ed.): *Ventricular Hypertrophy.* Academic Press, New York, 1971, p. 433.

7. Ross, J., Jr., and Braunwald, E.: Studies on Starling's law of the heart. IX. Effects of impeding venous return on performance of normal and failing human left ventricle. Circulation 30: 719, 1964.

8. Ross, J., Jr., and Braunwald, E.: The study of left ventricular function in man by increasing resistance to ventricular ejection with angiotensin. Circulation 29: 739, 1964.

9. Ross, J., Jr., Gault, J. H., Mason, D. T., Linhart, J. W., and Braunwald, E.: Left ventricular performance during muscular exercise in patients with and without cardiac dysfunction. Circulation 34: 597, 1966.

10. Mason, D. T., Spann, J. F., Jr., Zelis, R., and Amsterdam, E. A.: Comparison of inotropic state and compensatory mechanisms between patients with primary and secondary ventricular hypertrophy. Circulation 42: (Suppl. 3): 85, 1970.

11. Levine, H. J., Neill, W. A., Wagman, R. J., Krasnow, N., and Gorlin, R.: The effect of exercise on mean left ventricular ejection rate in man. J. Clin. Invest. 41: 1050, 1962.

12. Gorlin, R., Rolett, E. L., Yurchak, P. M., and Elliot, W. C.: Left ventricular volume in man measured by thermodilution. J. Clin. Invest. 43: 1203, 1964.

13. Gault, J. H., Ross, J., Jr., and Covell, J. W.: Left ventricular myocardial function in patients with aortic regurgitation determined by instantaneous tension-velocity-length relations. Circulation 36 (Suppl. 11): 118, 1967.

14. Spann, J. F., Jr., Buccino, R. A., Sonnenblick, E. H., and Braunwald, E.: Contractile state of cardiac muscle obtained from cats with experimentally produced ventricular hypertrophy and heart failure. Circ. Res. 21: 341, 1967.

15. Spann, J. F., Jr., Mason, D. T., and Zelis, R.: The altered performance of the hypertrophied and failing myocardium. Amer. J. Med. Sci. 258: 291, 1969.

16. Spann, J. F., Jr., Chidsey, C. A., Pool, P. E., and Braunwald, E.: Mechanism of norepinephrine depletion in experimental heart failure produced by aortic constriction in the guinea pig. Circ. Res. 17: 312, 1965.

17. Nair, K. G., Cutilletta, A. F., Zak, R., Koide, T., and Rabinowitz, M.: Biochemical correlates of cardiac hypertrophy. I. Experimental model: changes in

heart weight, RNA content, and nuclear RNA polymerase activity. Circ. Res. 23: 451, 1968.

18. Williams, J. F., Jr., and Braunwald, E.: Studies on digitalis. XI. Effects of digitoxin on the development of cardiac hypertrophy in the rat subjected to aortic constriction. Amer. J. Cardiol. 16: 534, 1969.

19. Covell, J. W., Braunwald, E., Ross, J., Jr., and Sonnenblick, E. H.: Studies on digitalis. XVI. Effects on myocardial oxygen consumption. J. Clin. Invest. 45: 1535, 1966.

20. Chidsey, C. A., Braunwald, E., and Morrow, A. G.: Catecholamine excretion and cardiac stores of norepinephrine in congestive heart failure. Amer. J. Med. 39: 442, 1965.

21. Chidsey, C. A., Braunwald, E., Morrow, A. G., and Mason, D. T.: Myocardial norepinephrine concentration in man: effects of reserpine and of congestive heart failure. New Engl. J. Med. 269: 653, 1963.

22. Pool, P. E., Covell, J. W., Levitt, M., Gibb, J., and Braunwald, E.: Reduction of cardiac tyrosine hydroxylase activity in experimental congestive heart failure. Circ. Res. 20: 349, 1967.

23. Spann, J. F., Jr., Sonnenblick, E. H., Cooper, T., Chidsey, C. A., Willman, V. L., and Braunwald, E.: Cardiac norepinephrine stores and the contractile state of heart muscle. Circ. Res. 19: 317, 1966.

24. Covell, J. W., Chidsey, C. A., and Braunwald, E.: Reduction of the cardiac response to postganglionic sympathetic nerve stimulation in experimental heart failure. Circ. Res. 19: 51, 1966.

25. Vogel, J. H. K., and Chidsey, C. A.: Cardiac adrenergic activity in experimental heart failure assessed with beta receptor blockade. Amer. J. Cardiol. 24: 198, 1969.

26. Mason, D. T., and Braunwald, E.: Studies on digitalis. X. Effects of ouabain on forearm vascular resistance and venous tone in normal subjects and in patients in heart failure. J. Clin. Invest. 43: 532, 1964.

27. Mason, D. T., and Zelis, R.: The function of the arterial and venous beds in congestive heart failure. Heart Bull. 17: 109, 1968.

28. Zelis, R., Mason, D. T., and Braunwald, E.: A comparison of the effects of vasodilator stimuli on the peripheral resistance vessels in normal subjects and patients with congestive heart failure. J. Clin. Invest. 47: 960, 1968.

29. Zelis, R., and Mason, D. T.: Compensatory mechanisms in congestive heart failure: the role of the peripheral resistance vessels. New Engl. J. Med. 282: 962, 1970.

30. Kramer, R. S., Mason, D. T., and Braunwald, E.: Augmented sympathetic neurotransmitter activity in the peripheral vascular bed of patients with congestive heart failure and cardiac norepinephrine depletion. Circulation 38: 629, 1968.

31. Zelis, R., Delea, C. S., Coleman, H. N., and Mason, D. T.: Arterial sodium content in experimental congestive heart failure. Circulation 41: 213, 1970.

32. Zelis, R., and Mason, D. T.: Diminished forearm arteriolar dilator capacity produced by mineralocorticoid-induced salt retention in man: implications concerning congestive heart failure and vascular stiffness. Circulation 41: 589, 1970.

33. Lee, G., Barnum, J., Zelis, R., Mason, D. T., Spann, J. F., Jr., and Amsterdam, E. A.: Diminished arteriolar dilator capacity produced by increasing tissue pressure: implications concerning "vascular stiffness" in congestive heart failure. Circulation 42 (Suppl. 3): 177, 1970.

34. Mason, D. T.: Control of the peripheral circulation in health and disease. Mod. Concepts Cardiovasc. Dis. 36: 25, 1967.

35. Zelis, R., Mason, D. T., and Braunwald, E.: Partition of blood flow to the cutaneous and muscular beds of the forearm at rest and during leg exercise in normal subjects and in patients with heart failure. Circ. Res. 24: 799, 1969.
36. Zelis, R., and Mason, D. T.: Comparison of reflex reactivity of skin and muscle veins in the human forearm. J. Clin. Invest. 48: 1870, 1969.
37. Epstein, S. E., Beiser, G. D., Stampfer, M., and Braunwald, E.: Role of the venous system in baroreceptor-mediated reflexes in man. J. Clin. Invest. 47: 139, 1968.
38. Zelis, R., Capone, R., Amsterdam, E. A., and Mason, D. T.: The concept of local determinants of venous volume: the role of nonadrenergic factors in the elevated venous tone of congestive heart failure. J. Clin. Invest. 50: 102a, 1971.
39. Gill, J. R., Jr., Mason, D. T., and Bartter, F. C.: Adrenergic nervous system in sodium metabolism: effects of guanethidine and sodium-retaining steroids in normal man. J. Clin. Invest. 43: 177, 1964.
40. Gaffney, T. E., and Braunwald, E.: Importance of the adrenergic nervous system in support of circulatory function in patients with congestive heart failure. Amer. J. Med. 34: 320, 1963.
41. Spotnitz, H., Sonnenblick, E. H., and Spiro, D.: Relation of ultrastructure to function in the intact heart. Sarcomere structure relative to pressure volume curves of intact left ventricles of dog and cat. Circ. Res. 18: 49, 1965.
42. Ross, J. Jr., Sonnenblick, E. H., Taylor, R. R., Spotnitz, H. M., and Covell, J. W.: Diastolic geometry and sarcomere lengths in the chronically dilated canine left ventricle. Circ. Res. 28: 49, 1971.
43. Wittels, B., and Spann, J. F., Jr.: Defective lipid metabolism in the failing heart. J. Clin. Invest. 47: 1787, 1968.
44. Sobel, B. E., Spann, J. F., Jr., Pool, P. E., Sonnenblick, E. H., and Braunwald, E.: Normal oxidative phosphorylation in mitochondria from the failing heart. Circ. Res. 21: 355, 1967.
45. Pool, P. E., Spann, J. F., Jr., Buccino, R. A., Sonnenblick, E. H., and Braunwald, E.: Myocardial high energy phosphate stores in cardiac hypertrophy and heart failure. Circ. Res. 21: 365, 1967.
46. Pool, P. E., Chandler, B. M., Spann, J. F. Jr., Sonnenblick, E. H., and Braunwald, E.: Mechanochemistry of cardiac muscle. IV. Utilization of high-energy phosphates in experimental heart failure in cats. Circ. Res. 24: 313, 1969.
47. Coleman, H. N., and Gunning, J. F.: Inefficient energy utilization in myocardial hypertrophy. Circulation 41 and 42 (Suppl. 3): 115, 1970.
48. Chandler, B. M., Sonnenblick, E. H., Spann, J. F., Jr., and Pool, P. E.: Association of depressed myofibrillar adenosine triphosphatase and reduced contractility in experimental heart failure. Circ. Res. 21: 717, 1967.
49. Gertz, E. Z., Hess, M. L., Lain, R. F., and Briggs, F. N.: Activity of the vesicular calcium pump in the spontaneously failing heart-lung preparation. Circ. Res. 20: 477, 1967.
50. Harigaya, S., and Schwartz, A.: Rate of calcium binding and uptake in normal animal and failing human cardiac muscle. Circ. Res. 25: 781, 1969.
51. Sulakhe, P. V., and Dhalla, N. S.: Excitation-contraction coupling in heart. VII. Calcium accumulation in subcellular particles in congestive heart failure. J. Clin. Invest. 50: 1019, 1971.
52. Epstein, S. E., Skelton, C. L., Levey, G. S., and Entman, M.: Adenyl cyclase and myocardial contractility. Ann. Intern. Med. 72: 561, 1970.
53. Gold, H. J., Prindle, K. H., Levey, G. S., and Epstein, S. E.: Effects of experimental heart failure on the capacity of glucagon to augment myocardial contractility and activate adenyl cyclase. J. Clin. Invest. 49: 999, 1970.

54. Sobel, B. E., Henry, P. D., and Robison, A.: Depressed adenyl cyclase activity in the failing guinea pig heart. Circ. Res. 24: 507, 1969.

55. Brostrom, M. A., Reimann, E. M., Walsh, D. A., and Krebs, E. G.: A cyclic 3',5'-AMP-stimulated protein kinase from cardiac muscle. Advan. Enzyme Regul. 8: 191, 1970.

56. Fanburg, B. L.: Recent studies on cardiac hypertrophy. Amer. Heart J. 81 (Suppl. 4): 447, 1971.

57. Scheur, J.: Metabolism of the heart in cardiac failure. Progr. Cardiovasc. Dis. 13: 24, 1970.

58. Meerson, F. Z., Alekhina, G. M., Aleksandrov, P. N., and Bazardjan, A. G.: Dynamics of nucleic acid and protein synthesis of the myocardium in compensatory hyperfunction and hypertrophy of the heart. Amer. J. Cardiol. 22: 337, 1968.

59. Morkin, E., and Ashford, T. P.: Myocardial DNA synthesis in experimental cardiac hypertrophy. Amer. J. Physiol. 215: 1409, 1968.

13

Treatment of the Failing Heart

WILLIAM LIKOFF, M.D.

Traditionally, heart failure is classified in a number of ways. Acute and chronic are temporal terms. The former applies when manifestations arise without clear warning and subside spontaneously or after treatment. The latter refers to an insistent disability of varying but progressive severity.

Although the heart usually fails as a unit, the expressions right and left ventricular failure commonly mark the chamber most involved. Physiological parameters also serve to qualify the syndrome as in heart failure with shock or high output failure.

However designated, heart failure is a clinical pattern which develops when cardiac output does not meet the metabolic demands of the total organism. Structural defects, myocardial weakness, or both are responisble. With time they lead to impaired contractile performance by adversely influencing the release and utilization of cardiac muscle energy.

GENERAL PRINCIPLES

Whenever treatment in any of the medical disciplines is reviewed, it is axiomatic that the principles from which specific measures have evolved be included. Nowhere in the vast complex of cardiovascular disorders is this more meaningful than for heart failure.

The first principle is to determine and, when possible, correct cause. Over the years, the list of remediable direct causes has been considerably enlarged. It now includes many congenital defects as well as those secondary to rheumatic activity, advanced grades of atrioventricular block, atrioventricular fistula, thyroid heart disease, hypertensive heart disease, and certain instances of coronary heart disease.

When the basic cause cannot be corrected, three principles guide management: (1) reduce the work load of the heart; (2) increase cardiac functional capacity; (3) control existing pathophysiological consequences of cardiac inadequacy.

153

Rest is foremost among the measures which reduce the work load of the heart. By diminishing pulse and respiratory rates as well as blood pressure, rest minimizes energy expenditure and helps restore the balance between output and metabolic needs. The extent and quality of rest depend upon the severity of failure. For those who are symptomatic with minimal activity, rest must be prolonged and complete, usually carried out in the sitting position either in a chair or bed. The decreased right heart filling which follows relieves pulmonary congestion and favors the accumulation of edema in the dependent extremities rather than the lungs. Regrettably prolonged immobilization predisposes to thromboembolism and perpetuates poor muscle tone, as well as inappropriate reactivity of the circulatory system.

Patients with modest manifestations of failure require less stringent restrictions, the work load being adequately reduced by modifying injudicious habits and senseless expenditures of energy. This also holds for those who experience failure following departure from normal exercise practices.

Since emotional stress produces hemodynamic changes akin to activity, mental rest is as important as physical in the treatment of failure. To this end, mild sedation and soporifics may be beneficial.

Extremes in heat and humidity, oversized meals, constipation, and nocturia increase cardiac work and should be avoided or eliminated if at all possible.

The functional capacity of the heart can be improved by increasing myocardial contractility. Digitalis is the primary agent in achieving this objective. It acts by modifying excitation-contraction coupling in a manner that increases ionic calcium at the contractile sites. Additionally, it slows heart rate by increasing the refractory period of the atrioventricular node and bundle of His and by increasing the sensitivity of the sinoatrial node and conduction system to vagal stimulation.

Digitalis is indicated in the treatment of all types of heart failure except, of course, when toxic reactions to the drug initiate or aggravate the clinical syndrome. The response to digitalis varies with a number of factors, including etiology of the heart disease, cardiac rhythm, severity of failure, and total therapeutic program. Hypertensive and rheumatic heart disease, for example, are more amenable than myocarditis or chronic cor pulmonale. Patients who have rapid ventricular responses to atrial flutter or fibrillation improve more readily than those with a normal sinus mechanism. If digitalis is administered with mild initial expressions of failure such as dyspnea, cough, unusual tachycardia, or an atrial gallop sound with effort, improvement is more rapid and complete than if it is withheld until manifestations of advanced decompensation appear. Finally, when rest, adequate sodium restriction, and appropriate diuretics are combined with digitalis, compensation is restored more effectively than when the drug is prescribed alone.

The remarkable properties of digitalis are counterbalanced by toxic reactions which, because of their serious and, at times, lethal effect, limit the clinical application of the drug. However, when proper guidelines are applied, chances of a misadventure are considerably reduced. Included among these regulations are the following.

1. Physicians should be thoroughly familiar with the clinical pharmacology of digitalis and its glycosides and should be experienced in using specific preparations. Without discrediting alternatives, it is clear that digoxin is eminently satisfactory for most patients. Digitoxin may be required occasionally and digitalis leaf even more infrequently.

2. Before instituting treatment, the patient's prior experiences with the medication should be known, including the amount and the date it was last taken, as well as sensitivity reactions.

3. Dose schedules must be individualized. Average rather than maximal doses are advisable. Decisions to omit or alter doses reside with the physician and should be based on all available clinical evidence rather than on isolated findings such as heart rate.

4. Digitalis toxicity is exceptionally common. Dietary restrictions, prolonged diuretic therapy, and associated diseases may increase the sensitivity of the myocardium to the drug by depleting potassium stores. Concurrent administration of certain drugs, particularly reserpine and guanethidine, also may predispose to digitalis toxicity.

5. Periodic examinations for toxicity including an electrocardiogram should take place whenever there is a commitment for a fixed dose schedule over a long interval.

6. Many of the manifestations of toxicity, including dysrhythmias and conduction disturbances, mimic the clinical symptoms and signs of a failing heart. Therefore, treatment for decompensation should not be instituted without eliminating the possibility that prior drug therapy caused the problem.

7. Digitalis toxicity varies in severity. The first and, at times, only treatment necessary is the discontinuance of the drug and of all measures such as diuretics and laxatives which deplete potassium. The ability to improve potassium levels by the administration of potassium salts or potassium-retaining diuretics does not replace the need to discontinue digitalis until all signs of toxicity have been abolished.

Digitalis therapy is based on an initial loading dose to achieve a therapeutic effect, followed by a subsequent daily maintenance dose to replace daily glycoside losses. The effects of the drug and its glycosides are determined by gastrointestinal absorption, hepatic metabolism and excretion, renal function, protein binding, potassium balance, and the myocardial response to a given myocardial concentration.

Gastrointestinal absorption of digoxin is approximately 85 per cent of the administered dose. Peak levels appear in the blood within 30 to 60 minutes. The drug is rapidly eliminated as an unchanged glycoside, mainly through the urine. When renal function is normal, digoxin has a short half-life of 1.6 days, permitting elective digitalization in approximately 8 days if patients are placed on a daily maintenance dose without an initial loading dose.

Whenever possible, oral administration of digoxin is preferred. Complete digitalization in 24 hours usually can be attained, with 2.5 mg. offered in a number of combinations of divided doses at 6- to 8-hour intervals. Usually intravenous digitalization is desired over a shorter interval and is accomplished with a total dose of 2 mg., administered in an initial dose of 0.75 mg., followed by additional doses of 0.25 to 0.5 mg. at 2-hour periods.

Gastrointestinal absorption of digitoxin is essentially complete. Peak levels do not appear in the blood short of 4 hours. Approximately 70 per cent of the drug is excreted as inactive metabolites in the urine. Altered renal function, therefore, has a lesser effect upon the likelihood of toxicity. Digitoxin has a long half-life of 5.75 days. Because elective digitalization requires approximately 1 month if patients are placed on a daily maintenance dose, a loading dose is essential for effective therapy.

Whether by oral or parenteral routes, the digitalizing dose of digitoxin is 1.2 to 2 mg. The maintenance dose varies from 0.1 to 0.2 mg.

A number of sympathomimetic amines, epinephrine, norepinephrine, and isoproterenol exhibit positive inotropism. None is considered equal or superior to digitalis or is advisable as the drug of choice for the treatment of chronic heart failure. The rational use of these agents when the heart fails depends upon their actions on alpha and beta adrenergic receptors and according to whether they act directly or indirectly for release of norepinephrine from sympathetic storage sites.

Isoproterenol, for example, acts on cardiac beta adrenergic receptors. It increases cardiac rate, stroke volume, amplitude of myocardial contraction, and coronary blood flow. It also decreases the mean afterload to contraction. When administered intravenously, myocardial irritability is increased and dysrhythmias may ensue. Isoproterenol should not be used in heart failure, except in acute states following myocardial infarction when a high degree of atrioventricular block is present and pacing is not possible. A dose of 1 to 2 mg. diluted in 200 cc. of 5 per cent glucose or distilled water is usually administered intravenously, with flow rates adjusted from 30 drops per minute depending upon clinical response. Isoproterenol may also be used in acute failure, mainly following myocardial infarction, when patients who are free of atrioventricular block fail to respond to digitalis.

Glucagon is prominent among other agents having positive inotropic effects. When administered intravenously to subjects with mild acute cardiac impairment, these effects are short-lived. Furthermore, they cannot be duplicated in patients with chronic heart failure.

The major pathophysiological consequences of heart failure devolve from sodium retention. Control of this fault resides with measures which limit intake and promote excretion.

Ingestion of 200 to 1000 mg. of sodium is permissible each day, depending upon the severity of the failure. This requires the elimination of salt in cooking and at the table, ordinary bread, crackers, cake, milk, cheese, cream, smoked and salt-cured meats and fish, seafood, canned vegetables and soups, pretzels, salted nuts, and most candies. It does allow for meat, fish, and poultry prepared without salt, fresh fruits and vegetables, unsalted butter and margarine, salt-free bread, and most beverages. Seasoning with salt substitutes containing potassium chloride and with pepper, onions, lemon, or spices helps to alleviate the unpalatability of the diet.

Although moderate impairment of water excretion occurs with even mild heart failure, restriction of the amount ingested is not usually required. This does not apply when there is gross edema and severe oliguria in spite of adequate diuretic therapy. In such cases, water intake must be restricted to 500 to 1000 cc.

Rest and sodium restriction often are sufficient to reduce the work of the heart and to control sodium retention. In most instances, however, digitalis must be added to the routine, along with diuretic agents. Included among the latter are a number which have simplified the control of heart failure by promoting brisk sodium excretion.

Thiazide diuretics are potent oral saluretics. They are useful in left, right, and combined failure, alone or in combination with other diuretics as well as with digitalis. Diuresis begins within 2 hours after a maximal therapeutic dose and continues for as long as 12 hours. A number of preparations are available. Dose schedules vary considerably since some are 10 to 250 times as potent as others in terms of milligram dosage. Major disadvantages include potassium depletion, accentuation of blood glucose in diabetics, suppression of uric acid excretion, and the fact that large doses over prolonged periods may cause azotemia by reducing extracellular volume and glomerular filtration. In spite of these handicaps, thiazides are reasonably safe, only occasionally producing serious side effects or toxic reactions.

Ethacrynic acid is a newer diuretic which can be administered orally or parenterally. Onset of action begins within minutes and persists for about 6 hours. It is equal to or surpasses the effectiveness of the thiazides in therapeutic doses of 50 to 100 mg. two to four times daily, administered orally. Uric acid excretion is diminished by the drug, resulting in abnormally elevated serum values. Potassium loss is an indirect effect dependent on aldosterone activity and can be prevented by simultaneous administration of spironolactone or triampterine.

When given in doses above 50 mg. intravenously, ethacrynic acid may produce deafness which may be permanent.

Furosemide, which closely resembles the thiazides chemically, can be administered orally and parenterally. It has a rapid onset of action which persists for 6 hours. Like the thiazides, it diminishes glucose tolerance and uric acid excretion. Potassium excretion is less than sodium and varies with aldosterone activity and urine volume. The average oral dose is 40 mg. once daily. Intravenously, maximal effect is usually obtained with 40 to 80 mg.

Organic mercurial compounds are effective diuretics, particularly when administered parenterally. Although their mechanism of action remains obscure, diuresis begins within 1 or 2 hours after injection, peaks in 4 to 8 hours, and persists for as long as 24 hours. Mercurial diuretics are indicated in all forms of congestive failure, particularly when edema is pronounced. As in the case with potent oral agents, repeated and vigorous diuresis with the mercurial diuretics may contribute to serious electrolyte imbalances.

Other diuretics are available but infrequently required. Potassium-sparing diuretics are useful in combating digitalis toxicity. The competitive antagonists such as spirolactones and aldactone have a slow onset of action which persists for several days after the drugs are discontinued. Those that function by direct interference with cellular enzymes, such as Dyrenium and Amiloride, have a rapid and quickly dissipated action.

Ammonium chloride has its major usefulness in portentiating the action of mercurial diuretics. Osmotic diuretics, such as mannitol and urea and xanthine derivates, are rarely used.

In addition to diuretics, a number of measures are generally helpful in relieving or modifying the pathophysiological consequences of heart failure. These measures include oxygen administered in high concentration to correct depressed peripheral oxygenation, antibiotics to prevent infection in congested lungs, and anticoagulants to reduce the frequency of thromboembolic episodes.

ACUTE MYOCARDIAL INFARCTION

Left ventricular failure is a common complication of acute myocardial infarction. Its presence implies severe, generalized impairment of coronary perfusion, extensive myocardial destruction, structural complications such as papillary muscle dysfunction, or any combination of these events.

Prompt treatment is required. Mild manifestations may respond rapidly and completely. In the more severely ill patient, the prognosis is extremely guarded, regardless of the measures utilized.

The question of using digitalis is constantly debated. In the main, the objections are based on the fact that the drug increases the likelihood of electrical dysfunction which is already a problem with infarction. In deference to this possibility, digitalis commonly is withheld when the manifestations of failure are relatively mild. If failure is gross, however, it should be administered unhesitantly, although dose schedules may be reduced to avoid an increase in automatism.

As already indicated, the sympathomimetic amine isoproterenol may prove helpful for heart failure complicating myocardial infarction when a high degree atrioventricular block is present; occasionally, it may be useful in the absence of block when digitalis has not been effective. The positive inotropic effect of glucagon may qualify this drug for use when digitalis is contraindicated or fails.

Devices to assist the circulation in subjects with acute infarction and heart failure are still experimental. Although there is evidence that they can provide help which cannot be obtained otherwise, the routine use of such methods in the management of the failing heart must await further progress and practice.

Over the years, a number of surgical procedures have been proposed for coronary heart disease. The most recent, bypass vein graft, appears to offer exceptional promise in that it is a simple, direct method of circumventing obstruction to coronary flow. Evidence suggests that the procedure may restore reasonable contractility to ischemic hypokinetic segments of the myocardium.

AFTER BETA ADRENERGIC BLOCKADE

Beta receptor blockade decreases heart rate, arterial pressure, and velocity of myocardial contraction, thereby diminishing the demand of the myocardium for oxygen. On the other hand, it prolongs the duration of the systolic ejection and increases ventricular dimensions. The latter changes tend to augment myocardial oxygen requirement. While the net change usually resulting from beta blockade is reduction in myocardial oxygen needs, heart failure can ensue in an unsound organ when negative inotropism outweighs the oxygen-sparing qualities of the drug.

Classic examples are encountered when propranolol is used as an antidysrhythmic or to control angina when the underlying cardiac defect is severe. Failure is variously expressed, depending upon the heart lesion and the magnitude of the functional disorder.

The first principle of treatment is to discontinue or reduce the dose of the drug. Salt restriction and diuretics hasten recovery. The positive inotropic effect of digitalis is mediated through mechanisms other than beta receptors. Hence the drug may be used both to prevent failure and to restore compensation more rapidly after blockade has been lifted.

AFTER OPEN HEART SURGERY

The likelihood of heart failure after open heart surgery depends upon the antecedent cardiac lesion, the severity of pre-existing functional impairment, and the operative and postoperative complications. Subjects with severe defects who have had failure in the past, those in whom the operation has been difficult or uncertain, and those with electrolyte imbalances, unusual blood loss, dysrhythmias, or thromboembolic issues obviously are more apt to be decompensated.

The fundamental requirement is to define and treat the cause. This requires information regarding preoperative status, surgery, physical condition, and laboratory findings.

Failure is said to be due to intrinsic cardiac disease when it occurs in spite of an adequate operation and in the absence of meaningful complications. Treatment consists of rest, salt restriction, and administration of diuretics and digitalis.

Failure to correct all significant lesions and the use of inappropriate prosthetics are the major technical errors leading to decompensation. At times, compensation may be restored without additional corrective surgery. However, when failure is profound and intractable, a second operation is required.

Finally, blood loss, electrolyte imbalance, and inadequate oxygenation are common correctable complications leading to heart failure. Specific measures should be applied prior to the use of diuretics and digitalis for the decompensation.

14

Newer Approaches in Diuretic Therapy for Refractory Cardiac Failure

JOHN H. LARAGH, M.D.

As with so many aspects of cardiac failure, the direct "lesion" in congestive heart failure is a consequence of inappropriate compensation. The sequence, of course, begins with degenerative changes in the myocardium, leading to incompetence of the cardiac pump. It can then be traced to decreased mean arterial pressure generated during cardiac contraction and, consequently, to reduced delivery of blood to the kidney. In some manner not yet fully understood, this reduction of renal blood flow is associated with a signal to the kidney to conserve sodium, and this conservation underlies the fluid retention which produces congestion in the lungs, liver, abdomen, and peripheral tissues.

As long as one keeps in mind that the original failure is myocardial, it is completely appropriate, and clinically quite pragmatic, to regard congestive heart failure as secondarily but dominantly a disease whose major determinant is the kidney. Equally, diuretics can be discussed as the key to any regimen for the management of congestive heart failure. Not that a theoretical basis is needed for assigning such primacy to the diuretics. Every clinician must be aware of the revolutionary improvement in our ability to manage and to understand disorders characterized by abnormal fluid accumulation and/or elevated blood pressure; an improvement that has resulted from the development of effective oral diuretic agents, starting with the introduction of chlorothiazide in 1958. Now, physicians treating congestive heart failure have available at least five different classes of diuretic agents (Fig. 14.1), each of which is capable of selectively interfering in a different way with the active transport mechanisms involved in tubular reabsorption and thereby promoting natriuresis and diuresis.

RENAL TRANSPORT

A brief review of the mechanisms of salt and water transport in the kidney is appropriate here as a context for subsequent discussion of the

161

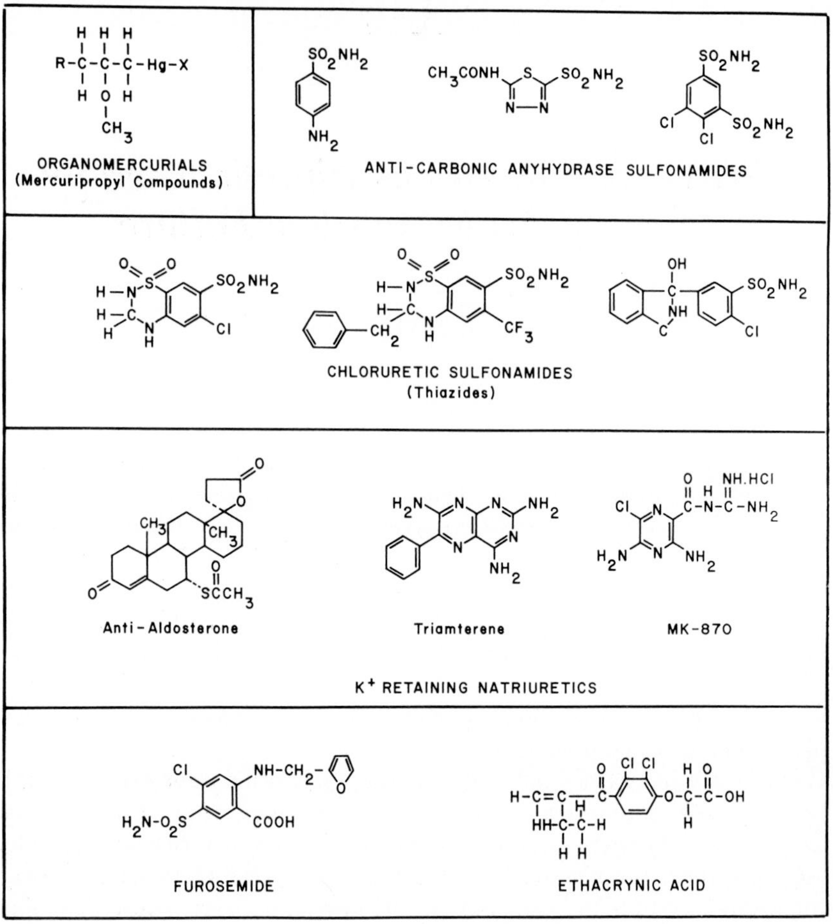

Fig. 14.1. Diuretic species.

selective action of different diuretics. The glomerular filtration rate in man is approximately 100 ml. per minute, with the resulting filtrate containing concentrations of sodium and other electrolytes equal to those found in plasma. Tubular reabsorption returns at least 99 per cent of the filtrate to the circulation, the remaining 1 per cent being excreted. Normally about 70 per cent of the filtrate is returned to the circulation by the proximal tubule in the form of an isotonic solution containing equivalent amounts of sodium and water. In other words, there is no dilution or concentration in conjunction with reabsorption from the proximal tubule, and water absorption in this region is secondary to activate sodium reabsorption. The permeability of the proximal tubular membrane to water permits passive isotonic reabsorption of water first into the interstitium and from there into the circulation. Because bicarbonate reabsorption from the proximal tubule follows sodium, 90 per cent or more of the bicarbonate in the filtrate may be reabsorbed at this site, so that bicarbonate reabsorption may exceed that of chloride.

The other major changes in composition occur distally in the nephron where the remaining 30 per cent of the filtrate is acted upon. The next reabsorption site is the renal medullary portion of the ascending loop of Henle. This portion of the nephron is impermeable to water. Therefore, although active sodium reabsorption takes place, returning anywhere from 15 to 30 per cent of the filtrate sodium to the body, an equivalent amount of water is not removed. The fluid remaining in the lumen therefore becomes dilute in terms of its concentration of sodium, chloride, and other electrolytes. Conversely, fluid on the interstitial side of the nephron, in the renal medulla, becomes hypertonic to plasma, generating the driving force for the eventual production of concentrated urine when the filtrate passes by again in the collecting ducts. The process of dilution continues as the dilute tubular fluid passes back into the renal cortex and as sodium reabsorption continues without equivalent water movement in the next portion of the nephron, still within the ascending limb of the loop of Henle. The passage of fluid through the distal convolution and the collecting duct then continues without osmotic equilibration with the hypertonic medullary interstitium, unless the kidney is under stress to retain water mediated by antidiuretic hormone (ADH) which acts to increase the water permeability of the descending limb and collecting ducts. ADH activity can result in a concentrated urine with approximately a 1,200 milliosmolal concentration of solutes, about four times the osmolality of plasma. In this way, large volumes of water with low concentrations of sodium are excreted. On the other hand, under the stress of water ingestion, dilution can occur which will produce urine with one-sixth the normal osmolality. In this manner, large volumes of water with low concentrations of sodium are excreted.

Essentially all diuretic agents function by affecting the processes of tubular reabsorption either directly or by inhibiting those hormones which regulate these processes. Because different agents affect different steps in the sequence, the physician not only has a choice which may be governed by definable physiological needs but he also has the opportunity to design a diuretic regimen which is rationally tailored to specific clinical problems. This is discussed below in terms of the specific diuretic agents now available. First, however, let us return to the concept that congestive heart failure represents an inappropriate compensation in response to derangement of the normal interactions between the heart and the kidney.

The obvious premise is that the initial fluid overload in congestive failure results from the failure of the heart as a pump, a failure which relates back to a basically mechanical defect, albeit one which probably has a biochemical basis: faulty performance by the muscle fibrils. Cardiac output is reduced as is the delivery of blood to the kidneys. This in turn reduces the kidney's capacity to excrete salt and therefore leads to the accumulation of water and to congestion, which then increases the demands on a cardiac pump that to start with lacked the ability to handle even normal demands.

The first question to be asked is why the reduction of blood flow in the kidney should lead to retention of salt and water? There is evidence suggesting that the kidney's functional incompetence is not simply the product of underperfusion. It has been shown that the renal tubules in affected persons are actually hyperactive: that they reabsorb relatively more of the filtered sodium than in normal individuals. In a sense, the kidney is responding as if there were a shortage of electrolytes in the circulation. It is not clear why this should be so, but it has been postulated that the reduced perfusion of such organs as the brain, the various endocrine glands, the heart, and the kidneys signals receptors in these organs into behaving as if there were an overall shortage of plasma volume (and of electrolytes) even though exactly the reverse is true. Therefore, signals are transmitted to the kidneys directing them to conserve salts. This is effected by an increased tubular sodium reabsorption and attendant fluid retention.

How can this vicious cycle of cardiac incompetence, decreased output and perfusion, salt conservation, fluid congestion, and exacerbated cardiac incompetence be broken? Certainly one could rationally concentrate on the underlying pathophysiological flaw by seeking to increase cardiac contractility and output. And indeed this is what is done whenever possible with digitalis and other inotropic drugs. However, we have learned in the past dozen years that, in patients whose cardiac failure is clinically manifested most conspicuously by edema, more consistent and often more dramatic results can be achieved by addressing our therapeutic attentions to the kidney disturbance. Thus the remarkably successful role played by diuretics.

ACTION OF DIURETIC AGENTS

Depending on the taxonomic criteria one uses, the different diuretic agents now available for the management of congestive heart failure and other edematous states can be subdivided in varied manners. Based on differences in their physiological effects, it is convenient to discuss them as five different groups, the organomercurials, the sulfonamide-carbonic anhydrase inhibitors, the oral chloruretic sulfonamide compounds of which the thiazides were the first and are still the foremost representatives, ethacrynic acid and furosemide, and the potassium-retaining diuretics, notably aldosterone antagonists (Fig. 14.1). For each of these groups, current concepts of their site and mode of action are discussed, thus laying the groundwork for a subsequent discussion of the rational design of diuretic regimens.

Organomercurials

From the discovery of their diuretic potential in the early 1900s for close to half a century, the organomercurials served as the only available and effective compounds for the removal of excess body fluid. This property of the mercurials was happened upon by physicians who used them in the treatment of syphilis and who observed the profound diuretic effect on some patients. The organomercurials remain the most effective of diuretic agents, the use of which is, of course, severely limited by the need for parenteral administration. In terms of the site of action, there is still no clear evidence as to whether the mercurials act by distal tubular blockade or by proximal tubular blockade, but it has been established that, at either site, they function primarily by inhibition of an isosmotic reabsorptive process. Mercurial agents do not significantly inhibit either urinary concentrating or diluting mechanisms.

Carbonic Anhydrase Inhibitors

The discovery of the diuretic value of carbonic anhydrase inhibitors in one sense ushered in the new age of diuretic therapy. These drugs were harbingers of the far more important things to come only a year or so after. Once again, progress came in the form of fortuitous fallout from another branch of chemotherapy. It was noted that patients with congestive heart failure receiving sulfanilamide for pneumonia often had impressive diureses. It was known that sulfanilamide was a carbonic anhydrase inhibitor and that the process of hydrogen ion secretion by the kidney was dependent on the carbonic anhydrase system. From these premises, it was decided to seek sulfonamide compounds more specifically tailored for their carbonic anhydrase inhibition, and these were developed. Although these carbonic anhydrase inhibitor diuretic drugs are still in use, their role has been somewhat limited by the rapid development of tolerance that characterizes patient reaction to them. The diuretics are generally effective for a day or two and then lose their potency in the person being treated. For this reason, the carbonic anhydrase inhibitors are best used intermittently and as adjuvants to other diuretics.

The mode of action and the site have been suggested above in the observation that the carbonic anhydrase inhibitors act by blocking an enzyme system which is necessary for the secretion of hydrogen ions by the kidney. These drugs act all along the nephron, primarily in the proximal tubule, by inhibiting the acidification of the urine. This serves to produce a natriuresis and a diuresis because the secretion of hydrogen ions into the tubular urine is accomplished by an exchange with sodium ions, which are then reabsorbed. By blocking acidification, sodium reabsorption is prevented.

Thiazides

If the discovery of the carbonic anhydrase inhibitors was the forerunner of the revolution in the management of congestive heart failure, then that revolution came into full force with the discovery and introduction of chlorothiazide. Here at last was a drug which could produce a potent diuresis and which was effective orally. Nor were any problems of refractoriness apparent with chlorothiazide. Now, of course, there are probably a score or more thiazide drugs on the market. Basically none of these analogues differs significantly from chlorothiazide. One may need a different number of milligrams of one analogue to achieve a dose equipotent with another and there may be some differences in duration of action, but essentially all of the thiazides are closely similar in their therapeutic capacity.

The sites of action of the thiazides have been quite well pinpointed as within the ascending limb of the loop of Henle and the distal convoluted tubule. They interfere with the dilution of urinary fluids that occurs in these portions of the nephron, and in this way they prevent the reabsorption of sodium and other electrolytes in the distal cortical convolutions. The result, of course, includes the inhibition of free water formation and the excretion of not only sodium and water but also of chloride, potassium, and other ions. The kaliuretic effect of the thiazides constitutes one of the problems in their use. Before discussing this, however, let us turn to newer compounds which resemble the thiazides in terms of their diuretic and electrolyte effects, but which are more powerful, ethacrynic acid and furosemide.

Ethacrynic Acid and Furosemide

Quantitatively, both of these newer agents exert a much greater effect than do the thiazides, probably because, in addition to their thiazide-like interference with diluting mechanisms in the distal cortical tubules, they also block sodium transport in the loop or ascending limb. Therefore, they depress urinary concentrating as well as urinary diluting activity.

Aldosterone Antagonists

The two basic effects of the adrenal hormone aldosterone on electrolytes are the promotion of sodium retention and the promotion of potassium excretion. It is this combination that tends to make the aldosterone antagonists ideal diuretics in a clinical context, when the effects sought by the physician are most likely to be sodium excretion and potassium retention. Three pharmacological agents have proved capable of effective aldosterone antagonism: spironolactone (Aldactone A), which is the most widely used, triamterene, and amiloride (MK 870), which is the most powerful of the three but which has not received Food and Drug Administration approval for general clinical use. All three of these agents act by competition for receptor sites at the distal renal tubule where the aldosterone-dependent exchange between sodium and potassium ions takes place. These compounds are therefore especially valuable in correcting potassium loss produced by the thiazides or by other diuretic species. Spironolactone is a true competitive inhibitor of endogenous aldosterone and has no action in the absence of this hormone. On the other hand, triamterene and amiloride can block the aldosterone-directed transport mechanism even in the absence of the hormone, and therefore they have the properties of a noncompetitive inhibitor. This means that the latter two drugs can still be effective even when endogenous aldosterone secretion is enormous.

In an important sense, Aldactone and other diuretics in its class approach the ideal in their mode of action and in their effects. It is true that they are not as powerful as the thiazides or as ethacrynic acid and furosemide as natriuretic agents. This is because aldosterone has only a minor influence on the total bulk electrolyte reabsorption by the tubule. But practically, a minor effect maintained over a sufficient time becomes a major effect. By administering Aldactone over, say, 3 or 4 weeks, one may actually induce a greater sodium and water loss than with more powerful natriuretic agents, even than with ethacrynic acid or furosemide. With the latter two drugs, there is a tendency on the part of the patient to develop resistance and rebound to the violence of action. There is something to be said for gradual smooth diuresis and, in many cases, impatience on the part of the physician or patient to see tangible results quickly may cause an inappropriate turning away from the aldosterone antagonists as the first diuretics to be tried.

WHAT IS AN IDEAL DIURETIC REGIMEN?

Obviously there is no single answer for this question. What should be stressed is the fact that different classes of diuretics act at least in part on different sites in the renal tubules, thus affecting qualitatively different transport mechanisms. By taking advantage of this selectivity, the clinician may choose a particular diuretic to correct any particular derangement in the blood electrolytes of the patient. There are many practical illustrations of the combined use of diuretics to achieve maximal efficacy. In fact, the only two classes that cannot be used effectively in combination are the organomercurials and the carbonic anhydrase inhibitors since the latter may block the effects of the mercurials by preventing acidification of the urine.

In designing a regimen, the physician must also take into account the fact that, with the thiazides and ethacrynic acid and furosemide, there is a tendency to develop some degree of refractoriness. These drugs tend to be most powerful in the first few days of administration, becoming somewhat less effective subsequently. This is one of the reasons why many of us have advocated intermittent programs in which "resting periods" are allowed. Not only will this type of program provide recovery time for the drug action, but it will also permit restoration of the electrolyte imbalance that commonly occurs with diuretics. For example, if a patient is receiving thiazides, there will be some potassium loss and therefore some danger of hypokalemia. If, on the other hand, the regimen prescribes a 3-day period of taking the drug, followed by 3 days of rest, the patient may replenish his potassium from natural food sources such as fruit and meat which are abundantly provided with ionic potassium.

The two main arguments against intermittent therapy are, first, that such regimens are inconvenient for the patient and for the physician, an argument which I think can be dismissed offhand, and second, that a smooth, even diuretic effect is lost. It is true that, with intermittent regimens, the patient's weight may fluctuate to a greater extent, climbing during the off periods, then dropping sharply when the drug is reintroduced. And I would agree that this is not as desirable as a daily blockade but, on balance, I believe that the advantages of intermittent therapy outweigh the disadvantage.

One major exception to this evaluation would apply to the aldosterone antagonists. These can only be effective on a continuous basis since the object of therapy is to attain high enough blood levels to create a chronic blockade of potassium loss. For this reason we are beginning to feel increasingly that, to treat any difficult patient, the best approach is to start with spironolactone or triamterene, then to add one of the thiazides or ethacrynic acid or furosemide intermittently. Such a program can maintain an even baseline effect while at the same time preventing potassium depletion.

In many patients, of course, thiazides alone will work, and they will do the diuretic job when administered on an intermittent basis. If we start with thiazides and they prove inadequate, our next step is to add an aldosterone antagonist, which we give chronically while using the thiazides intermittently. If this still fails to produce adequate diuresis, we will substitute one of the two more powerful agents, ethacrynic acid or furosemide, for the thiazide. In rare cases, with very sick patients, none of these regimens may be effective. As a last resort in such cases, we give volume expanders such as mannitol or albumen, together with cortisone. The purpose of this last maneuver is to correct the poor forward delivery from the heart and consequent underperfusion of the arterial tree that may occur in serious congestive heart failure. By increasing the perfusion of the kidney, the physician may provide a more favorable environment for the action of the diuretics and thereby increase their efficacy. Cortisone seems to make a specific contribution to the enhancement of renal blood flow. Obviously, such an approach cannot be used on an outpatient basis and, in fact, by definition it is appropriate only to a desperately ill, hospitalized individual.

THE ILLOGIC AND HAZARDS OF POTASSIUM THERAPY

It should be noted that, in describing these various regimens, no mention is made of using potassium supplementation in the form of potassium salts. We have never advocated such supplementation for ambulatory patients because the amounts of potassium chloride required for correction can be dangerous by virtue of toxicity to the heart and because of a tendency to cause ileal ulceration. We believe that hyperkalemia is far more threatening to the cardiac patient than hypokalemia. Potassium salts are far more potent physiological and pharmacological agents than is generally recognized even by those who are aware that these salts can be and have been used to induce cardiac arrest.

THERAPY AND RENAL MECHANISMS

In any review of a field as rapidly developing as that of diuretic therapy one must be concerned with the physiological implications as well as with the therapeutic criteria. It is therefore significant that, in the more than a dozen years in which oral diuretics have been available, we have used these agents not only for their primary purpose, the dissipation of edema, but also as an extremely valuable tool for the dissection of renal tubular transport mechanisms. Many of the facts cited to explain the sites and mechanisms of action of the various classes of diuretic have actually been learned from observing these drugs in action and then reasoning backwards. We have also made a substantial beginning toward understanding the intrarenal transport mechanisms for the regulation of sodium reabsorption at a perhaps more basic level, that is to say, in terms of control by signals arising extrarenally. The effects of chlorothiazide and other diuretics on the release of renin and on aldosterone secretion might also involve extrarenal signals. Solution of the problem of how diuretic-induced depletion of electrolytes and fluid triggers increased renin and then aldosterone secretion could, for example, go a long way toward unraveling the delicately entwined mechanisms for sodium and blood pressure homeostasis. These are but examples of the type of problem which can be productively approached through close study of the roles being played by diuretics. We are in the particularly happy position of being able to pursue such studies while at the same time providing our patients with the immense and often lifesaving benefits of the very agents through which increased knowledge will come.

This study was supported by Grants HE-01275 and HE-05741 from the United States Public Health Service.

REFERENCES

1. Laragh, J. H.: The proper use of newer diuretics: diagnosis and treatment. Ann. Intern. Med. 67: 606, 1967.
2. Laragh, J. H., Heinemann, H. O., and Demartini, F. E.: Effect of chlorothiazide on electrolyte transport in man. Its use in the treatment of edema of congestive heart failure, nephrosis and cirrhosis. J. A. M. A. 166: 145, 1958.
3. Laragh, J. H.: Hormones and the pathogenesis of congestive heart failure: vasopressin, aldosterone, and angiotensin. II. Further evidence for renal-adrenal interaction from studies in hypertension and in cirrhosis. Circulation 25: 1015, 1962.
4. Laragh, J. H.: The mode of action and use of chlorothiazide on renal excretion of electrolytes and free water. Amer. J. Med. 26: 843, 1959.
5. Cannon, P. J., Heinemann, H. O., Stason, W. B., and Laragh, J. H.: Ethacrynic acid. Effectiveness and mode of diuretic action in man. Circulation 31: 5, 1965.
6. Stason, W. B., Cannon, P. J., Heinemann, H. O., and Laragh, J. H.: Furosemide, a clinical evaluation of its diuretic action. Circulation, 34: 910, 1966.

15

Mechanisms of Cardiac Arrhythmias

YOSHIO WATANABE, M.D., AND
LEONARD S. DREIFUS, M.D.

Both clinical and electrophysiological studies have suggested certain basic concepts in the genesis of cardiac arrhythmias.[1-4] For clinical purposes, classification of cardiac arrhythmias is usually based on the origin of impulses (supraventricular or ventricular) and their mode of appearance (premature systole, tachycardia, flutter, fibrillation, etc.). From the electrophysiological standpoint, on the other hand, the genesis of cardiac arrhythmias is often divided into (1) disturbances of impulse formation, (2) disturbances of conduction, and (3) a combination of both (Table 15.1).

It is obvious that certain arrhythmias appearing in the atria disturb cardiac dynamics very little, while the same mechanism occurring in the ventricles could be disastrous. Hence, clinical implication of the same electrophysiological derangement is not always identical. However, both identification and therapy of cardiac arrhythmias must still be predicated on a precise understanding of the underlying mechanisms. It is the purpose of this review to disucss some of the more important concepts among those listed in Table 15.1.

DISTURBANCES OF IMPULSE FORMATION

Automaticity

The term automaticity refers to the ability of certain cardiac fibers to generate an impulse of their own. This ability appears to be characteristic of the specialized cardiac fibers, which are found in the sinoatrial (SA) node, intra-atrial conducting system, atrioventricular (AV) node, His bundle, bundle branches, and peripheral Purkinje system.[3] On the other hand, ordinary atrial and ventricular fibers do not possess automaticity and are called nonspecialized myocardial fibers. An automatic fiber can spontaneously and gradually lose its resting potential to reach the threshold

171

Table 15.1

Genesis of cardiac arrhythmias

I. Disturbances of impulse formation
   A. Automaticity
      1. physiological alterations
      2. enhanced automaticity
      3. depressed automaticity
   B. Other mechanisms of impulse formation
      1. oscillation
      2. afterpotentials
      3. local potential difference
         a. asynchronous repolarization
         b. partial depolarization
II. Disturbances of impulse conduction
   A. Simple conduction block
      1. refractory tissue
         a. dissimilar action potential duration and excitability between fiber types
         b. interference of two impulses
      2. decremental conduction
      3. inhomogeneous conduction
   B. Unidirectional block and re-entry
      1. unidirectional block and re-entry in the AV junction
      2. local block and microre-entry
III. Combined disturbances of impulse formation and conduction
   A. Parasystole
   B. Ectopic rhythms with exit block
IV. Fibrillation

level. This gradual decrease in the resting potential is called diastolic depolarization, which is the actual mechanism of automaticity.

The most important factor which modifies the cycle length of an automatic fiber is the slope of diastolic depolarization,[5] although the levels of maximal diastolic potential and the threshold potential also play a role. An increase in the slope of diastolic depolarization in SA nodal fibers will bring the transmembrane potential to the threshold more rapidly and accelerate the sinus rhythm.

On the other hand, a shift of the pacemaker from the SA node to other specialized fibers with less automaticity may result from a sinus slowing or failure of the sinus impulses to activate such fibers, as a "latent" pacemaker now finds enough time to continue its slow diastolic depolarization until the threshold is reached. These beats are termed AV junctional or His-Purkinje escape beats and are beneficial in that ventricular asystole is prevented. Several types of "AV nodal rhythm" with dependent activation of the atria and the ventricles have been shown to originate from automatic fibers located in specific regions of the AV junction.[6]

If the slope of diastolic depolarization in automatic fibers outside the SA node becomes abnormally steep, these fibers may eventually take over the control of the atrial and/or ventricular excitation. Such enhanced automaticity in ectopic sites may result from ischemia, hypokalemia, or excess cardiac glycosides. It is most likely that many instances of self-sustaining ectopic tachycardias result from increased automaticity, while the role of this mechanism in the production of isolated premature beats (extrasystoles) is unknown, except in the presence of a parasystolic rhythm.

DISTURBANCES OF IMPULSE CONDUCTION

Of the various mechanisms causing failure of impulse propagation, the one most classically invoked is the presence of refractory tissue ahead of the advancing wave of excitation. This condition may occur at a junction of two fiber groups with dissimilar excitability or duration of refractoriness. It has been demonstrated that the action potential duration becomes progressively prolonged from the atrial fibers through the AN, N, and NH regions of the AV node,[7] His bundle, bundle branches, and more peripheral Purkinje fibers.[5] Thus, at any junction of two specialized conducting tissues, the distal fibers usually have a longer effective refractory period and may fail to respond to high frequency of the proximal fibers.[2] Failure of AV conduction in the presence of extremely rapid atrial rhythms (*e.g.*, atrial flutter) or of an early atrial premature systole may occur on this basis. Complete failure of propagation of a premature atrial impulse at the level of the right bundle branch, where the action potential duration is significantly longer than in the left bundle branch or in the more proximal fiber has been demonstrated.[8, 9] A new concept of the "gate" mechanism in peripheral Purkinje fibers,[10] where the duration of refractoriness is the longest, undoubtedly emerged from the above observations and might prove valuable in explaining certain ventricular arrhythmias.

Another factor causing refractoriness or a state of nonresponsiveness in tissues ahead of the excitation front is the interference of two impulses within the AV conducting system. Indeed, interference by return conduction (reciprocation) within the lower regions of the AV junction has been demonstrated.[11] Interfering impulses due to either automaticity or reciprocation could be concealed and may not be apparent on the clinical electrocardiogram.

Recently, increasing attention has been given to the phenomenon of decremental conduction in cardiac tissues.[12, 13] In some cardiac fiber groups, the action potential amplitude and the rate of depolarization are progressively decreased from cell to cell, and the resultant stimulus becomes weaker and less effective in the course of transmission. Under these conditions, excitation of more distal fibers may depend on the number of participating proximal fibers. Finally, the impulse may fade out when the integrated stimulus strength becomes insufficient to cause a propagated response in more distal and still excitable fibers.

In the AV node, especially in the N region,[14] the fibers show a lower level of membrane resting potential and a significantly slower rate of depolarization than atrial or ventricular fibers, even under physiological conditions. Factors known to depress AV conduction such as acetylcholine,[13, 15] digitalis glycosides,[7, 16] or lowered potassium concentration[17] tend to further decrease the rate of depolarization in these fibers and to slow conduction. Varying degrees of step formation preceding the more rapid depolarization phase are commonly observed.[14, 15] Finally, the step fails to develop a full-sized action potential, resulting in a local response, and propagation does not proceed more distally. Thus, an increased decrement in these regions of the AV junction may explain some of the AV conduction disturbances. It is to be noted that this type of conduction block is not the result of refractoriness or loss of excitability in the fibers distal to the excitation front.[13] The concept of inhomogeneous conduction[18] is closely related to the phenomenon of decremental conduction, but it has certain advantages in explaining some aspects of abnormal AV transmission.

Normally, successful conduction through the AV nodal tissue occurs with rather synchronous activation of fibers in the AN and the N regions and a smooth excitation front invading the NH region. When the rate of depolarization is decreased and conduction is further slowed, particularly in the critical N region of the AV node, the spread of excitation in this region becomes inhomogeneous. Such inhomogeneity of conduction could manifest itself as two or more functionally separate portions of tissue, some of which show a relatively rapid conduction. Increasing decrement in all portions or in the slower conducting portions alone can cause further fractionation of the wave front, leading to the failure of propagation. Intranodal conduction block, including the instances with classic Wenckebach periodicity, can be explained on this basis.[11]

The above concept was supported by Janse, who demonstrated that an atrial wave front coming from the interatrial septum excited the atrial margin of the AV node asynchronously, resulting in inhomogeneous conduction and functional longitudinal dissociation within the node.[19] The possible importance of this mechanism in the presence of atrial fibrillation was also pointed out.

On the other hand, if the more rapidly conducting portions are selectively depressed by either a forward or retrograde impulse, slower spread of excitation in this portion may result in a synchronized or smoother wave front. Then, an unexpected, successful AV or VA transmission in the presence of advanced degrees of block may ensue. This phenomenon has been described as a variety of supernormal AV or VA conduction.[20]

The importance of decremental conduction in Purkinje fibers, as a result of either incomplete repolarization[8, 21] (during the relative refractory period) or diastolic depolarization,[22, 23] has also been emphasized. It has been implied that a sufficient reduction in transmembrane potential can change propragation from all-or-none to decremental conduction.[3] These observations are quite valuable in the explanation of certain clinical and experimental arrhythmias.

Unidirectional Block and Re-entry

Local block with microre-entry has long been invoked in the genesis of various ectopic rhythms.[24] The term microre-entry implies a small geometrical arrangement of the re-entry pathway, as contrasted with the classic concept of circus movement in the explanation of atrial flutter.[25, 26] The phenomenon was first demonstrated by Schmitt and Erlanger[27] in 1928, utilizing isolated myocardial strips. In this instance, asymmetrical depression of conductivity resulting from localized compression of the muscle initially engendered different conduction velocities in one direction versus the other. These alterations culminated in the block of an impulse spreading into one region of the tissue and re-entry of the same impulse to this region from the distal end of a blocked area (Fig. 15.1, left). Hence, this condition is analogous to the functional, longitudinal dissociation observed in the AV node.[18]

In contrast, anatomic rather than functional separation of two pathways facilitating re-entry is illustrated in Fig. 15.1, right. The mechanism

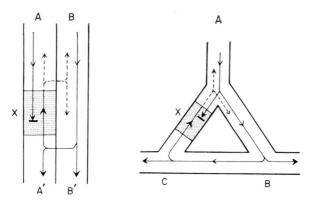

FIG. 15.1. Schematic representation of re-entry movement. The left diagram corresponds to functional longitudinal dissociation of cardiac tissue into two parallel portions. Unidirectional block is present at X. Re-excitation of the initially depolarized area is shown by dotted lines. The right diagram illustrates anatomically separate pathways causing re-entry. AB and AC could represent ramifications of a peripheral Purkinje fiber, and BC could represent ventricular myocardium. (Reproduced from Watanabe, Y., and Dreifus, L. S : Amer. Heart J. 76: 114, 1968.[4])

which prevents forward transmission of an impulse but permits subsequent retrograde conduction through the depressed area is most likely dissimilar degrees of decrement depending on the direction of transmission (unidirectional block). That such an anatomic arrangement of fibers can actually be found at junctions between peripheral branches of the Purkinje system and the ventricular myocardium has been pointed out by Hoffman.[3] Hoffman has also suggested another possible mechanism of reexcitation in a similar model.[3] If forward conduction across region X (Fig. 15.1, right) is markedly slowed and retrograde transmission is blocked, the peripheral tissue (BC) initially depolarized through the faster conducting pathway (AB), after the expiration of its refractory period, may be discharged for a second time by the slowly spreading forward impulse through AC.

In all of these models of re-entry, either within the AV junction or at any other portions of the myocardium, re-excitation of some fibers may cause a coupled premature systole, which obviously requires an initiating beat. When an appropriate electrophysiological condition is present, the previously generated premature systole may act as another initiating beat, and a self-sustaining arrhythmia may ensue.[3] There is general agreement that two factors, *i.e.*, a decreased conduction velocity and a shorter refractory period, favor the development of re-entry. The actual size of a re-entry pathway, less than 2 mm., was observed in the AV junction.[18]

In contrast to microre-entry as discussed above and seen in the fibrillatory state, large circus movement can be identified in some varieties of atrial flutter[26, 28] and also in the circulation of the excitation wave along the normal AV transmission system and accessory pathways during Wolff-Parkinson-White tachycardia.[29, 30]

COMBINED DISTURBANCES OF IMPULSE FORMATION AND CONDUCTION

Certain cardiac arrhythmias result from combined disturbances of impulse formation and conduction. However, many varieties of clinical arrhythmias, such as atrial tachycardia with block, result from separate electrophysiological events occurring at two different sites, *e.g.*, ectopic impulse formation in the atria and conduction block in the AV junction. In contrast, parasystole and ectopic rhythms with exit block are produced by close interaction or association of these disturbances (impulse formation and conduction) in a localized region of the myocardium, and hence they deserve special comments.

In order to explain the mechanism of protection of a parasystolic rhythm, Scherf[31] postulates a high inherent frequency of firing (often 300 per minute or higher) at the site of impulse formation, which keeps the pacemaker refractory to the invading excitation front. However, alternative mechanisms such as protection (entrance) block surrounding the ectopic pacemaker are also possible.[1, 32] This zone of protection block must have the characteristics of unidirectional block, since it prevents the entrance of the sinus or other impulses into the pacemaking region while permitting the exit of impulses from this area. However, the concomitant presence of exit block has to be postulated in some instances in which an expected ectopic beat fails to appear despite its apparent timing outside the refractory period of the surrounding cardiac tissues.

It has been known that a lower level of resting potential could cause a slow conduction velocity or even decremental conduction. This situation may occur in any portions of the specialized conducting system when automaticity is enhanced and the membrane potential is significantly reduced by diastolic depolarization.[22, 23] Then it is quite possible that increased automaticity in a group of specialized fibers may create an ectopic pacemaker but, at the same time, may make propagation of impulses through this region more difficult. This mechanism may cause both entrance and exit block. Characteristics of parasystole and ectopic rhythms with exit block can thus be explained on one and the same basis of diastolic depolarization. Exit block from an ectopic pacemaker frequently shows Wenckebach phenomenon, resulting in a very complex arrhythmia.[33]

FIBRILLATION

In spite of exhaustive studies, the mechanisms of atrial and ventricular fibrillation are still subject to great controversy, and more sophisticated approaches are necessary to identify the precise sequence of events. The pathophysiology of both atrial and ventricular fibrillation appears similar, while it is rather widely accepted that the mechanisms which initiate the fibrillatory state and those sustaining this arrhythmia are not necessarily the same.[34] At least for the maintenance of fibrillatory state, numerous areas of microre-entries as a result of conduction disturbances are now considered the most likely mechanism.[35, 36]

Studies utilizing microelectrodes in the presence of established atrial or ventricular fibrillation have revealed that almost complete electrical disorganization of the respective chambers is present.[35, 37, 38] However, some degree of synchrony may be observed between fibers separated by a distance of less than 1 mm.[37] It is also abundantly clear that a shortened refractory period must necessarily be present for disorganized fibers to undergo rapid, repetitive discharge.

In order to explain such cellular disorganization with unifocal impulse formation, it has been argued that, with a high frequency of stimulation, some fibers fail to respond to every impulse, and islands of refractory tissue cause an irregular spread of excitation.[39] Indeed, this mode of initiation of asynchrony is quite possible. However, once irregular spread of excitation is invoked, it automatically implies local conduction disturbances, and the probability of microre-entry is inescapable. Similarly, the theory of multifocal impulse formation alone fails to explain certain characteristics of fibrillation,[40-42] and hence, the postulation of local conduction disturbances with possible microre-entry, or a combination of this mechanism with disturbances of impulse formation, appears to give the most plausible explanation for cellular disorganization.[35, 37, 38]

In both clinical and experimental fibrillation, several initiating mechanisms have been identified. The first type is characterized by rapid onset of fibrillation with one or two premature systoles early in the repolarization phase of a previous ventricular (or atrial) excitation (Fig. 15.2). Such onset of ventricular fibrillation was termed the R on T phenomenon by Smirk and Palmer.[43] The very early premature systole falling in the "vulnerable period"[44] produced varying degrees of incomplete depolarization in different fibers as a result of variations of the duration of refractoriness.[38] Local conduction block is thus prevalent, and the slow, irregular spread of excitation with multiple regions of microre-entry causes asynchrony between fibers. It should be clearly stated that the genesis of early premature systoles could be attributed to disturbances of either impulse formation or conduction. Shortening of the action potential duration with asynchronous repolarization of adjacent fibers appears as a rather common predisposing factor for this type of fibrillation.

In some instances, ventricular fibrillation may be initiated by a ventricular premature systole with a long coupling interval (Fig. 15.3) or even by an idioventricular escape beat. However, these initiating beats are usually followed by one or more premature beats with progressively shorter coupling intervals and subsequent disorganization as in the first variety (Fig. 15.4). It is possible that abnormal spread of excitation of an ectopic impulse may facilitate the production of a very early premature systole, especially in a more severely diseased or vulnerable heart. In these instances, generation

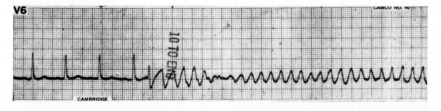

Fig. 15.2. Sinus rhythm is present at the left hand portion of the strip. An early ventricular premature beat only on the apex of the T wave of the fourth sinus beat engenders a run of ventricular tachycardia, followed by ventricular fibrillation.

of a local potential difference as a result of inhomogeneity of the myocardium with asynchronous repolarization may well be the cause of a very short coupling interval.

Initiation of ventricular fibrillation by these mechanisms appears more prevalent in the presence of a prolonged Q-Tc or Q-U interval. This condition may be seen in profound ischemia, with drug therapy such as quinidine

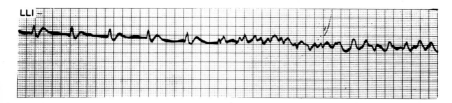

FIG. 15.3. Lead 1. Following the fifth QRS of junctional origin, a late ventricular premature systole engenders ventricular fibrillation. Although the beat is premature, it falls after the full inscription of the T wave.

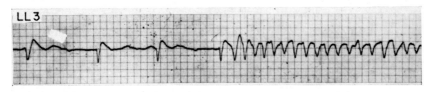

FIG. 15.4. Lead 3. Atrial fibrillation is present with second degree AV block. Following a long diastolic interval (fourth QRS complex), a premature ventricular systole engenders ventricular fibrillation.

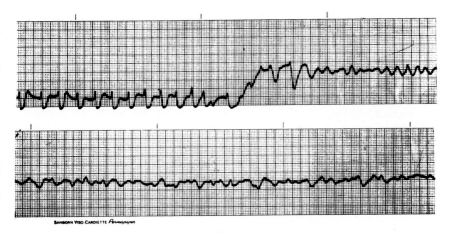

FIG. 15.5. Lead 2. Following a prolonged period of ventricular tachycardia, there is a gradual deterioration of the contour of the QRS, and ventricular fibrillation ensues.

or procaine amide, and with hypokalemia. Prolongation of the Q-Tc interval may be associated with a more non-uniform ventricular repolarization and a longer vulnerable period, which would facilitate disorganization of excitation.

In still another variety, gradual transition from a sustained period of tachycardia to fibrillation (Fig. 15.5) is usually preceded by (1) the development of prominent electrical alternation of some fibers, accompanied by a further decrease in the rate of depolarization in the majority of fibers,[37-38] and (2) fluctuations of the relative timing of depolarization in individual fibers.[38] These observations imply the development of local block and variation in the spread of excitation from beat to beat. High frequency of stimulation apparently exaggerates the inhomogeneity of the myocardium, which causes a non-uniform shortening of the refractory period and enhances a local block.

SUMMARY

Some of the current concepts on the electrophysiological basis of cardiac arrhythmias have been reviewed. Although significant progress has been made in our understanding of arrhythmias through these and other studies, the precise mechanisms of certain rhythm disturbances still remain unknown. Further investigations of these mechanisms will undoubtedly clarify the inconsistencies and close important gaps in our knowledge of cardiac arrhythmias, on which therapeutic approaches must be based.

This study was supported in part by Grant HE-011281 from the National Institutes of Health.

REFERENCES

1. Katz, L. N., and Pick, A.: *Clinical Electrocardiography, Part I: The Arrhythmias.* Lea & Febiger, Philadelphia, 1956.
2. Hoffman, B. F., and Cranefield, P. F.: The physiological basis of cardiac arrhythmias. Amer. J. Med. 37: 670, 1964.
3. Hoffman, B. F.: The electrophysiology of heart muscle and the genesis of arrhythmias. In Dreifus, L. S., and Likoff, W. (eds.): *Mechanisms and Therapy of Cardiac Arrhythmias,* Grune & Stratton, Inc., New York, 1966, p. 27.
4. Watanabe, Y., and Dreifus, L. S.: Newer concepts in the genesis of cardiac arrhythmias. Amer. Heart J. 76: 114, 1968.
5. Hoffman, B. F., and Cranefield, P. F.: *Electrophysiology of the Heart.* McGraw-Hill Book Company, Inc., New York, 1960.
6. Watanabe, Y., and Dreifus, L. S.: Sites of impulse formation within the atrioventricular junction of the rabbit. Circ. Res. 22: 717, 1968.
7. Watanabe, Y., and Dreifus, L. S.: Electrophysiologic effects of digitalis on A-V transmission. Amer. J. Physiol. 211: 1461, 1966.
8. Hoffman, B. F., Moore, E. N., Stuckey, J. H., and Cranefield, P. F.: Functional properties of the atrioventricular conduction system. Circ. Res. 13: 308, 1963.
9. Moore, E. N.: Microelectrode studies on concealment of multiple premature atrial responses. Circ. Res. 18: 660, 1966.

10. Myerberg, R. J., Gelband, H., and Hoffman, B. F.: Functional characteristics of the gating mechanism in the canine A-V conducting system. Circ. Res. 28: 136, 1971.
11. Watanabe, Y., and Dreifus, L. S.: Second degree atrioventricular block. Cardiovasc. Res. 1: 150, 1967.
12. Hoffman, B. F., Paes de Carvalho, A., de Mello, W. C., and Cranefield, P. F.: Electrical activity of single fibers of the atrioventricular node. Circ. Res. 7: 11, 1959.
13. Cranefield, P. F., Hoffman, B. F., and Paes de Carvalho, A.: The effect of acetylcholine on single fibers of the atrioventricular node. Circ. Res. 7: 19, 1959.
14. Paes de Carvalho, A.: Cellular electrophysiology of the atrial specialized tissues. In Paes de Carvalho, A., de Mello, W. C., and Hoffman, B. F. (eds.): *The specialized Tissues of the Heart*, Elsevier Press, Inc., Amsterdam, 1962, p. 115.
15. Matsuda, K., Hoshi, T., and Kameyama, S.: Action of acetylcholine and adrenaline upon the membrane potential of the atrioventricular node (Tawara). Tohoku J. Exp. Med. 68: 16, 1958.
16. Watanabe, Y., and Dreifus, L. S.: Interactions of lanatoside C and potassium on atrioventricular conduction in rabbits. Circ. Res. 27: 931, 1970.
17. Watanabe, Y., and Dreifus, L. S.: Interactions of quinidine and potassium on atrioventricular transmission. Circ. Res. 20: 434, 1967.
18. Watanabe, Y., and Dreifus, L. S.: Inhomogeneous conduction in the A-V node. A model for re-entry. Amer. Heart J. 70: 505, 1965.
19. Janse, M. J.: Influence of the direction of the atrial wave front on A-V nodal transmission in isolated hearts of rabbits. Circ. Res. 25: 439, 1969.
20. Watanabe, Y., and Dreifus, L. S.: Mechanisms of supernormal A-V conduction. Fed. Proc. 25: 635, 1966.
21. Van Dam, R. T., Moore, E. N., and Hoffman, B. F.: Initiation and conduction of impulses in partially depolarized cardiac fibers. Amer. J. Physiol. 204: 1133, 1963.
22. Weidmann, S.: *Elektrophysiologie der Herzmuskelfaser*. Hans Huber, Bern, 1956.
23. Singer, D. H., Lazzara, R., and Hoffman, B. F.: Interrelationships between automaticity and conduction in Purkinje fibers. Circ. Res. 21: 537, 1967.
24. MacWilliam, J. A.: Fibrillar contraction of the heart. J. Physiol. 8: 298, 1887.
25. Lewis, T.: *Mechanism and Graphic Registration of Heart Beat*. Shaw and Sons, Ltd., London, 1925.
26. Rosenblueth, A., and Garcia Ramos, J.: Studies on flutter and fibrillation. Amer. Heart J. 33: 677, 1947.
27. Schmitt, F. O., and Erlanger, J.: Directional differences in the conduction of impulse through heart muscle and their possible relation to extrasystolic and fibrillatory contractions. Amer. J. Physiol. 87: 326, 1928.
28. Rytand, D. A., Toole, J. G., and Weinreb, I.: Circus movement in atrial flutter. Circulation 34 (Suppl. 3): 204, 1966.
29. Durrer, D., Schoo, L., Schuilenburg, R. M., and Wellens, H. J. J.: The role of premature beats in the initiation and the termination of supraventricular tachycardia in the Wolff-Parkinson-White syndrome. Circulation 36: 644, 1967.
30. Dreifus, L. S., Nichols, H., Morse, D., Watanabe, Y., and Truex, R.: Control of recurrent tachycardia of Wolff-Parkinson-White syndrome by surgical ligature of the A-V bundle. Circulation 38: 1030, 1968.
31. Scherf, D.: Zur Entstehungsweise der Extrasystolen und der extrasystolischen Allorhythmien. Ztschr. Ges. Exp. Med. 51: 816, 1926.
32. Kaufmann, R., and Rothberger, C. J.: Beitrag zur Kenntnis der Entstehungsweise der extrasystolischen Allorhythmien. Ztschr. Ges. Exp. Med. 5: 349, 1917.

33. Dreifus, L. S., Katz, M., Watanabe, Y., and Likoff, W.: Clinical significance of disorders of impulse formation and conduction in the atrioventricular junction. Amer. J. Cardiol. 11: 384, 1963.

34. Moe, G. K., and Abildskov, J. A.: Atrial fibrillation as a self-sustaining arrhythmia independent of focal discharge. Amer. Heart J. 58: 59, 1959.

35. Sano, T., Tsuchihashi, H., and Shimamoto, T.: Ventricular fibrillation studied by the microelectrode method. Circ. Res. 6: 41, 1958.

36. Moe, G. K., Rheinboldt, W. C., and Abildskov, J. A.: A computer model of atrial fibrillation. Amer. Heart J. 67: 200, 1964.

37. Hogancamp, C. E., Kardesch, M., Danforth, W. H., and Bing, R. J.: Transmembrane electrical potentials in ventricular tachycardia and fibrillation. Amer. Heart J. 57: 214, 1959.

38. Watanabe, Y., and Dreifus, L. S.: Mechanisms of ventricular fibrillation. Jap Heart J. 7: 110, 1966.

39. Scherf, D.: The mechanism of flutter and fibrillation. Amer. Heart J. 71: 273, 1966.

40. Matsuda, K., Hoshi, T., and Kameyama, S.: Effects of aconitine on the cardiac membrane potential of the dog. Jap. J. Physiol. 9: 419, 1959.

41. Nahum, L. H., and Hoff, H. E.: Production of auricular fibrillation by application of acetyl-β-methycholine to localized regions on the auricular surface. Amer. J. Physiol. 129: 428, 1940.

42. Burn, J. H.: Ion movement and cardiac fibrillation. Proc. Roy. Soc. Med. (London) 50: 725, 1957.

43. Smirk, F. H., and Palmer, D. G.: A myocardial syndrome. With particular reference to the occurrence of sudden death and premature systoles interrupting antecedent T waves. Amer. J. Cardiol. 6: 620, 1960.

44. Wiggers, C. J., and Wégria, R.: Ventricular fibrillation due to a single localized induction and condenser shocks applied during the vulnerable phase of ventricular systole. Amer. J. Physiol. 128: 500, 1940.

16

Office Management of Cardiac Arrhythmias

ARTHUR M. MASTER, M.D.

In the months of May, June, and July 1970, we kept a record of all of the patients we examined in whom we detected any disturbances in cardiac rate or rhythm, e.g., tachycardia, premature contractions, bradycardia or heart block. Of 100 such patients, 31 were classified as having paroxysmal auricular tachycardia (PAT) alone or associated with other disturbances of rhythm, 24 as having ventricular premature contractions (VPC), 14 as having auricular premature contractions (APC), 13 as having APC associated always with VPC, 7 as having sinus bradycardia (SB), and a miscellaneous group of 11, consisting of 5 with heart block, 2 with constant auricular fibrillation, 2 with this irregularity which was always paroxysmal, and 2 with paroxysmal auricular fibrillation which finally became constant. As indicated in Tables 16.1 to 16.6, these findings were usually associated with other cardiac irregularities or with slow or fast rhythm, although at times each was the sole disturbance.

In the description to each of the first five tables, the check marks should really be ditto marks. They refer to the caption placed vertically above them, and their frequency is indicated by the number to the left of them in the first column of the table.

In Table 16.1, we have listed the incidence of PAT or simple paroxysmal tachycardia (PT). The PT was not the type that lasted days, caused heart failure, or required hospitalization, but it was the most frequent disorder we discovered. This came as rather a surprise, but it was substantiated. These patients were for the most part persons we examined repeatedly, and the presence of cardiac disorders was corroborated on many occasions. They were seen in the office, they were ambulatory, and the PT was their chief complaint, the signal reason for their visit. The heart rate was 150 per minute, confirmed by our own electrocardiograms and by those taken by referring doctors and documented by detailed questioning. I would drum my knuckles on the desk top at different speeds and ask the patient to tell me when the rate was similar to his heart rate; the patient would always

183

Table 16.1. *Paroxysmal tachycardia (31 cases), alone or combined with other arrhythmias**

PT	VPC	APC	SB	Aur. Fib.	P. Aur. Fib.	P. Aur. Flut.
31	16	9	5	4	3	2
10	(1 SAB)					
7	√	(1 Multiform, 3 bigeminy, 1 salvo)				
3	√	√	√			
2	√	√				
2	√					
1	√	√		√	√	√
1	√	√			√	
1	√			√		√
1	√		√			
1				√	√	
1	(Carotid sinus, syncope)		√			
1				√		

* Check mark refers to the irregularity vertically above in the first row of the table. The numbers in the left column represent the frequency with which that particular arrhythmia was found.

pick a very fast rate, from 140 to 180 per minute. Often the patient knew his rate. When the tachycardia appeared, the patient would lie down, relax, and take tranquilizers until the episode ceased. Sometimes he stopped it himself by applying pressure to one side of his neck or by taking a deep breath and holding it, but usually the tachycardia ran its course from a very few minutes to hours.

PT was found in 31 patients. In 10, it was the only disturbance but, as shown in Table 16.1, it was associated with VPC in 16 patients, with APC in 9, with SB in 5, with auricular fibrillation in 4, with paroxysmal auricular fibrillation in 3, and with true paroxysmal auricular flutter in 2 patients. At times, three, four, and even five different arrhythmias were discovered in the same patient, in addition to the paroxysmal tachycardia. The more numerous these different cardiac disorders in the same patient, the fewer the number of patients affected. Thus, there was only one patient with paroxysmal tachycardia, VPC, APC, paroxysmal auricular fibrillation, and paroxysmal auricular flutter.

In 7 patients, the PT was associated with VPC alone, in 3 with VPC, APC, and SB (less than 60 beats per minute), in 2 with VPC and APC, and in 2 others with APC alone. There were a few patients with multiple other irregularities.

After PT, the most frequent arrhythmia was VPC, detected in 24 patients

Table 16.2. *Ventricular premature contractions (24 cases) alone or combined with other arrhythmias*

VPC	Aur. Fib.	P.Aur. Fib.
24	3	1
2 0	(1 salvo, 1 mult.+bigeminy)	
3	✓	
1		✓

Table 16.3. *Auricular premature contractions (14 cases) alone or combined with other arrhythmias*

APC	Aur. Fib.	P.Aur. Fib.	Aur. Flut.
14	2	1	1
11	(1 bigeminy, 1 bigeminy+SAB, 1 bigeminy+salvo, 1 carotid sinus + syncope)		
1	✓	✓	
1	✓		
1	(rate controlled)		✓

(Table 16.2). In 20 patients, this was the only irregularity. In 1 of these patients there was a salvo of three VPCs in succession, and in another patient, multiform and bigeminal types were observed. In 3 patients, auricular fibrillation was present permanently, and in 1 patient paroxysmal auricular fibrillation was present permanently.

The next most frequent arrhythmia encountered was APC, which was discovered in 14 patients (Table 16.3). In 11, it was the sole disturbance, but in 1 patient it was associated with a bigeminy, in another with a bigeminy and salvos of VPCs, and in another with carotid sinus sensitivity and syncope. One patient showed both auricular fibrillation and paroxysmal auricular fibrillation which became chronic, 1 had permanent auricular fibrillation, and 1 had an auricular flutter.

The next most common arrhythmia, found in 13 patients, was the combination of APC and VPC, which were always observed together (Table 16.4). In 9 patients, this combination was the only disturbance, but in 4 it was associated with bigeminy of VPC and in 1 with a bigeminy and salvos of VP beats. Four others each had other irregularities in addition to the combination of APC and VPC.

From patients with rapid ventricular or normal heart rates, we now come to 7 patients with sinus bradycardia, *i.e.*, heart rates of 60 per minute or less (Table 16.5). This was the sole cardiac disturbance in 3 patients, but in the other 4 it was associated with APC or VPC and, in one of these, with APC and paroxysmal auricular fibrillation which finally became permanent.

There were 5 patients with heart block (HB). One patient had complete HB of congenital origin; in the other 4 HB was partial. Two patients had chronic auricular fibrillation alone, 2 were subject to paroxysmal auricular fibrillation which became permanent, 2 developed paroxysmal auricular fibrillation which became chronic, and 1 patient had partial HB with supraventricular premature contractions (Table 16.6).

The most common form of therapy, utilized in 21 instances, was the elimination of all drinks and food from the diet that contained caffeine (*e.g.*, coffee, tea, "Cokes," Seven-Up, coffee ice cream, and "diet" or low calorie drinks that contain caffeine for stimulation). Adherence to this practice alone was frequently successful in abolishing the cardiac disturb-

Table 16.4. *Combination of APC and VPC, always together (13 cases)*

APC	VPC	PT	Aur. Fib.	P.Aur. Fib.	Aur. Flut.	P.Aur. Flut.	VT
13	13	2	1	2	1	1	1
9	√	(4 bigeminy, 1 bigeminy + salvo)					
1	√						√
1	√				√	√	
1	√	√		√			
1	√	√	√	√			

Table 16.5. *Sinus bradycardia (7 cases) either alone or in combination with other irregularities*

SB	APC	VPC	Aur. Fib.	P.Aur. Fib.
7	1	3	1	1
3				
1	√			
2		√		
1	√		√	√

Table 16.6. *Miscellaneous group of arrhythmias (11 cases)*

5	HB (2 partial, 1 VPC-SB-syncope, 1 VPC, 1 congenital)
2	Aur. Fib.
2	P.Aur. Fib.
2	P.Aur. Fib.→ Aur. Fib.
1	PC

ance. For patients taking diuretics, those agents which cause or enhance arrhythmias and even tachycardia, particularly those containing thiazides, were changed to those that had no such propensities or only in a minor way (*e.g.*, furosemide, ethacrynic acid). If the diuretic contained only a small amount of thiazide, potassium was supplemented in a liquid vehicle or in potassium-containing foods such as tomatoes, bananas, fruits and fruit juices, dried apricots, and dried prunes. Potassium was always given in a liquid preparation further diluted with water. Potassium chloride was never given by itself because it is so indigestible and causes gastric irritation. The actual fruit rather than the juice was preferable, since the latter, too, is indigestible, and stomach distention could aggravate the arrhythmia. In cases of heart failure, the electrolytes were watched carefully, particularly the potassium content of the blood.

The next most frequent type of therapy employed was digitalis, which was prescribed in 20 patients. Here, too, in some instances the drug was supplemented with potassium in the form of a liquid drug or food containing it.

Frequently diuretics and digitalis were given together but, in the absence of heart failure, digitalis was prescribed to control the ventricular rate in auricular fibrillation or auricular flutter, or in an endeavor to transform the irregularity to a normal sinus rhythm.

In 18 patients we prescribed quinidine, usually because of premature contractions but also on a more or less permanent basis to prevent paroxysmal tachycardia, fibrillation, or flutter.

Propranolol was dispensed to 16 patients but only because these patients also had angina pectoris. For an antiarrhythmic agent, we found other preparations more valuable.

Chlordiazepoxide (Librium) was prescribed to 16 patients for the management of tachycardia or arrhythmia if these were associated with alarm and nervousness.

Before initiating treatment, every effort was made to determine the cause of the rate or rhythm disorder. Excessive cigarette smoking was a factor 12 times, and proved by the disappearance of the cardiac disorder when smoking was stopped and its reappearance when smoking was resumed. Liquor was found to be the cause of PAT or paroxysmal auricular fibrillation in 7 patients. The disorder in these 7 patients was always controlled when the patient "went on the wagon" or drastically curtailed his drinking. Usually one or two drinks a day played no role.

Procaine amide was prescribed in 9 patients for premature contractions or maintenance of a regular sinus rhythm. Quinidine was usually our first choice for the treatment of these disturbances but, in patients sensitive to this agent, procaine amide was substituted.

The use of potassium alone was found to help curtail these disturbances.

It was never prescribed first for a simple irregularity, but it made possible the continuance of digitalis or a thiazide diuretic or both. It was prescribed in one of the many more or less palatable liquid forms on the market, and a teaspoonful or tablespoonful of the preparation itself was always taken in water.

Atropine was administered in 5 patients with either HB or SB in whom the slow ventricular rate produced dizziness, feelings of faintness, or actual syncope (1 patient). It was given orally in the amount of $\frac{1}{150}$ or $\frac{1}{100}$ grain q.i.d., whichever caused a little dryness in the mouth. In 2 of our patients with complete HB, the insertion of a permanent pacemaker was necessary.

In patients with the slow ventricular rate, the consumption of coffee, tea, and other caffeine-containing drinks was often encouraged. In 2 patients, this step alone helped to increase the heart rate. One was a patient with congenital complete HB and the other a patient with SB of about 35 beats per minute and no actual symptoms.

Dilantin, 100 mg. q.i.d., helped in 3 patients with ventricular premature beats, one of whom was subject to epileptic seizures.

The frequency of PT as the signal complaint and the fact that many irregularities occurred in the same patient were enlightening. I had not expected this.

Many years ago I made it a practice to teach the patient how to feel his pulse and to count his pulse rate. I demonstrated it to the patient on his own radial pulse. The small area on the wrist right next to the hand between the outer border of the wrist and the first obvious tendon was palpated first on my wrist and then on the patient's own. He was advised to press lightly or with moderate force, with index and middle fingers, until he felt the pulse beat best. With practice, the patient can report how many irregularities occur per minute. In fact he can learn, in the average case, how much quinidine or procaine amide to use to regulate it. This procedure is particularly important for the patient who is not aware of his cardiac irregularities, which often may consist of numerous premature beats, or even salvos of them. He is told that the irregularity in his pulse rate has significance. The interesting point is that the patient does not mind taking his pulse. In fact, he is pleased to cooperate. He rather likes the idea of helping the doctor and is not fearful in the least.

17

The Effect of Cardiovascular Drugs on Atrioventricular and Intraventricular Conduction

ANTHONY N. DAMATO, M.D.

The recording of His bundle activity in man has permitted a more precise assessment of atrioventricular (AV) conduction.[1-11] One important application of this technique is in the evaluation of various cardiac drugs on AV conduction. The technique is safe and relatively simple to perform.[1] A tripolar electrode catheter is percutaneously inserted into a femoral vein and fluoroscopically positioned in the region of the tricuspid valve. The proximal terminals are formed into bipolar leads which are led into the AC input of an electrocardiograph (ECG) preamplifier. The recordings are made at filter frequency settings of 40 to 500 Hz. at fast paper speeds (100 to 200 mm. per sec.). The bipolar intracardiac recordings consist of an atrial electrogram (A) from the low atrial septal region, a His deflection (H), and a ventricular electrogram (V) (Fig. 17.1).

The interval from the onset of the low atrial septal electrogram to the onset of the His deflection (A-H interval) is a measure of AV nodal conduction time. The interval from the onset of the His deflection to the onset of ventricular depolarization (H-V interval) is a measure of His-Purkinje conduction time. Since most cardiac drugs affect sinus rate, a more precise assessment of a drug's action is obtained by maintaining a constant atrial rate with a bipolar atrial pacing catheter. Furthermore, by programming atrial extrasystoles, the effect of a particular drug on the relative, functional, and effective refractory periods of various portions of the conduction system can also be studied.

This report deals with the effects of several of the more commonly used cardiac drugs on AV nodal and His-Purkinje conduction times. A knowledge of these effects can at times be important in the selection of a drug for the treatment of a cardiac rhythm disturbance. In addition, this knowledge may help explain certain post-treatment phenomena.

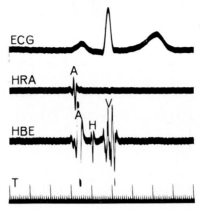

FIG. 17.1. The tracings from the top downward are electrocardiographic lead 1. HRA, a bipolar electrogram recorded from the high right atrium; HBE, a bipolar His bundle electrogram recording in which A is a bipolar electrogram recording from the low atrial septal region, H is the bundle of His deflection, and V is the ventricular electrogram. The A-H interval as recorded on the HBE tracing is a measure of AV nodal conduction, while the H-V interval is a measure of conduction within the His-Purkinje system. T, time base in which the large deflections equal 100 msec. and the smaller deflections equal 10 msec.

ATROPINE

Atropine produces an increase in the sinus rate. In addition, atropine enhances AV nodal conduction and has little or no effect on conduction within the His-Purkinje system. The effects of atropine on AV nodal conduction are illustrated in Figure 17.2. The top panel illustrates the control period in which the right atrium was stimulated at a rate of 120 per min. AV nodal conduction as measured by the SH interval was 277 msec., while conduction within the ventricular specialized conduction system (H-V interval) measured 33 msec. The effects of 1 mg. of atropine injected intravenously are illustrated in the bottom panel of Figure 17.2. At the same paced heart rate, atropine markedly shortened AV nodal conduction time. The S-H interval decreased to 145 msec., while the H-V interval remained unchanged. It is the enhancement of AV nodal conduction which makes atropine a useful agent in the treatment of Type I second degree AV block (AV nodal Wenckebach phenomenon). The Type I second degree AV block which may occur during acute diaphragmatic myocardial infarctions is generally a transient phenomenon. In most instances, 1:1 AV conduction can be established with the use of small doses (0.5 to 1.0 mg.) of atropine. Occasionally, the increase in sinus rate produced by atropine may exceed the capacity of the AV node to transmit impulses to the ventricles, and a Type I AV block is converted to a high degree (2:1) AV block.

The positive chronotropic effect of atropine on the sinoatrial pacemaker,

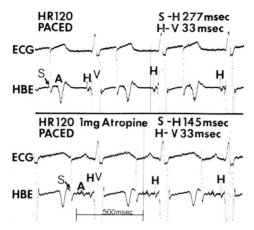

Fig. 17.2. The effects of atropine on AV nodal and His-Purkinje conduction. S denotes the stimulus artifact delivered to the right atrium at a rate of 120 per min. Atropine shortened AV nodal conduction time from 277 to 145 msec. (Modified from Damato *et al.*, Circulation 39: 287, 1969.[3])

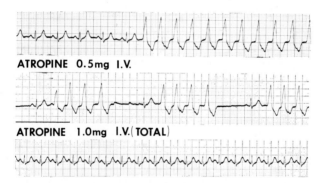

Fig. 17.3. In the top panel, a sinus rhythm is suddenly interrupted by a ventricular tachycardia at a rate of approximately 130 per min. The middle panel was recorded following the administration of 0.5 mg. of atropine. Following 1 mg. of atropine (bottom panel), the atrial rate was increased sufficiently to override the ventricular tachycardia. I.V., intravenous administration.

along with its enhancing effect on AV nodal conduction, makes this drug useful in overriding some ventricular tachycardias. This is illustrated in Figure 17.3. In the top panel, sinus rhythm is suddenly interrupted by the onset of a ventricular tachycardia at a rate of approximately 130 per min. The middle panel was recorded following the administration of 0.5 mg. of atropine. As shown in the bottom panel, 1:1 AV conduction resulted when 1 mg. of atropine accelerated the atrial rate above the firing rate of the idioventricular pacemaker.

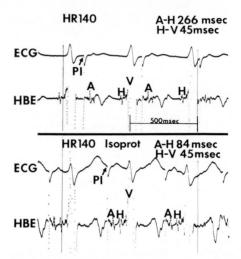

FIG. 17.4. In the top panel, atrial pacing at 140 per min. produced a variable but prolonged A-H interval of approximately 266 msec. At the same paced heart rate (HR), isoproterenol (Isoprot) markedly shortened the A-H interval to 84 msec. (Modified from Damato *et al.*, Circulation 39: 287, 1969.[3])

ISOPROTERENOL

The effects of isoproterenol on AV nodal and His-Purkinje conduction are similar to those of atropine. Isoproterenol enhances AV nodal conduction and has little or no effect on conduction within the bundle branch-Purkinje system. This is illustrated in Figure 17.4. In the top panel, atrial pacing at a rate of 140 per min. produced a slightly variable but markedly prolonged AV nodal conduction time of 266 msec. Conduction time from the bundle of His to the onset of ventricular depolarization (H-V interval) measured 45 msec. Following the infusion of isoproterenol at a rate of 4 μg. per min., AV nodal conduction was markedly shortened to 84 msec. with no effect on the H-V interval.

DIGITALIS

The arrhythmogenic properties of digitalis are well known. Equally well known are the effects which digitalis has on AV nodal conduction. This latter effect makes digitalis a useful antiarrhythmic agent, as in the treatment of atrial fibrillation with a rapid ventricular response. Figure 17.5 depicts the effects of digitalis on AV nodal conduction. For illustrative purposes, the results of an animal experiment are shown. Similar results have been demonstrated in man. In the top panel, the AV nodal conduction time prior to digitalis was 84 msec. Following the administration of digitalis, as shown in the bottom panel, the A-H interval at the same heart rate

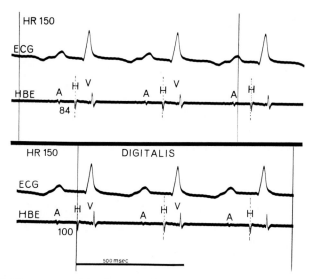

F𝚒𝚐. 17.5. The top panel is the control period. The bottom panel was recorded following the infusion of digitalis, which prolonged AV nodal conduction time from 84 to 100 msec. The H-V interval remained unchanged.

increased to 100 msec. The H-V interval remains constant. In atrial fibrillation, digitalis slows the ventricular rate by causing greater concealment of impulses within the AV node.

PROPRANOLOL

The beta adrenergic blocking agent, propranolol, has effects on AV conduction which are qualitatively similar to those of digitalis. Propranolol produces AV nodal conduction delay and has little or no effect on intraventricular conduction. Figure 17.6 is representative of 10 clinical studies in which the effects of intravenous propranolol (7 to 10 mg.) were measured. Like digitalis, propranolol also causes greater concealment of atrial impulses within the AV node and thereby slows the ventricular rate during acute atrial fibrillation.

ALPRENOLOL

Alprenolol is also a beta adrenergic blocking agent which affects AV conduction in man in a manner similar to that of propranolol. In Figure 17.7, the top panel was recorded prior to and the bottom panel following the intravenous administration of 15 mg. of alprenolol. In the control period, the A-H and H-V intervals were 260 and 50 msec., respectively. Alprenolol produced high degree (2:1) AV block. The nonconducted atrial

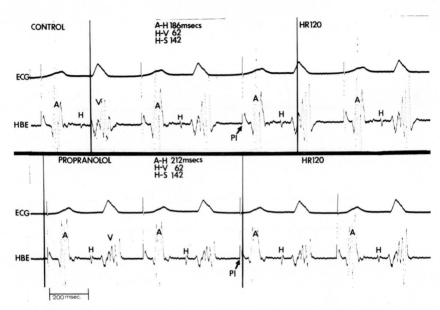

Fig. 17.6. The effect of intravenous propranolol (0.1 mg. per kg. of body weight) on AV conduction. At a similar atrial rate of 120 per min., propranolol prolonged AV nodal conduction from 186 to 212 msec. (Modified from Berkowitz *et al.*, Circulation 40: 855, 1969).

impulses were blocked proximal to the bundle of His. This drug, like propranolol, has no significant effect on His-Purkinje conduction time as measured by the H-V interval. In a clinical study of 20 patients, we have observed that the effective dose of alprenolol is approximately twice that of propranolol.

LIDOCAINE

Probably the most commonly used antiarrhythmic agent for the treatment of ventricular arrhythmias is lidocaine. The drug can be injected intravenously as a 50- to 150-mg. bolus. Recently Rosen and associates studied the effects of 2 per cent lidocaine on AV nodal and intraventricular conduction in 10 patients.[8] The results of these studies demonstrated that lidocaine had minimal effects on AV nodal conduction time as measured by the A-H interval. In all patients, lidocaine had no effect on His-Purkinje conduction time (H-V interval). Figure 17.8 is a recording obtained from a patient who had received a total dose of 150 mg. of lidocaine. The top panel is the control, and the bottom panel was recorded following administration of lidocaine. The A-H and H-V intervals were unaffected by lidocaine.

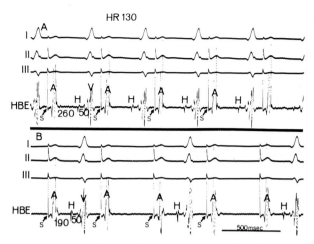

FIG. 17.7. The effects of alprenolol (beta adrenergic blocking agent) on AV conduction. In the control period, the A-H and H-V intervals at a paced atrial rate of 130 per min. measured 260 and 50 msec., respectively. Following the intravenous infusion of 20 mg. of alprenolol (bottom panel), 2:1 AV block occurred at the same paced atrial rate. The nonconducted atrial impulses were blocked proximal to the bundle of His.

PROCAINAMIDE

Rosen and associates have evaluated the effects of procainamide (200 to 500 mg.) in 15 patients requiring antiarrhythmic therapy for atrial and ventricular arrhythmias.[9] The effects of procainamide on AV nodal conduction were variable. In nine subjects, AV nodal conduction time increased by varied amounts. Four subjects showed no significant change in conduction, and one patient developed a significant decrease in AV nodal conduction following administration of the drug. The effects of procainamide on conduction within the His-Purkinje system were more consistent. In 13 of 15 subjects, H-V prolongation occurred which was between 8 and 33 per cent of control values. In two subjects, intraventricular conduction was not affected by the drug. Procainamide's effect on His-Purkinje conduction time is in contrast to other commonly used antiarrhythmic agents, such as lidocaine, propranolol, and diphenylhydantoin. The latter drugs do not significantly alter intraventricular conduction.

The prolongation of intraventricular conduction time by procainamide probably contributes in part to this drug's antiarrhythmic action. Reentrant ventricular arrhythmias can result when a unidirectional conduction delay or block exists in a Purkinje muscle region. By further slowing intraventricular conduction, procainamide may cause the propagating impulse to be completely blocked within the re-entrant circuit and thereby

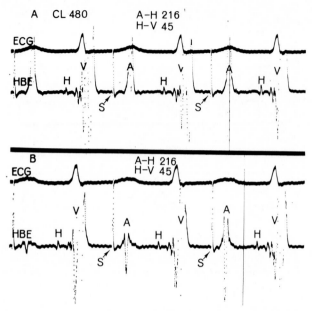

FIG. 17.8. Lidocaine, 150 mg., had no effect on AV nodal or His-Purkinje conduction time as measured by the A-H and H-V intervals. CL, control.

abolish the re-entrant rhythm. On the other hand, prolongation of intraventricular conduction by procainamide may create re-entrant circuits which in turn can result in serious ventricular arrhythmias.

DIPHENYLHYDANTOIN

The usefulness of diphenylhydantoin in the treatment of cardiac arrhythmias was first established in 1950.[12] Since that time, the drug has been shown in several clinical and experimental studies to be effective in abolishing cardiac arrhythmias resulting from various causes.[13-15] The effects of diphenylhydantoin on AV nodal and His-Purkinje conduction were studied in 15 subjects, who received intravenous doses between 250 to 1000 mg.[7] In 12 subjects, diphenylhydantoin produced a shortening of the A-H interval, and in three subjects the drug had no effect on AV nodal conduction time. Diphenylhydantoin has been shown to counteract the AV nodal conduction delay produced by digitalis. Diphenylhydantoin would appear to be a more useful drug in the treatment of digitalis-induced ventricular arrhythmia, especially when the latter has also produced significant AV nodal delay. In none of the 15 subjects studied did diphenylhydantoin produce a prolongation of intraventricular conduction time. Thus, diphenylhydantoin appears less likely to result in re-entrant ventricular arrhythmias.

This work was supported in part by the Federal Health Program Service, United States Public Health Service Project Py 71-1 and National Institutes of Health Projects HE 11829 and HE 12536.

REFERENCES

1. Scherlag, B. J., Lau, S. H., Helfant, R. H., Berkowitz, W. D., Stein, E., and Damato, A. N.: Catheter technique for recording His bundle activity in man. Circulation 39: 13, 1969.
2. Damato, A. N., Lau, S. H., Berkowitz, W. D., Rosen, K. M., and Lisi, K. R.: Recording of specialized conducting fibers (A-V nodal, His bundle, and right bundle branch) in man using an electrode catheter technique. Circulation 39: 435, 1969.
3. Damato, A. N., Lau, S. H., Helfant, R. H., Stein, E., Patton, R. D., Scherlag, B. J., and Berkowitz, W. D.: A study of heart block in man using His bundle recordings. Circulation 39: 287, 1969.
4. Lau, S. H., Damato, A. N., Berkowitz, W. D., and Patton, R. D.: A study of atrioventricular conduction in atrial fibrillation and flutter in man using His bundle recordings. Circulation 30: 71, 1969.
5. Damato, A. N., and Lau, S. H.: Clinical value of the electrogram of the conduction system. Progr. Cardiovasc. Dis. 12: 119, 1970.
6. Berkowitz, W. D., Wit, A. L., Lau, S. H., Steiner, C., and Damato, A. N.: The effects of propranolol on cardiac conduction. Circulation 40: 855, 1969.
7. Damato, A. N., Berkowitz, W. D., Patton, R. D., and Lau, S. H.: The effects of diphenylhydantoin on atrioventricular and intraventricular conduction in man. Amer. Heart J. 79: 51, 1970.
8. Rosen, K. M., Lau, S. H., Stein, E., and Damato, A. N.: The effects of lidocaine on atrioventricular and intraventricular conduction in man. Amer. J. Cardiol. 25: 1, 1970.
9. Rosen, K. M., Lau, S. H., Stein, E., Wit, A. L., and Damato, A. N.: The effects of procainamide on atrioventricular and intraventricular conduction, unpublished observations.
10. Wit, A. L., Weiss, M. B., Berkowitz, W. D., Rosen, K. M., Steiner, C., and Damato, A. N.: Patterns of atrioventricular conduction in man. Circ. Res. 27: 345, 1970.
11. Narula, O. S., Cohen, L. S., Samet, P., Lister, J. W., Scherlag, B., and Hildner, F. J.: Localization of A-V conduction defects in man by recording of the His bundle electrogram. Amer. J. Cardiol. 25: 228, 1969.
12. Harris, A. S., and Kokernot, R. H.: Effects of diphenylhydantoin sodium (Dilantin sodium) and phenobarbital sodium upon ectopic ventricular tachycardia in acute myocardial infarction. Amer. J. Physiol. 163: 505, 1950.
13. Conn, R. D.: Diphenylhydantoin sodium in cardiac arrhythmias. New Engl. J. Med. 272: 277, 1965.
14. Mercer, E. N., and Osborne, J. A.: Current status of diphenylhydantoin in heart disease. Ann. Intern. Med. 67: 1084, 1967.
15. Bigger, T. J., Schmidt, D. H., and Kutt, H.: Relationship between the plasma level of diphenylhydantoin sodium and its antiarrhythmic effects. Circulation 38: 363, 1968.

18

The Treatment of Coronary Thrombosis since Herrick

PAUL D. WHITE, M.D.

On December 6, 1912, James B. Herrick of Chicago published in the *Journal of the American Medical Association* one of the most important medical papers ever written, entitled "Clinical Features of Sudden Obstruction of the Coronary Arteries."[1] It was the lead article, and yet for a decade or more it remained unrecognized. As a friend and student of Herrick, I once asked him about this delay; his answer was that he never knew why. Even his own colleagues and students in Chicago were slow to grasp its significance. I suggest three reasons: first and most important, coronary thrombosis was not nearly the common disease it has slowly become since; second, it was a new idea to clinicians, although well known to pathologists for a good many decades before the days of the clinical-pathological conference, and like many new ideas, it was slow to be accepted; and third, there were very few science writers in those days.

I have reread this paper and was interested to find Herrick so far ahead of his time. For background, let me quote his first few sentences and a few paragraphs which reveal the fact that he realized that survival was often dependent on the existence or development of an adequate anastomotic and collateral coronary circulation which, even in those days with no surgical and very little medical therapy, allowed complete recovery to take place spontaneously, that is, by nature. The only measures that were used routinely were opiate for pain and shock, and rest in bed with nursing care. And now I quote:

Obstruction of a coronary artery or of any of its large branches has long been regarded as a serious accident. Several events contributed toward the prevalence of the view that this condition was almost always suddenly fatal. Parry's writings on angina pectoris and its relation to coronary disease, Jenner's observations on the same condition centering about John Hunter's case, Thorvaldsen's tragic death in the theater in Copenhagen with the finding of a plugged coronary, sharply attracted attention to the relation between the coronary and sudden death. . . .

But there are reasons for believing that even the largest branches of the coronary arteries may be occluded—at times acutely occluded—without resulting death, at least without death in the immediate future. Even the main trunk may at times be obstructed and the patient live. It is the object of this paper to present a few facts along this line, and particularly to describe some of the clinical manifestations of sudden yet not immediately fatal cases of coronary obstruction. . . .

One may conclude, therefore, from a consideration of the clinical histories of numerous cases in which there has been careful autopsy control, from animal experiments and from anatomic study, that there is no inherent reason why stoppage of a large branch of a coronary artery, or even of a main trunk, must of necessity cause sudden death. Rather may it be concluded that while sudden death often does occur, yet at times it is postponed for several hours or even days, and in some instances a complete, i.e., functionally complete, recovery ensues. . . .

The variations in the results are to be accounted for in part by variations in the freedom with which anastomosing branches occur. . . . The condition of the remaining vessels as to patency and presence of sclerosis must play an important part in deciding how much they are capable of doing in the way of compensatory nutrition to the anemic myocardium; the strength of the heart itself, as determined, perhaps, by old valvular or myocardial disease, would also have its influence. And presumably a sudden overwhelming obstruction, with comparatively normal vessels, would be followed by a profounder shock than the gradual narrowing of a lumen through sclerosis which has accustomed the heart to this pathologic condition and has perhaps caused collateral circulation through neighboring or anastomosing vessels to be compensatorily increased. The influence of the vessels of Thebesius is also not to be overlooked in this connection; compensatory circulation through these accessory channels may be of considerable importance in nourishing areas of heart muscle poorly supplied by sclerotic or obstructed arteries.

Let me end these significant quotations with the last paragraph of all; which deals with treatment: in particular, absolute rest and the use of digitalis. We may ourselves still fear too much to use digitalis in desperate cases when congestive heart failure has been set off by the acute episode. The danger of arrhythmia from digitalis can usually be controlled without omitting the help that digitalis brings.

If these cases [of severe coronary thrombosis] are recognized, the importance of absolute rest in bed for several days is clear. It would also seem to be far wiser to use digitalis, strophanthus or their congeners than to follow the routine practice of giving nitroglycerin or allied drugs. The hope for the damaged myocardium lies in the direction of securing a supply of blood through friendly neighboring vessels so as to restore so far as possible its functional integrity. Digitalis or strophanthus, by increasing the force of the heart's beat, would tend to help in this direction more than the nitrites. The prejudice against digitalis in cases in which the myocardium is weak is only partially grounded in fact. Clinical experience shows this remedy of great value in angina, and especially in cases of angina with low blood pressure, and these obstructive cases come under this head. The timely use of this remedy may occasionally in such cases save life. Quick results should also be sought by using it hypodermically or intravenously. Other quickly acting heart remedies would also be of service.

Speaking of digitalis brings me to the two interesting cases reported by S. A. Levine and C. L. Tranter in the *American Journal of the Medical Sciences*[2] without, incidentally, any mention of Herrick, whose classic paper of 1912 was still largely unrecognized. The article by Levine and Tranter was entitled "Infarction of the Heart Simulating Acute Abdominal Conditions." The abdominal pain in those two cases was undoubtedly the result of acute distension of the liver from serious congestive failure due to massive myocardial infarction, found in both cases at autopsy. The first of the two cases was actually explored surgically and died on the table, while the second, seen in consultation by the surgeons, was considered too ill for immediate operation and died the next day in serious heart failure and with complete atrioventricular block. Whether digitalization of these patients could have helped them seems unlikely, but myocardial failure of lesser degree might well respond.

In 1916 I was called to see a surgeon from Ohio who was visiting in the summer one of his Boston surgical friends on our North Shore of Long Island. His specialty was gall bladder surgery, and he had made a diagnosis of an acute attack in himself confirmed by his host. The reason why I was called was that he had developed an unusual complication of acute pericarditis and I was a young doctor just beginning an interest in cardiology. This finding seemed very odd at the time to all of us, but I suppose in retrospect now that he too had suffered acute congestion of the liver when his heart failed. But he, in contrast to the cases of Levine and Tranter, slowly recovered and returned home. However, his electrocardiogram taken back at home showed what we now recognize as a typical coronary pattern, and he died within a year. This was before Pardee had published his electrocardiographic sign of the "coronary T wave" in 1920.

It was only in the 1920s that we began to see and recognize coronary thrombosis as a disease susceptible of treatment. Some patients died quickly, as now, before they ever reached the hospital. As a matter of fact, we often felt that it was best to leave them at home for, with nursing care more available in those days, many completely recovered with avoidance of the physical and emotional stress of transportation to the hospital where, in those times, little could be done for them that could not be done at home. I believe that in that decade I took care of about half of my patients with coronary thrombosis at home, sharing the responsibility with the family doctor.

I was called to see my first case at home in January 1921 by my father, a family physician, after I had been in practice as a pioneer specialist in cardiovascular diseases for about 6 months. The patient was very ill and lived only about 10 days. Most of those early cases were severe, doubtless in part because of the fact that we were missing at least some of the more mildly afflicted patients, especially if they were younger. Most of my early cases were in their 60s, some were over 70, a few were in their 50s, and a rare patient was in his 40s. Of a random group of 12 of the cases in the early 1920s, 10 were men and only 2 were women.

We treated most of them by rest in bed for 3 weeks, although some other doctors often doubled or tripled such a sentence. The shorter length of this complete rest was later justified by our study in the 1930s of the speed of healing of myocardial infarction[3] and still later by the study on the frequency of rupture of the heart wall through a fresh myocardial lesion in psychotic patients during the first 10 days of their illness.[4] We noted that another few weeks of convalescence with the patient allowed to get up and around often sufficed before a return to part-time work in the course of 6 to 8 weeks altogether. We also found that a 3rd month of physical and emotional rehabilitation was often helpful if it could be arranged. When however, there was much concern in the patient's mind about his business or other important matters, we did, as also later in President Eisenhower's case, allow during the 2nd week (after the 1st week of sedation) some slowly increasing contact with the outside world by phone, letters, or visitor. This we discovered as a rule to be good therapy.

The entertaining debate between the proponents of the chair treatment of acute coronary cases and those who advocated bed rest began in the 1930s. It finally boiled down to the recognition by both sides that the orthopneic position was best, indeed essential, for a minority of cases with pulmonary congestion due to left ventricular failure, and that in all cases the heart in its recovery would have less work to do if the body position was not horizontal but rather placed with thorax and head in a sloping position above the horizontal. At that time, complete rest for the first 2 weeks could be best secured in an adjustable bed such as had to be contrived until the new type of hospital bed was invented. I well recall importing in the 1920s from England several of the heavy and clumsy Lewis "chair beds" for use by my coronary cases at the Massachusetts General Hospital. One other comment should be added, namely, that for bowel evacuation the sitting position is easiest for the patient's heart and equanimity, and therefore very early in our experience we allowed the use of the bedside commode but with the patient being lifted or at least supported with great care in the process.* One of my patients did, however, expire on such a commode, an event that was much more common with the use of the bedpan.

---

* President Eisenhower during his acute heart attack in 1955 blessed all of us, his doctors, for permitting him to be carried daily by two strong hospital orderlies to his bathroom for his bowel evacuations.

Through the years, there has been much experimentation with the diet in acute coronary thrombosis, but of course there cannot be the same rules for all. There are many factors to be considered, including the severity of the illness, the presence or absence of congestive failure, diabetes, gout, or hypercholesterolemia, the state of nutrition, including obesity, the food habits, and the liking of the individual. With very ill patients, I used to start with the Karell diet, consisting of four feedings a day of 200 cc. of skimmed milk each, and low in calories, fat, and sodium. For fat patients, the several weeks in the hospital offer an invaluable opportunity to reduce weight. A small amount of whiskey or wine according to taste daily has made the long hospital stay endurable for some patients, but I never permitted the use of tobacco.

And now as to medicines. I have already spoken of opiates and digitalis as having been prescribed when needed and I do not recall harmful results from the moderate use of either. Later on, when the modern, more effective diuretics came into use, I have often used them helpfully instead of digitalis or to supplement a smaller dosage thereof and, as a matter of fact, the mercurial diuretics for parenteral use were available earlier, even as far back as the late 1920s. I began to use quinidine sulphate when needed for arrhythmia early in the 1920s. It helped some patients and so, for 10 years or more, I kept it up more or less routinely in the dosage of 0.2 gram (3 grains) three or four times a day. But finally I gave up its routine use because I could not decide that it had reduced the mortality. During this period, I also tried the effect of epinephrine injected by a long needle through the precordial chest wall directly into the heart for cardiac standstill with or without ventricular fibrillation but, as I recall, I never resuscitated a single one of a score or more such patients. We used sedatives and hypnotics as seemed to be needed before the days of the more modern tranquilizers. In my review, I do not find that oxygen was easily available at first, but by the 1930s we employed it by mask or tent as needed for the sickest patients. The tent supplied a cooler, less humid atmosphere which in itself was beneficial to many patients. In recent decades, oxygen has become a more or less routine treatment, with considerable benefit in congested patients.

A word should be added about anticoagulants for coronary thrombosis. Anticoagulants entered the therapeutic field in the 1940s in the form of heparin and the dicoumarin derivatives. There has been all along considerable difference of opinion about their value but, based on the slight statistical evidence in its favor, I have continued to use Coumadin during the first 2 months after the event of coronary thrombosis and have omitted it thereafter if all goes well, unless there is frequent and serious angina pectoris or the patient refuses to follow my advice to control his obesity, to stop smoking, to establish a program of adequate physical activity, and to reduce to a minimum excessive stress, both physical and emotional. Certainly a part of the value of the anticoagulant is in preventing leg vein or other stasis thrombosis elsewhere during the weeks of physical rest.

Finally, in the early 1930s, we began seriously to undertake an organized effort to rehabilitate our patients with coronary thrombosis as we had done with our young people with acute and chronic rheumatic heart disease 10 years earlier. This was 20 years or more before we were faced in 1955 with the greatest challenge of all in the person of President Eisenhower. I have the impression nowadays that at times we may be overdoing our efforts of returning to full program, both physical and mental, some older patients who do not need to run or jog a few miles a day for their health. They can perhaps best walk into old age. Just recently, Vannevar Bush, the great engineer of World War II fame, asked me if I didn't think that we needed less physical exercise as we grew older, and that perhaps at his age he needed none at all. I am inclined to think him nearer right than those who keep urging us all to continue a strenuous exercise program until we drop. I dare say that there is a happy mean, and with that I shall stop.

REFERENCES

1. Herrick, J. B.: Clinical features of sudden obstruction of the coronary arteries. J. A. M. A., 59: 2015, 1912.
2. Levine, S. A., and Tranter, C. L.: Infarction of the heart simulating acute abdominal conditions. Amer. J. Med. Sci. 160: 57, 1918.
3. Mallory, K., White, P. D., and Salcedo-Salgar, J.: The speed of healing of myocardial infarction. Amer. Heart J. 18: 647, 1939.
4. Jetter, W. W., and White, P. D.: Rupture of the heart in patients in mental institutions. Ann. Intern. Med. 21: 783, 1944.

19

The Changing Coronary Care Unit

SYLVAN LEE WEINBERG, M.D., AND
JACQUES J. COL, M.D.

The coronary care unit (CCU) dates from 1962. Its beginnings were modest. In the simplest terms, it had three components: first, a group of patients likely to have acute rhythm disturbances: patients with acute myocardial infarction; second, equipment to detect and treat these arrhythmias; and third, people able to use the equipment effectively.

Figure 19.1 shows how small indeed was the early coronary care unit in relation to the total problem of acute coronary disease as represented by the heartlike structure. The first units were small, comprising three to four beds. The patient's stay was brief, usually 3 to 5 days. These units, however, quickly proved capable of obtaining the limited objective of treating rhythm disturbances in acute myocardial infarction. The mortality of hospitalized patients with acute infarction dropped from about 30 per cent to 15 to 20 per cent.[1-8]

The character of the unit began to evolve almost with its creation. What started as a coronary care unit soon became a part of the coronary care movement. We are in the midst of that movement today. One of the first changes was in the role of the nurse. She became the eyes, ears, and hands of the physician who could not be at the bedside at all times. She learned to recognize arrhythmias, to use drugs, and to use the defibrillator. Without her participation in this manner, the coronary care units did not improve the mortality.[5, 9, 9a, 9b] A new industry arose, teaching the nurse the methodology of coronary care.

Emphasis in the unit changed from defibrillation to prevention of fibrillation. "Aggressive management" was the watchword of the day.[6, 10, 11] The unit became a place to prevent arrhythmias and to avoid rather than respond to catastrophe. Inevitably, the units began to expand in size as more physicians became aware of them and as the demand for surveillance of suspected infarction increased. As it became apparent that disaster lurked

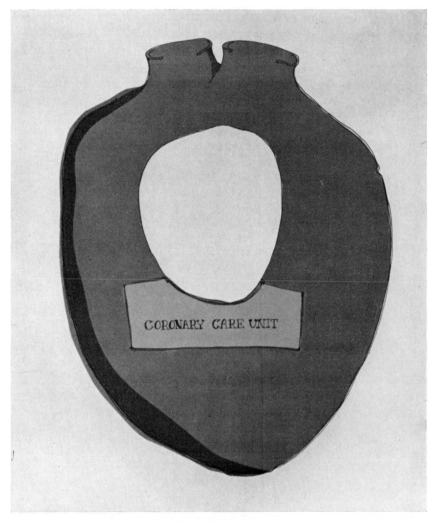

FIG. 19.1. A representation of the early coronary care unit in relation to the total problem of acute coronary disease.

in the first moments and hours of infarction, more beds were needed for the "suspect infarction."

Figure 19.2 uses the format of a gameboard to illustrate a total coronary care system. This represents a concept of the ultimate for which a hospital and a community might strive. The lower part of the diagram shows an expanded coronary care unit which became necessary as indications for surveillance broadened. In a well-functioning unit, approximately one-half of the admissions would prove to have myocardial infarction.[4, 6] This mini-

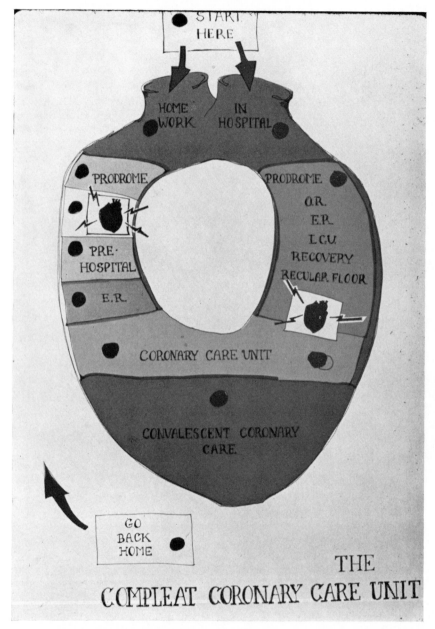

Fig. 19.2. A conceptional diagram of the ultimate coronary care system which is currently in an evolutionary stage.

mized the chance of missing an infarction but increased the size of the unit. The lower part of the diagram in Figure 19.2 shows the appearance of a second unit, a convalescent unit, which became part of the coronary care movement.

Even as hospitals rushed to install monitors and defibrillators and to train nurses, the coronary care unit was being described as part of an overall system of coronary care rather than a finite entity unto itself.[12-15] Effective implementation of the system depended on getting patients into it quickly and, as evidenced by the stepdown or convalescent unit, interest began to develop in the fate of the patient who left the coronary care unit.

The left side of Figure 19.2 shows one channel of entry into the system, which at present poses enormous problems to the coronary care movement. The diagram illustrates the challenge to put under surveillance and treatment all patients with acute coronary disease, whether they are at home, at work, or in the hospital emergency room.

Flying squads and monitored ambulances are in a developmental stage.[12, 16, 17] No attempt is made here to assess their role except to say that the ultimate reduction of mortality depends on getting patients with acute infarction under surveillance in a far shorter time than is currently being done.[18] Great delay still occurs in the emergency room of the best hospitals, where a frontier for improving the coronary care system still exists.

The right side of Figure 19.2 shows a second important and, as yet, underdeveloped channel of input into the coronary care system. This channel lies within the hospital itself. Patients in areas which we might consider to be safe, such as surgical suites, recovery rooms, and intensive care areas, even now suffer unrecognized prodromes of early infarction and impending infarction. The best coronary care unit is not complete until the areas shown in Figure 19.2 are properly staffed and instrumented and able to recognize and treat acute coronary problems. In other words, the coronary care unit must extend far beyond the limited concept of 1962. Thus, in the "Compleat Coronary Care Unit," a patient may enter from the outside world or from the hospital world, proceed through the various phases, and ultimately go home again.

In considering the fundamental concept of the coronary care unit as a comprehensive system of coronary care, looking whence the patient came and where the patient goes, a further analysis of the so-called stepdown or convalescent coronary care unit is required. Since 1962, most major and perhaps most of the smaller hospitals in this country have succeeded in developing coronary care units. In general, they are doing a good job in dealing with arrhythmias in the context in which the coronary care unit was originally constituted. To achieve this end, budgets are strained as pressures rise to equip hospital emergency rooms, recovery rooms, and operating suites as already described. The obligation to provide extensive stepdown and intermediate care areas, therefore, is a burden which cannot be undertaken without hard evidence that the facility will provide a major contribution to better care and patient survival.[11, 13, 15]

A review of coronary care statistics may help to define what may be expected from the stepdown or convalescent unit. Table 19.1 shows the deaths which have occurred at the Good Samaritan Hospital in Dayton, Ohio, among 590 patients with myocardial infarction after transfer from the coronary care unit before the establishment of a convalescent or stepdown area. These patients were observed during a 4-year-period beginning in 1966. Of the 590 patients, a total of 93 died. Seventeen patients died after leaving the CCU. Our institution has a 10-bed unit, in which the average stay is approximately 9 days. The design and operational aspects of the Unit have been described elsewhere.[4, 19] Table 19.2 focuses on the 17 post CCU deaths, which theoretically might have been prevented by a stepdown unit. Among these patients, 8 died with degenerative disease which, at present, probably no monitoring would avail. Nine patients died suddenly. These were found dead in bed in most instances, as many patients were throughout general hospitals prior to the advent of the coronary care unit.

Table 19.3 indicates the average length of the CCU stay among these patients and their day of death. Table 19.4 shows that, among 9 who died suddenly, 7 had abnormal conduction disturbances, 6 had intraventricular (IV) defects, and 1 had an atrioventricular conduction defect. This rather striking incidence of IV conduction disturbances in patients with sudden

Table 19.1. *In-hospital survival, acute myocardial infarction*

Total cases	Deaths	
	In CCU	Post CCU
590	73	17

Table 19.2. *Post CCU deaths, acute myocardial infarction*

Deaths among 514 patients dismissed from CCU	Degenerative pump syndrome	Sudden death
17	8	9

Table 19.3. *Average day of death of 17 patients among 514 dismissed from CCU*

	Sudden (9)	Degenerative (8)
Days in CCU	13	10
Day of Death	23	23

Table 19.4. *Mode of death of 17 patients among 514 dismissed from the CCU*

	Sudden (9)	Degenerative (8)
Abnormal conduction	7	4
Intraventricular	6	3
Atrioventricular	1	1

Table 19.5. *Patients with acute transmural myocardial infarction:*
effect of conduction disturbances

	No. patients	Total mortality	CCU mortality	Post CCU mortality
Total	158	(31) 19.6%	(23) 14.5%	(8) 5%
No conduction defect	105	(12) 11.4%	(10) 9.5%	(2) 1.9%
Conduction defect	53	(19) 35.8%	(13) 24.5%	(6) 11.3%
Intraventricular conduction defect	40	(17) 42.5%	(12) 30%	(5) 12.5%

Table 19.6. *Patients with acute transmural myocardial infarction:*
effect of previous infarction

	No. patients	Total mortality	CCU mortality	Post CCU mortality
Total	158	(31) 19.6%	(23) 14.5%	(8) 5%
No previous infarction	116	(16) 13.7%	(12) 10.3%	(4) 3.4%
Previous infarction	49	(15) 35.7%	(11) 26.1%	(4) 9.5%

death led us to review, in detail, some 158 patients with acute transmural myocardial infarction, as seen in Table 19.5. In this group, the total mortality was approximately 20 per cent, 15 per cent in the CCU, and 5 per cent after the CCU. Among those with no conduction disturbances, the mortality was 11, 10, and 2 per cent, respectively. Where a conduction defect occurred there was a 36 per cent overall mortality, 25 per cent in the CCU, and 11 per cent after CCU. Among the group with IV conduction disturbances alone, mortality was even higher: 43 per cent, 30 per cent in the CCU, and 13 per cent post CCU.

Table 19.6 considers this group of 158 patients from another point of view, with and without previous infarction. A striking difference in mortality is noted. If no infarction had occurred, 14 per cent overall mortality occurred. This rose to 36 per cent if there had been a previous infarction. Table 19.7 makes a further analysis of these patients. There were 90 patients with no previous infarction and no conduction disturbances. Among them the mortality was 10 per cent; 8 per cent died in the CCU and 2 per cent outside the CCU. However, when combining previous infarction with conduction disturbances, a mortality of 46 per cent is seen.

The purpose of this approach is to try to determine whether there are certain criteria among patients with myocardial infarction which would place them in a higher risk group and which would constitute an indication for prolonged monitoring and for establishing priorities among post CCU patients for monitoring in convalescent or stepdown units. Thus far, it would seem that patients with a history of previous infarction and with IV conduction disturbances are at high risk and in greater danger of sudden death post CCU.

Another factor of major importance in determining the risk of mortality is location of infarction. Of the nine patients who died suddenly post CCU, seven had anterior infarction. Table 19.8 illustrates the mortality related to location among the 158 patients with infarction. Anterior and inferior infarction appeared with almost equal incidence. Mortality for the anterior group is 26 per cent and, for the inferior group, 12 per cent. The anterior group had a slightly higher post CCU mortality. Table 19.9 shows that the presence of previous infarction and anterior location produces a mortality of 43 per cent. However, inferior infarction superimposed on a previous lesion has only a 20 per cent mortality, which is approximately the same as for all cases in the series (Table 19.5). It is interesting that anterior infarction with no previous history of infarction has nearly the same mortality as an inferior lesion with a prior history of infarction. Among 59

Table 19.7. *Patients with acute transmural myocardial infarction (MI): combined effect of previous myocardial infarction and conduction disturbances*

	No. patients	Total mortality	CCU mortality	Post CCU mortality
Total	158	(31) 19.6%	(23) 14.5%	(8) 5%
No Previous MI, no conduction disturbances	90	(9) 10%	(7) 7.8%	(2) 2.2%
Previous MI and conduction disturbances	24	(11) 45.8%	(7) 29.1%	(4) 16.6%

Table 19.8. *Patients with acute transmural myocardial infarction: effects of localization*

	No. patients	Total mortality	CCU mortality	Post CCU mortality
Total	158	(31) 19.6%	(23) 14.5%	(8) 5%
Anterior	78	(20) 25.6%	(14) 17.9%	(6) 7.6%
Inferior	74	(9) 12.1%	(7) 9.5%	(2) 2.6%

Table 19.9. *Combined effects of previous myocardial infarction (MI) and localization*

	No. patients	Total mortality	CCU mortality	Post CCU mortality
Anterior location and previous MI	23	(10) 43.5%	(6) 26%	(4) 17.4%
Inferior location and previous MI	15	(3) 20%	(3) 20%	
Anterior location, no previous MI	55	(10) 18.2%	(8) 14.5%	(2) 3.6%
Inferior location, no previous MI	59	(6) 10.2%	(4) 6.8%	(2) 3.4%

Table 19.10. *Patients with transmural infarction: combined effect of localization and conduction defect*

	No. patients	Total mortality	CCU mortality	Post CCU mortality
Total	158	(31) 19.6%	(23) 14.5%	(8) 5%
Anterior MI and conduction defect	27	(12) 44.4%	(7) 25.9%	(8) 18.5%
Anterior MI and no conduction defect	51	(6) 11.7%	(5) 9.8%	(1) 1.9%
Inferior MI and conduction Defect	22	(4) 18.2%	(3) 13.6%	(1) 4.5%
Inferior MI and no conduction defect	53	(5) 9.4%	(4) 7.5%	(1) 1.8%

patients with no previous infarction, the inferior lesion has a mortality of 10 per cent.

Table 19.10 combines the influence of location and the presence of a conduction defect. With anterior infarction and a conduction defect, the mortality is again quite high: 44 per cent. With an inferior lesion and a conduction defect, the mortality is approximately that of the overall group.

Anterior and inferior infarction without conduction disturbances have a relatively low mortality, 12 and 9 per cent, respectively. In considering the mortality of these two locations overall, the anterior lesion has a higher mortality of more than 2 to 1 (26 and 12 per cent, Table 19.8). Each location with a previous infarction shows more than a 2 to 1 increase in mortality (44 and 20 per cent, Table 19.9). The inference would therefore seem to be that the factor which contributes heavily to the increase in mortality in anterior infarction overall and in the presence of previous infarction is that of an IV conduction disturbance.

Table 19.11 shows the mortality considering all three factors: location, presence of previous infarction, and conduction defects. Among 13 patients

Table 19.11. *Mortality in 158 patients with transmural infarction: combined effect of previous myocardial infarction* (*MI*), *conduction defect, and localization*

	No. patients	Total mortality	CCU mortality	Post CCU mortality
Total	158	(31) 19.6%	(23) 14.5%	(8) 5%
Anterior location, previous MI, conduction defect	13	(7) 53.8%	(3) 25%	(4) 30.8%
Anterior location, no previous MI, no conduction defect	41	(4) 9.8%	(3) 7.3%	(1) 2.4%
Inferior location, previous MI, conduction defect	8	(2) 25%	(2) 25%	
Inferior location, no previous MI, no conduction defect	45	(4) 8.7%	(3) 6.5%	(1) 2.2%

with this combination, there is the highest mortality in the series: 54 per cent. Of the 7 in this group who died, 4 died after leaving the coronary care unit, even though the average stay was 9 days. The least deadly situation among those with infarction is an inferior lesion without previous infarction and without conduction disturbance. Among 45 such cases, the mortality is less than 9 per cent.

The reduction in mortality to be achieved from a convalescent or so-called stepdown unit will have to be judged individually in each hospital. For example, in an institution with a relatively large CCU and where a longer CCU stay can be permitted, many of the high risk patients will be retained in this area past the more critical period, and therefore the need for a convalescent area will be somewhat reduced. As an illustration: among 158 of our patients with infarction, 31 died. Eight of these died after leaving the CCU. However, among the 23 CCU deaths, 10 occurred after the 5th day. In a hospital where the CCU stay is only 5 or 6 days, the losses post CCU will appear to be much higher than our series. It is obvious that these additional 10 deaths would not be improved by a post CCU facility in an institution with a very short stay, since they died under surveillance in a CCU. The hard facts are that, in our series of patients with myocardial infarctions, 514 were dismissed from the coronary care unit after a stay of approximately 9 days. Among these, 17 died; 9 died suddenly and were therefore considered amenable to possible salvage by stepdown unit care. At least 2 of these had extension of infarction and probably would not have been helped by extended monitoring. The residue of patients (7 out of 514) dismissed who might potentially be saved is very small. Based on mortality statistics alone, it may not be defensible to monitor every patient through-out the course of hospitalization for infarction.

It must be emphasized, however, that there may be other advantages which accrue from a convalescent unit than those of reducing in-hospital mortality. These may result from a more comprehensive pre-discharge evaluation of the patient who has had a myocardial infarction. An example might be the study of his response to activity, particularly in terms of his propensity toward ectopic rhythms. This information may influence management of the patient after he leaves the hospital in terms of antiarrhythmic therapy. From the observations made on the patient during the convalescent phase in a properly equipped convalescent unit, projections may be made for angiographic studies in the near term.

Evaluation of the patient's metabolic and lipid status late in the convalescent phase may also govern post-discharge dietary and medical therapy. It is during the convalescent phase also when the acute situation has subsided that the education of the patient with regard to activity, diet, and recognition of warning symptoms may be carried out, thus contributing materially to his chances for survival. In general, the ultimate contribution of the stepdown unit may lie in a more comprehensive approach to the patient, rather than in the improvement of in-hospital survival statistics.

In summary, the coronary care unit has become a coronary care system no longer limited to intensive management and monitoring during the first few days following myocardial infarction.

It is possible to define post myocardial infarction risk factors related to higher mortality and greater chance for sudden death. Among these are previous infarction, intraventricular conduction disturbances, and anterior location of infarction. Analysis of patients for these and other factors may help to define a group in whom protracted surveillance can contribute to increasing survival. The data, however, do not permit unlimited enthusiasm for what the most comprehensive convalescent area may accomplish in terms of overall in-hospital survival following myocardial infarction.

Acknowledgment: The authors wish to express their appreciation to Sylvia Stevens, Research Assistant, Coronary Care Unit, Good Samaritan Hospital, for invaluable assistance in the compilation of the data presented and in the preparation of this manuscript, and to Joan Weinberg for the design and execution of Figures 19.1 and 19.2.

REFERENCES

1. Day, H. W.: An intensive coronary care area. Dis. Chest 44: 423, 1963.
2. Brown, K., MacMillan, R., Scott, J., *et al.*: Coronary care—an intensive care center for acute myocardial infarction. Lancet 2: 349, 1963.
3. Day, H. W.: Effectiveness of an intensive coronary care area. Amer. J. Cardiol. 15: 51, 1965.
4. Weinberg, S. L.: Should your hospital have a coronary care unit? Hosp. Pract. 2: 6, 1967.
5. MacMillan, R. L., Brown, K. W. G., *et al.*: Changing perspective in coronary care. Amer. J. Cardiol. 20: 451, 1967.

6. Lown, B., Fakhro, A. M., *et al.*: The coronary care unit. J. A. M. A. 199: 156, 1967.
7. Lawrie, D. M., Greenwood, T. W., Goddard, M., *et al.*: A coronary care unit in the routine management of acute myocardial infarction. Lancet 109: 1967.
8. Marshall, R. M., Blount, S. G., and Brenton, E.: Acute myocardial infarction: influence of a coronary care unit. Arch. Intern. Med. 122: 472, 1968.
9. Mounsey, P.: Intensive coronary care. Amer. J. Cardiol. 20: 475, 1967.
9a. Killip, T., and Kimball, J. T.: Treatment of myocardial infarction in a coronary care unit. Amer. J. Cardiol. 20: 457, 1967.
9b. Oliver, M. F., Julian, D. G., and Donald, K. W.: Problems in evaluating coronary care units. Amer. J. Cardiol. 20: 465, 1967.
10. Kimball, J. T., and Killip, T.: Aggressive treatment of arrhythmias in acute myocardial infarction: procedures and results. Progr. Cardiovasc. Dis. 8: 1967.
11. Meltzer, L. E.: The present status and future direction of intensive coronary care. Cardiovasc. Clin. 1 (Suppl. 2) 177, 1969.
12. Grace, W. J.: The mobile coronary care unit and the intermediate coronary care unit in the total systems approach to coronary care. Chest 58: 4, 1970.
13. Grace, W. J.: Acute myocardial infarction: the course of the illness following discharge from the coronary care unit. Chest 59: 1, 1969.
14. Lown, B., and Ruberman, W.: The concept of precoronary care. Mod. Concepts Cardiovasc. Dis. 39: 97, 1970.
15. Weinberg, S. L.: Complacency in coronary care. Dis. Chest 56: 273, 1969.
16. Pantridge, J. G., and Geddes, J. A.: A mobile intensive care unit in the management of myocardial infarction. Lancet 2: 271, 1967.
17. Pantridge, J. F., and Adgey, A. A. J.: Prehospital coronary care: mobile coronary care unit. Amer. J. Cardiol. 24: 666, 1969.
18. Moss, A. J., Wynar, B., and Goldstein, S.: Delay in hospitalization during the acute coronary period. Amer. J. Cardiol. 24: 659, 1969.
19. Weinberg, S. L.: The current status of instrumentation systems for the coronary care unit. Progr. Cardiovasc. Dis. 11: 1, 1968.

20

Present Status of Glucagon and Bretylium Tosylate

EZRA A. AMSTERDAM, M.D., EDWARD J. MANSOUR,
M.D., JAMES L. HUGHES, III, M.D., JOSEPH A.
BONANNO, M.D., RASHID A. MASSUMI, M.D.,
ROBERT ZELIS, M.D., AND
DEAN T. MASON, M.D.

Among recent developments in cardiovascular pharmacology, considerable attention and investigation have been devoted to two promising new drugs: glucagon and bretylium tosylate. Glucagon, a positive inotropic agent acting through a mechanism distinct from those of digitalis and the catecholamines, has been evaluated for its potential in the treatment of the failing heart. Bretylium has been found promising, in early studies, in suppressing ventricular ectopic rhythms and, in addition, has attracted interest because of its positive inotropic effect on the myocardium, a unique property of an antiarrhythmic agent.

GLUCAGON

Glucagon, a polypeptide hormone produced by the alpha cells of the pancreas, is composed of 29 amino acids and has a molecular weight of 3400.[1] An immunologically identical substance, enteroglucagon, is present in the gastrointestinal tract and shares some biological properties with glucagon.[2] Although it is best known for its hyperglycemic and glycogenolytic activity,[1, 3, 4] glucagon possesses a variety of endocrine actions, exerts diverse influences on substrate metabolism, and also has certain nonmetabolic effects. Recently, the positive cardiac inotropic action of glucagon has been demonstrated experimentally and extended to clinical evaluation in the treatment of cardiac pump failure in man.

It is now known that glucagon produces a number of its physiological effects by acting through the adenyl cyclase-cyclic $3',5'$-adenosine monophosphate (cyclic-AMP) system. This enzyme system has been recognized as the mediator of many of the effects of hormones on cells and is thus an important regulator of metabolic and physiological processes.[5] Glucagon activates adenyl cyclase, a membrane-bound particulate fraction of the cell, which enhances formation of cyclic-AMP from adenosine triphosphate. Cyclic-AMP in turn stimulates phosphorylase activity, with production of glucose 1-phosphate from glycogen.[5] The hyperglycemic effect of glucagon is thus produced by its activation of hepatic adenyl cyclase, resulting in stimulation of cyclic-AMP with resultant glycogenolysis and increased output of hepatic glucose.[5, 6] Likewise, it has been shown that the positive inotropic action of glucagon is related to its stimulation of myocardial cyclic-AMP.[7, 8]

Metabolic and Extracardiac Effects

Glucagon is released in response to hypoglycemia and, through its physiological effects, counters this state.[9] Its augmentation of blood glucose is effected by, in addition to stimulation of glycogenolysis in the liver,[10] gluconeogenesis through hepatic conversion of amino acids to glucose.[11] Release of the hormone is suppressed by hyperglycemia.[3] Glucagon further directly influences metabolism by its lipolytic action, mobilizing fat and increasing free fatty acid levels through hydrolysis of triglycerides to free fatty acids by activation of lipase.[3] Oxidation of free fatty acids is stimulated and, by increasing their availability, the hormone may additionally promote gluconeogenesis.[12]

Glucagon has broad effects on endocrine regulation in directly stimulating the release of a number of hormones[3]: insulin, catecholamines, growth hormone, thyroid hormone, parathyroid hormone, and thyrocalcitonin. It also inhibits gastrointestinal motility, suppresses secretion of gastric juice and digestive enzymes, and causes hypokalemia after an initial increase in serum potassium, the alterations of this electrolyte paralleling the changes in blood glucose.[3]

Cardiovascular Effects

Experimental Studies

Glucagon has been demonstrated in experimental studies to have a potent positive inotropic effect on the myocardium. Enhanced myocardial performance is manifested in isolated cardiac muscle by increases in tension development[13, 14] and maximal velocity of contractile element shortening (V_{max}),[15] the index of contractility. In intact animals, glucagon augments myocardial contractile force[14, 15] and left ventricular dp/dt,[14, 16] the rate of rise of ventricular pressure. Cardiac output is increased,[13, 17, 18] and the hormone also has a positive chronotropic effect[13, 14, 18] and reduces peripheral vascular resistance.[14, 19]

Laboratory investigation has distinguished a number of potentially important characteristics of the cardiac actions of glucagon. The positive inotropic effect is independent of endogenous catecholamine stores and intact beta adrenergic receptors, and thus the augmented cardiac contractile performance of isolated myocardium and intact animals is unaffected by reserpine[13-15] and beta adrenergic blockade.[14] Most experimental studies indicate that glucagon, unlike the traditional positive inotropic agents such as the catecholamines, does not produce atrial or ventricular irritability,[14, 20] and it can further enhance cardiac performance in the presence of other positive inotropic therapy such as full doses of digitalis without provoking arrhythmias.[14] Further, the drug has been shown to possess antiarrhythmic activity in relation to the ectopic rhythms associated with experimentally induced digitalis toxicity.[20]

The effect of glucagon on the electrophysiological properties of the heart include increased rate of sinoatrial node discharge,[21, 22] increased velocity of atrioventricular conduction,[21-23] and absence of increased ventricular automaticity,[21, 23] although findings contrary to the latter have been reported.[22] The positive chronotropic effect has been demonstrated to be direct by its manifestation after injection of glucagon into the sinus node artery.[24] In addition to its enhancement of atrioventricular (AV) conduction in normal animals, glucagon reverses propranolol-induced depression of AV conduction.[21, 25] Further, during atrial pacing in dogs, a decrease in the time interval from pacing impulse to His bundle spike has been demonstrated.[21] The salutary action of glucagon in digitalis-induced arrhythmias in animals has been attributed to overdrive suppression, enhanced AV conduction, and shift of potassium from extracellular to intracellular localization.[20]

In its overall action on the coronary circulation in experimental animals, glucagon is a secondary coronary vasodilator, producing its effects on coronary circulatory dynamics through augmentation of myocardial contractile state and mechanical effort and thereby of cardiac oxygen requirements.[3] In investigations utilizing the isolated heart[26] and intact animal,[17, 18, 27] glucagon lowers coronary vascular resistance and increases myocardial oxygen consumption and coronary blood flow. Myocardial oxygen extraction has been variable, rising[18] or remaining unaltered.[17] Of interest is the finding that increase in coronary blood flow after glucagon is independent of elevation of heart rate.[27]

In experimental myocardial infarction in dogs, administration of glucagon has resulted in improvement in impaired hemodynamic function. Thus, glucagon augmented cardiac output, blood pressure, and left ventricular dp/dt while it decreased the elevated left ventricular end diastolic pressure.[29, 30] Further, during cardiogenic shock, glucagon, in conjunction with intra-aortic balloon counterpulsation, produced a rise in arterial blood pressure, whereas balloon counterpulsation alone had no effect.[30]

Studies in Man during Cardiac Catheterization

Investigation of the positive contractile actions of glucagon has been extended to its evaluation in man during diagnostic cardiac catheterization. A dose of 3 to 5 mg. or 50 mcg. per kg. administered intravenously over 3 to 5 minutes is usually utilized.[31-37] The onset of action occurs in 1 to 3 minutes, effect is maximal in 5 to 10 minutes, and duration is 10 to 20 minutes.[31, 32] The effect of glucagon in augmenting myocardial performance in man has been less consistent and of considerably less magnitude than in experimental investigations. Thus, in a study of the effects of the drug in canines and in man, it was found that cardiac output after glucagon rose 65 per cent in the animals, compared with 22 per cent in human subjects.[17] Further, while elevations in cardiac output[31-34, 37] following glucagon administration have been observed in some series, little or no effect has been documented in others.[35, 36] In addition, it has been reported that glucagon failed to raise cardiac output during exercise in patients with fixed rate pacemakers.[38] Glucagon has generally produced an increase in heart rate[31-33, 38] and in left ventricular dp/dt.[31, 32, 34] Its peripheral circulatory effects are manifested by a decrease in systemic vascular resistance.[33, 34, 37] Blood pressure may be increased[32, 33] or unchanged[36] by glucagon, and stroke volume[32-36] and left ventricular end diastolic pressure[32, 34, 35] are generally unaltered. In accord with experimental findings, glucagon enhances cardiac performance in man in the presence of digitalis,[32] and ventricular irritability was not produced by the hormone in these studies.[32]

Studies of the influence of glucagon on coronary circulatory dynamics in man confirm its effect as a secondary vasodilator. Thus, coronary blood flow and myocardial oxygen consumption are increased while myocardial oxygen extraction is unaltered.[17, 39] Further, in one study of patients with coronary artery disease, glucagon administration was associated with a marked improvement in myocardial lactate metabolism.[40]

The hyperglycemic, hypokalemic effect of glucagon is a consistent finding in man,[3] and nausea and vomiting have been relatively common.[3]

Clinical Application in Cardiac Pump Dysfunction

Utilization of glucagon in the treatment of cardiac disease and hemodynamic failure has yielded inconsistent results. In therapeutic trials, glucagon has been administered intravenously in a dose of 1 to 10 mg.[41, 42] and 1 to 7.5 mg. per hour in a continuous infusion.[43-47] Administration in the early postoperative period to patients undergoing cardiac surgery has variably produced no changes in cardiac output and stroke volume[48] and modest increases of up to 14 and 10 per cent, respectively.[41, 42]

The use of glucagon in patients with congestive heart failure has produced variable results. In five patients with acute myocardial infarction[37] and two patients with myocardial infarction shock,[49] cardiac output after 2 to 5 mg. of the hormone was augmented significantly. Glucagon administration in patients with congestive heart failure of diverse etiologies has been predominantly associated with improvement in some series,[43-45] as manifested by clinical course, but has lacked general efficacy in others.[46, 47]

In order to define clearly the therapeutic status of a new positive inotropic drug, it is important that it be systemically evaluated by detailed hemodynamic studies and by comparison with conventional agents in the same patients. Although there has been relatively little investigation directly comparing the therapeutic effects of glucagon with those of other cardiosupportive drugs, several such studies have been performed. Thus, glucagon has been compared to norepinephrine in patients with acute myocardial infarction and left ventricular failure. Glucagon (70 mcg. per kg.) increased cardiac output by 23 per cent without a significant change in the tension-time index (TTI), whereas norepinephrine increased cardiac output 16 per cent with an associated increase of 15 per cent in TTI.[50] The greater increment in cardiac output after glucagon concomitant with a lower TTI resulted from the latter agent's reduction of systemic vascular resistance, in contrast to the increase in resistance following norepinephrine, and suggests improvement in cardiac pump function at a lower cost in myocardial oxygen needs with glucagon. However, in another clinical study of the use of glucagon in patients with left ventricular failure associated with myocardial infarction, the same investigators found, in association with a 25 per cent increase in cardiac output produced by the hormone,[51] a significant rise in TTI.

The effects of glucagon and dopamine on urine production and excretion of sodium and potassium were compared in a group of patients with congestive heart failure.[52] Although significant diuretic effects and electrolyte excretion were produced by glucagon, these were of relatively short duration, were inconsistently sustained with repeated administration of the hormone, and were only 23 and 15 per cent of the magnitude of the effect of dopamine on sodium excretion and urine flow, respectively. Further, in more than half of the patients, glucagon induced vomiting, and in one patient a serious episode of ventricular ectopic rhythm resulted after administration of the hormone.

We have evaluated the efficacy of glucagon in patients with severely impaired myocardial performance and compared it with that of traditional inotropic agents.[53] Sixteen patients with cardiac pump failure received glucagon and either isoproterenol, norepinephrine, or metaraminol for comparative hemodynamic evaluation. Eight patients were in cardiogenic shock following acute myocardial infarction, and eight demonstrated severe con-

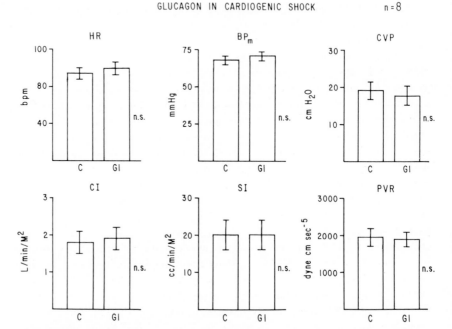

GLUCAGON IN CARDIOGENIC SHOCK   n = 8

FIG. 20.1. Hemodynamic effects of glucagon (Gl), 50 mcg. per kg., in eight patients with shock associated with acute myocardial infarction. C, control; bpm, beats per minute; HR, heart rate; BP_m, mean blood pressure; CVP, central venous pressure; CI, cardiac index; SI, stroke index; PVR, peripheral vascular resistance; n.s., not significant.

gestive heart failure of varying etiologies. Glucagon was administered intravenously in a dose of 50 mcg. per kg., resulting in a total dose of 3 to 5 mg. which was given over a period of approximately 3 minutes. Values for heart rate, mean intra-arterial blood pressure, central venous pressure, cardiac index, stroke index, and peripheral vascular resistance before and after glucagon in the shock patients are shown in Figure 20.1. No significant changes resulted after glucagon in any of these hemodynamic functions. Administration of glucagon to eight patients in congestive heart failure, in whom left ventricular end diastolic pressure was also determined, likewise produced no significant alterations in their cardiovascular function (Fig. 20.2).

The effects of glucagon during a continuous intravenous infusion of 1 mg. every 10 minutes were also determined in six patients from both groups with cardiac pump failure. Control cardiac output of 2.2 liters per minute per m^2 was essentially unaltered 5 minutes after the single administration of 50 mcg. per kg. of glucagon, nor was there a significant change after 10 minutes of continuous infusion of glucagon. Similarly, there was no effect on heart

GLUCAGON IN CHF   n = 8

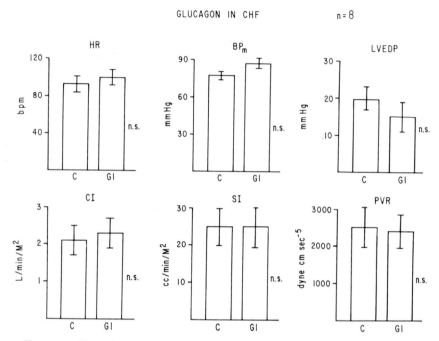

FIG. 20.2. Hemodynamic effects of glucagon (Gl), 50 mcg. per kg., in eight patients with congestive heart failure (CHF). LVEDP, left ventricular end diastolic pressure. (See Fig. 20.1 for other abbreviations.)

rate, mean intra-arterial blood pressure, stroke index, or peripheral vascular resistance.

The hemodynamic effects of glucagon were also compared with those of isoproterenol in four patients (three with congestive heart failure and one with cardiogenic shock) and with norepinephrine or metaraminol in two patients with cardiogenic shock. Again it was found that alterations in hemodynamic function were small and considerably less than those produced by the catecholamines (Fig. 20.3). Differences were especially marked in the comparative effects of glucagon and norepinephrine on blood pressure, +5 and +33 per cent, respectively, and of glucagon and isoproterenol on cardiac index, +4 and +48 per cent, respectively. In addition, isoproterenol and norepinephrine had more marked effects on heart rate and the former agent exerted a more potent dilator effect on peripheral resistance vessels than did glucagon. Thus, after the administration of single doses of glucagon, single doses of glucagon coupled with continuous infusion and comparison of the hemodynamic effects of glucagon with those of sympathomimetic amines, all in patients with cardiac pump failure, it was found that favorable effects on myocardial function after glucagon were relatively

GLUCAGON AND SYMPATHOMIMETIC AMINES IN CARDIAC PUMP FAILURE

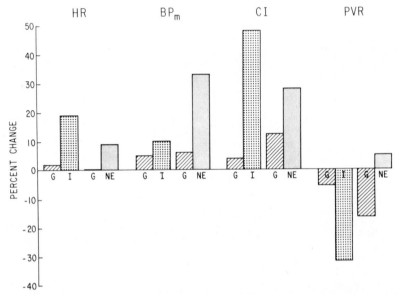

FIG. 20.3. Comparative effects of glucagon (Gl) and sympathomimetic amines (SA) (norepinephrine, one patient; metaraminol, one patient; isoproterenol, four patients) in six patients with cardiac pump failure. (See Fig. 20.1 for other abbreviations.)

small and inconsistent. Further, the effects of the sympathomimetic amines were considerably greater in improving myocardial performance than were those of glucagon.

Side effects attributable to glucagon have generally been considered of relatively minor consequence. This has been thought especially true of arrhythmias, based on the lack of arrhythmogenic potential of glucagon in animal studies,[14, 20, 21, 23] in man during cardiac catheterization,[32] and in its clinical application in the low cardiac output state.[43-45, 47] Indeed, the hormone has demonstrated beneficial effects on arrhythmias both experimentally[20, 21] and clinically.[45, 47] However, several studies suggest that, albeit unusual, ventricular irritability may be produced by glucagon. Thus, increased ventricular automaticity after glucagon has been demonstrated in the dog[22] and in man.[52] Nausea is a common effect of glucagon, occurring in one-third of patients receiving the hormone,[3] and nausea and vomiting limit its use in some patients. Elevation of blood glucose and decrease in serum potassium have been consistently produced by glucagon, but these metabolic alterations have not been inordinate nor have they been of clinical significance.[3] However, the hazards of hypokalemia dictate attention to this potential complication.

Mechanism of Cardiac Inotropic Action

Recent investigations of the mechanism of the positive inotropic action of glucagon may provide some clarification of the lack of correlation between the salutary effects of the hormone in animal studies and its inconsistent actions in man with cardiac decompensation. As previously noted, glucagon augments production of cyclic-AMP in cardiac tissue by activation of adenyl cyclase.[7, 10] It has been further suggested that the fundamental mechanism of the positive inotropic effect of glucagon is its promotion of increased sarcotubular calcium stores through activation of the adenyl cyclase-cyclic-AMP system[7] and that it shares this mechanism with the catecholamines. However, glucagon, unlike the catecholamines, produces these subcellular effects independent of beta adrenergic receptor stimulation.[7] In contrast with the ability of glucagon to enhance myocardial contractility in normal cardiac tissue, this capacity of the hormone is markedly diminished in cardiac muscle from animals with chronic congestive heart failure.[7, 8] Associated with this loss by glucagon of positive contractile action is failure to increase myocardial adenyl cyclase activity under these conditions. By contrast, in these studies, inotropic response and augmentation of adenyl cyclase activity by catecholamines are unaffected by heart failure, although diminished activation of adenyl cyclase by norepinephrine in heart failure has also been reported.[54] Current investigations, while not ultimately defining the basis for the altered inotropic capacity of glucagon in the normal and failing heart, provide a possible basis for the observed inconsistencies in the clinical effectiveness of the drug in patients with cardiac disease. Continuing observation relating clinical results of glucagon therapy to etiology and duration of cardiac decompensation may further clarify these findings. Further, the alteration of contractile capacity of glucagon is related only to chronic heart failure and has not been observed in acute cardiac decompensation.[7, 8] In this regard, it is of interest that, in several clinical series, patients with chronic heart failure were less responsive to glucagon than were those in whom cardiac decompensation was more acute.[42, 45-47]

The defect responsible for the loss of inotropic potency of glucagon in chronic heart failure remains undefined, although several possibilities have been suggested, such as alteration in the interaction between glucagon and its cellular binding site, uncoupling of the interaction between glucagon and adenyl cyclase, or production of a specific glucagon inhibitor.[7]

Conclusion

At the present time, the use of glucagon in heart disease is advocated by some workers for (1) cardiac failure induced by beta adrenergic blocking agents, (2) further enhancement of contractile performance in the presence of other positive inotropic agents, and (3) inotropic support when other agents have failed. Advantages of the drug include its relative lack of serious side effects. However, because of its generally modest and shortlived effects in augmenting cardiac performance in man and the availability of more potent therapeutic agents, glucagon presently occupies a limited place in the treatment of cardiac pump failure in man.

BRETYLIUM

Bretylium tosylate is a sympathetic nerve blocking agent introduced into clinical medicine more than a decade ago as an antihypertensive agent.[55] Because of the rapid development of tolerance to its antihypertensive effect, however, bretylium proved unsuccessful in the treatment of hypertension, and its use in this capacity was discontinued. Subsequent investigations have demonstrated that the drug possesses antiarrhythmic and inotropic activity of considerable interest and potential clinical importance.

Experimental Studies

Adrenergic Blocking Effect

Bretylium has been shown experimentally to possess sympathetic blocking activity by preventing release of the neurotransmitter norepinephrine from peripheral adrenergic nerve terminals.[56] Bretylium does not cause depletion of norepinephrine from sympathetic nerves,[57] and it has no effect on adrenergic receptor function.[56, 58] Sympathetic pre- and postganglionic nerve conduction, initially considered to be impaired by the drug,[56] has been found to be unaffected,[59] as are impulse transmission by sympathetic ganglia[60] and release of catecholamines from the adrenal medulla.[56] The effects of circulating or infused epinephrine and norepinephrine are not blocked but are augmented following bretylium as after denervation.[56, 61] The drug accumulates in adrenergic nerve endings,[62] initially causing release of norepinephrine,[59, 63, 64] followed by prevention of its uptake,[65] the latter action accounting for the enhanced effects of circulating, direct-acting catecholamines.[56, 61]

Cardiovascular Effects

In isolated cardiac tissue,[56] isolated intact heart,[66, 67] and intact animals,[61, 68] bretylium has a positive inotropic action. This effect has been noted to persist, albeit to a lesser degree, following prior depletion of endogenous catecholamines by reserpine[66] or cardiac denervation.[67] Our studies[69] of the effect of bretylium on myocardial contractile function, carried out on isolated, supported right ventricular cat papillary muscles, demonstrated significant increases in maximal contractile element velocity (V_{max}) and tension development (Fig. 20.4). As in previous investigations,[66, 68]

PAPILLARY MUSCLE
RESPONSE TO BRETYLIUM

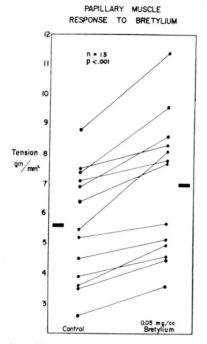

FIG. 20.4. Effect of bretylium on peak isometric tension in isolated cat right ventricular papillary muscles.

the enhanced contractility produced by bretylium was only partially attenuated by interference with sympathetic nervous function. This effect of bretylium was obtained in isolated papillary muscles from animals pretreated with reserpine and also in papillary muscles subjected to beta adrenergic blockade with propranolol.[69] These data indicate that the positive inotropic action of bretylium results from the combined effects of catecholamine release and an intrinsic effect of the drug itself. However, it has also been proposed from recent studies that the contractile actions of bretylium are entirely inherent and dependent on catecholamine release.[70] Bretylium has also been shown to possess a positive chronotropic effect.[56, 61, 66, 67] Blood pressure is initially increased[56, 66, 67] but may subsequently be reduced to hypotensive levels[56, 61] by bretylium. Occasionally there is an initial vasodepressor effect.[61]

Antiarrhythmic and Electrophysiological Effects

Experimentally, bretylium possesses antiarrhythmic activity against both atrial and ventricular arrhythmias. Initially reported as effective in experimental atrial fibrillation,[71] the drug was subsequently found to prevent electrically induced ventricular fibrillation[72] and ventricular fibrillation following experimental myocardial infarction.[73] Bretylium was found more effective in raising the electrical ventricular fibrillation threshold than quinidine, procainamide, lidocaine, diphenylhydantoin, and propranolol.[68] Further, bretylium induced spontaneous defibrillation after electrically induced ventricular fibrillation.[68]

Although the precise mechanism of its antiarrhythmic action is unclear, the effects of bretylium on the cellular electrophysiology of the myocardium have been elucidated by experimental studies. Bretylium possesses certain actions which differ from those of the usual antiarrhythmic agents and in addition, lacks several of their commonly held properties.[74, 75] It has been emphasized that the major antiarrhythmic drugs—quinidine, procainamide, diphenylhydantoin, xylocaine, and propranolol—share two effects on Purkinje fiber preparations which may, in large part, account for their efficacy in cardiac rhythm disorders: (1) decrease in automaticity resulting from suppression of phase 4 depolarization and (2) prolongation of the effective refractory period relative to the duration of the action potential.[74, 75] These properties are not possessed by bretylium.[74, 75] Indeed, bretylium increases automaticity in spontaneously discharging canine Purkinje fibers.[74, 75] This effect appears to result from bretylium-induced release of norepinephrine from sympathetic nerve endings and is absent when bretylium is applied to canine Purkinje fibers after reserpine pretreatment[74, 75] or in the presence of beta adrenergic blockade.[74]

These experimental studies provide several possible bases for the antiarrhythmic action of bretylium. The drug prolongs the duration of both the action potential and effective refractory period in Purkinje fibers without altering the relation of the two and without decreasing conduction velocity.[74, 75] In these actions, it differs significantly from the usual antiarrhythmic drugs. In addition to the differential effects of the latter agents on action potential duration and effective refractory period, conduction velocity in Purkinje fibers is reduced by quinidine, procainamide, and propranolol[75, 76] and is either unaffected or increased by diphenylhydantoin[77] and xylocaine.[77-79] The effective refractory period of atrial and ventricular myocardium in intact dogs is also increased by bretylium.[80] Although not a consistent effect, bretylium may produce hyperpolarization, or an increase in the resting transmembrane potential, of Purkinje fibers[74, 75, 81, 82] and thereby an increase in the rate of phase 0 depolarization (dV/dt).[83] This results in enhanced conduction velocity[74] since the latter is largely a direct function of dV/dt.[84] Thus, the antiarrhythmic actions of bretylium may be the result of (1) prolongation of the refractory period and (2) hyperpolarization. The first effect has been generally identified with abolition of ventricular arrhythmias.[85] The second action, by effecting an increase in conduction velocity, may terminate arrhythmias produced by abnormalities of conduction such as re-entry phenomena and decremental conduction.[84] It is of interest that prolongation of the effective refractory period appears to be a direct effect of bretylium and is not related to its alteration of adrenergic function. On the other hand, intact adrenergic neurohumeral function is necessary for the hyperpolarizing effect of bretylium which apparently is produced indirectly by catecholamine release.[74] In this regard, it has been suggested that catecholamines may have antiarrhythmic effects based on their hyperpolarizing action.[84] Thus, the antiarrhythmic activity of bretylium may be the result of a combination of direct and indirect actions. It has also been suggested that, in its action against re-entry arrhythmias, bretylium may decrease the effective refractory period in contrast to the prolongation noted above.[81] Studies utilizing high doses of bretylium (10 mg. per kg.) in intact canines have shown a negative chronotropic effect and increase in atrioventricular conduction time by the drug.[80] It is of interest and possible clinical significance that, under experimental conditions, prior administration of quinidine diminished the effectiveness of bretylium in raising the ventricular fibrillation threshold to electrically induced fibrillation.[80]

Clinical Application in Arrhythmias

Initial clinical evaluation of bretylium has demonstrated its effectiveness in the treatment of a variety of ventricular arrhythmias of differing etiologies. However, contrasting findings and untoward actions of the drug have also been reported. Thus, in several series of patients with acute myocardial infarction, bretylium administration has been associated with alleviation and prevention of ventricular ectopic beats,[86-88] ventricular tachycardia,[86, 88, 89] and ventricular fibrillation.[80-86] Bretylium has also been of value as adjunctive therapy in achieving electrical defibrillation which could not be accomplished by countershock alone.[86, 90, 91] Further, long-term control of recurrent ventricular tachycardia has been reported with oral bretylium.[92] At variance with this evidence of the therapeutic efficacy of bretylium is a report of its lack of effectiveness in controlling ventricular ectopic rhythms in acute myocardial infarction.[93] It is of interest, however, that bretylium was associated with a reduction in the frequency of supraventricular arrhythmias in these patients. Further, bretylium was ineffective in preventing recurrent fibrillation in a patient in whom the arrhythmia was subsequently controlled by ventricular pacing.[94]

Bretylium has been successfully utilized in the control of arrhythmias associated with cardiac valve replacement. Thus, prophylactic, preoperative administration of the drug was associated with a significant reduction in postoperative arrhythmias[95] and resulted in successful abolition of both atrial and ventricular arrhythmias in over 90 per cent of patients.[95] Further, the drug was particularly helpful in achieving postoperative defibrillation after elective fibrillation had been utilized for surgery.

In addition to our investigation of bretylium in isolated cardiac tissue,[69]

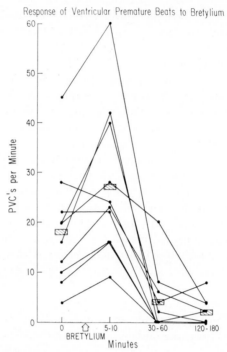

FIG. 20.5. Antiarrhythmic action of bretylium (5 mg. per kg. intravenously) in 10 patients with premature ventricular beats (PVC's). The shaded rectangles indicate group mean number of PVC's at each time interval.

we have evaluated its effects on arrhythmias and cardiac performance in man.[96] In the control of arrhythmias, we have utilized the drug both therapeutically and prophylactically. Bretylium was administered (5 mg. per kg. intravenously or intramuscularly) in 13 patients with ventricular ectopic beats which were unresponsive to one or more of the commonly employed antiarrhythmic agents., *i.e.*, xylocaine, procainamide, quinidine, and diphenylhydantoin. Clinical diagnoses included acute myocardial infarction, coronary artery disease without recent infarction, digitalis toxicity, and cardiomyopathy. The results following bretylium administration in these patients are depicted in Figure 20.5. In 10 of the 13 episodes of premature ventricular contractions, there was a marked decrease in ectopic beats after bretylium. The mean number of premature ventricular beats decreased from 18 per minute before bretylium to two per minute at 2 to 3 hours after treatment. However, it was also noted that, in eight patients, prior to alleviation of premature ventricular beats there was an increase in their number which occurred 5 to 10 minutes after administration of bretylium. Although this increase in ventricular automaticity was an alarming finding, it was tran-

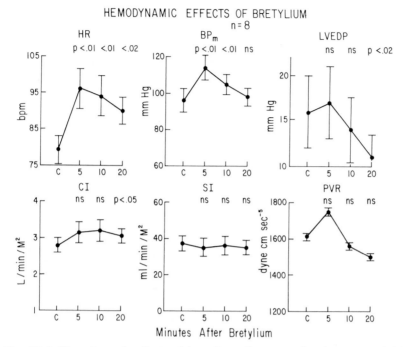

HEMODYNAMIC EFFECTS OF BRETYLIUM

Fig. 20.6. Hemodynamic effects of bretylium (5 mg. per kg. intravenously) in eight patients. LVEDP, left ventricular end diastolic pressure. (See Fig. 20.1 for other abbreviations.)

sient and without further consequences. The antiarrhythmic effects were usually manifest within 30 minutes and endured for 3 to 12 hours. Bretylium was also utilized as prophylactic therapy in five patients with recurrent ventricular tachycardia. In these patients, bretylium was highly successful in preventing recurrence of the arrhythmia.

We have also evaluated the effects of bretylium on cardiac performance in patients during diagnostic catheterization (Fig. 20.6). The drug produced significant increases in cardiac index, heart rate, and mean intra-arterial blood pressure. Left ventricular end diastolic pressure, elevated prior to bretylium, fell to normal. The effects on stroke index and peripheral resistance were not significant during the 20-minute period of observation. Maximal contractile element velocity (V_{max}), not depicted in Figure 20.6, rose significantly in all patients during the first 20 minutes after bretylium administration. Analysis of the effects of bretylium on cardiac performance may be considered in terms of data from isolated cardiac muscle preparations and intact man. Thus, it appears that the early enhancement of left ventricular performance produced by bretylium is the result of (1) a combination of norepinephrine release from sympathetic nerve terminals and

(2) a direct action of the drug. The early positive inotropic effect and also the increase in ventricular automaticity are consistent with release of norepinephrine, an action demonstrated in experimental studies.[59, 63, 64] The delayed hypotensive effect, a relatively frequent, untoward occurrence after bretylium, results from peripheral sympathetic nerve blockade after initial catecholamine release. The resultant decrease in peripheral vascular resistance, if inordinate, can significantly reduce systemic blood pressure. Hypotension, occurring in 88 per cent of patients in our clinical studies, was the most common untoward effect of bretylium. In over 50 per cent of the patients, systolic blood pressure decreased more than 20 mm. Hg, despite maintenance of bed rest in the supine position. However, pressor therapy was not required in these patients, and no complications resulted from the hypotension which abated within 24 hours. As noted above early increase in ventricular ectopic beats following bretylium administration, not reported previously, was observed in 50 per cent of patients in our clinical trial. Untoward subjective symptoms such as agitation, headache, nausea and, less commonly, vomiting, occurred in approximately one-third of the patients and were less than 24 hours in duration.

Present clinical experience with bretylium has indicated that hypotension is both the most common and most important side effect produced by the drug[88, 90-93, 96] and may occasionally limit its use. Thus, in one study of bretylium in patients with acute myocardial infarction, the drug was withdrawn from more than one-third of the group because of the development of hypotension.[93] This effect, although accentuated with orthostasis,[86, 87, 92, 93] is not uncommon in supine patients.[86, 88, 92, 93] Further, hypotension has been produced by oral bretylium therapy.[92] Nausea and vomiting, as in our experience,[96] have been relatively frequent but transient.[86, 88, 90, 93, 95]

There is little clinical information regarding the effect of bretylium on AV conduction in patients with and without heart block. On the basis of current data, bretylium does not tend to produce or augment any degree of heart block or intraventricular conduction abnormality. In clinical studies, the drug has been variably reported to have no effect on the PR, QRS, and QT intervals,[88] to increase the PR interval slightly,[96] and to abolish second degree heart block of the Wenckebach type.[86]

Conclusion

Initial clinical evaluation of the adrenergic blocking drug bretylium suggests that it may be effective in the treatment and prevention of cardiac arrhythmias, particularly those of ventricular origin. Bretylium differs from the usual antiarrhythmic drugs in the mechanism of its antiarrhythmic action and its possession of a positive inotropic effect on the myocardium. Its side effects and some reports of ineffectiveness indicate the necessity for further evaluation to determine its therapeutic efficacy and the clinical significance of its potentially advantageous properties.

REFERENCES

1. Lawrence, A. M.: Glucagon in medicine: new ideas for an old hormone. Med. Clin. N. Amer. 54: 183, 1970.
2. Samols, E., Tyler, J., Megysei, C., and Marks, V.: Immunochemical glucagon in human pancreas, gut, and plasma. Lancet 2: 727, 1966.
3. Kones, R. J., and Phillips, J. H.: Glucagon: present status in cardiovascular disease. Clin. Pharmacol. Ther. 12: 427, 1971.
4. Foa, P. P.: Glucagon, the hyperglycemic glycogenolytic hormone of the pancreas. Advan. Intern. Med. 6: 29, 1954.
5. Sutherland, E. W., Robison, G. A. and Butcher, R. W.: Some aspects of the biological role of adenosine 3',5'-monophosphate (cyclic AMP). Circulation 37: 279, 1968.
6. Sutherland, E. W., and Rall, T. W.: The relation of adenosine-3',5'-phosphate and phosphorylase to the action of catecholamines and other hormones. Pharmacol. Rev. 12: 265, 1960.
7. Epstein, S. E., Skelton, C. L., Levey, G. S., and Entman, M.: Adenyl cyclase and myocardial contractility. Ann. Intern. Med. 72: 561, 1970.
8. Gold, H. J., Prindle, K. H., Levey, G. S., and Epstein, S. E.: Effects of experimental heart failure on the capacity of glucagon to augment myocardial contractility and activate adenyl cyclase. J. Clin. Invest. 49: 999, 1970.
9. Unger, R. H., Ohneda, A., Valverde, I., Eisentraut, A. M., and Exton, J.: Characterization of the responses of circulation glucagon-like immunoreactivity to intraduodenal and intravenous administration of glucose. J. Clin. Invest. 47: 48, 1968.
10. Sokal, J. E.: Glucagon—an essential hormone. Amer. J. Med. 41: 331, 1966.
11. Garcia, A., Williamson, J. R., and Cahill, G. F.: Studies on the perfused rat liver. II. Effect of glucagon on gluconeogenesis. Diabetes 15: 188, 1966.
12. Williamson, J. R.: Mechanism for the stimulation in vivo of hepatic gluconeogenesis by glucagon. Biochem. J. 101: 11C, 1966.
13. Farah, A., and Tuttle, R.: Studies on the pharmacology of glucagon. J. Pharmacol. Exp. Ther. 129: 49, 1960.
14. Glick, G., Parmley, W. W., Wechsler, A. S., and Sonnenblick, E. H.: Glucagon—its enhancement of cardiac performance in the cat and dog and persistence of its inotropic action despite beta receptor blockage with propranolol. Circ. Res. 22: 789, 1968.
15. Lucchesi, B. R.: Cardiac actions of glucagon. Circ. Res. 22: 777, 1968.
16. Regan, T. J., Lehan, P. H., Henneman, D. H., Behar, A., and Hellems, H. K.: Myocardial metabolic and contractile response to glucagon and epinephrine. J. Lab. Clin. Med. 63: 638, 1964.
17. Manchester, J. H., Parmley, W. W., Matloff, J. M., Keidtke, A. J., LaRaia, P., Herman, M., Sonnenblick, E. H., and Gorlin, R.: Effects of glucagon on myocardial oxygen consumption and coronary blood flow in man and in dog. Circulation 41: 579, 1970.
18. Rowe, G. G.: Systemic and coronary hemodynamic effects of glucagon. Amer. J. Cardiol. 25: 670, 1970.
19. Glick, G.: Comparison of the peripheral vascular effects of glucagon, norepinephrine, isoproterenol and dopamine. Clin. Res. 18: 307, 1970.

20. Cohn, K. E., Agmon, J., and Gamble, O. W.: The effect of glucagon on arrhythmias due to digitalis toxicity. Amer. J. Cardiol. 25: 683, 1970.
21. Steiner, C., Wit, A. L., and Damato, A. N.: Effects of glucagon on atrioventricular conduction and ventricular automaticity in dogs. Circ. Res. 24: 167, 1969.
22. Kipski, J. I., Kaminsky, D. M., Donoso, E., and Friedberg, C. K.: The electrophysiological properties of glucagon on the normal canine heart. Amer. J. Cardiol. 23: 124, 1969.
23. Lucchesi, B. R., Stutz, D. R., and Winfield, R. A.: Glucagon: its enhancement of atrioventricular nodal pacemaker activity and failure to increase ventricular automaticity in dogs. Circ. Res. 25: 183, 1969.
24. Whitehouse, F. W., and James T. N.: Chronotropic action of glucagon on the sinus node. Proc. Soc. Exp. Biol. Med. 122: 823, 1966.
25. Whitsitt, L. S., and Lucchesi, B. R.: Effects of beta-receptor blockade and glucagon on the atrioventricular transmission system in the dog. Circ. Res. 23: 855, 1968.
26. Moir, T. W., and Nayler, W. G.: Coronary vascular effects of glucagon in the isolated dog heart. Circ. Res. 26: 29, 1970.
27. Bache, R. J., McHale, P. H., Curry, C. L., Alexander, J. A., and Greenfield, J. C., Jr.: Coronary and systemic hemodynamic effects of glucagon in the intact unanesthetized dog. J. Appl. Physiol. 29: 769, 1970.
28. Deleted in proof.
29. Manchester, J. H., Parmley, W. W., Matloff, J. M., and Sonnenblick, E.: Beneficial effects of glucagon in canine experimental myocardial infarction and shock. Clin. Res. 17: 252, 1969.
30. Matloff, J. M., Parmley, W. W., Manchester, J. H., Berkovits, B., Sonnenblick, E., and Harken, D. E.: Hemodynamic effects of glucagon and intraaortic balloon counterpulsation in canine myocardial infarction. Amer. J. Cardiol. 25: 675, 1970.
31. Klein, S. W., Morch, J. E., and Mahon, W. A.: Cardiovascular effects of glucagon in man. Can. Med. Ass. J. 98: 1161, 1968.
32. Parmley, W. W., Glick, G., and Sonnenblick, E. H.: Cardiovascular effects of glucagon in man. New Engl. J. Med. 279: 12, 1968.
33. Linhart, J. W., Barold, S. S., Cohen, L. S., Hildner, F. J., and Samet, P.: Cardiovascular effects of glucagon in man. Amer. J. Cardiol. 22: 706, 1968.
34. Williams, J. F., Childress, R. H., Chip, J. N., and Border, J. F.: Hemodynamic effects of glucagon in patients with heart disease. Circulation 39: 38, 1969.
35. Greenberg, B. H., McCalister, B. D., and Frye, R. L.: Hemodynamic effects of glucagon in patients with coronary artery disease at rest and during mild supine exercise. Clin. Res. 17: 243, 1969.
36. Greenberg, B. H., Tsakiris, A. G., Moffitt, E. A., and Frye, R. L.: The hemodynamic and metabolic effects of glucagon in patients with chronic valvular heart disease. Mayo Clin. Proc. 45: 132, 1970.
37. Murtagh, J. G., Binnion, P. F., Lal, S., Hutchison, K. J., and Fletcher, E.: Haemodynamic effects of glucagon. Brit. Heart J. 32: 307, 1970.
38. Ashley, W. W., Kaminsky, D. M., Lipski, J. I., Weisenseel, A. C., Donoso, E., and Friedberg, C. K.: Hemodynamic effects of glucagon in patients with fixed rate pacemakers. Amer. J. Cardiol. 25: 82, 1970.
39. Goldschlager, N., Robin, E., Cowan, C. M., Leb, G., and Bing, R. J.: The effect of glucagon on the coronary circulation in man. Circulation 40: 829, 1969.
40. Bonrassa, M. G., Eibar, J., and Campeau, L.: Effects of glucagon on myocardial

metabolism in patients with and without coronary artery disease, Circulation 42: 53, 1970.

41. Sonnenblick, E. H., Parmley, W. W., and Matloff, J.: Hemodynamic effects of glucagon after prosthetic valve replacement. Circulation 37 (Suppl. 6): 183, 1968.

42. Vaughn, C. C., Warner, H. R., and Nelson, R. M.: Cardiovascular effects of glucagon following cardiac surgery. Surgery 67: 204, 1970.

43. Brogan, E., Kozonis, M. C., and Overy, D. C.: Glucagon therapy in heart failure. Lancet, 1: 482, 1969.

44. VanderArk, C. R., and Reynolds, E. W.: Clinical evaluation of glucagon by continuous infusion in the treatment of low output states. Amer. Heart J. 70: 481, 1970.

45. Wilcken, D. E. L., and Lvoff, R.: Glucagon in resistant heart failure and cardiogenic shock. Lancet 2: 1315, 1970.

46. Nord, H. J., Fontanes, A. L., and Williams, J. F., Jr.: Treatment of congestive heart failure with glucagon. Ann. Intern. Med. 72: 649, 1970.

47. Kones, R. J., and Phillips, J. H.: Glucagon in congestive heart failure. Chest, in press.

48. Gregory, J., Mueller, H., Gnoj, J., Ayres, S., Giannelli, S., and Conklin, E.: Effects of glucagon on cardiovascular dynamics and myocardial metabolism in the low output state. Clin. Res. 17: 243, 1969.

49. Eddy, J. D., O'Brien, E. T., and Singh, S. P.: Glucagon and haemodynamics of acute myocardial infarction. Brit. Med. J. 4: 663, 1969.

50. Diamond, G., Forrester, J., Danzig, R., Parmley, W. W., and Swan, H. J. C.: Acute myocardial infarction in man. Comparative hemodynamic effects of norepinephrine and glucagon. Amer. J. Cardiol. 27: 612, 1971.

51. Diamond, G., Forrester, J., Danzig, R., Parmley, W. W., and Swan, H. J. C.: Hemodynamic effects of glucagon during acute myocardial infarction with left ventricular failure in man. Brit. Heart J. 33: 290, 1971.

52. Simanis, J., Goldberg, L. I.: The effects of glucagon on sodium, potassium, and urine excretion in patients in congestive heart failure. Amer. Heart J. 81: 202, 1971.

53. Amsterdam, E. A., Zelis, R., Spann, J. F., Jr., Hurley, E. J., and Mason, D. T.: Comparison of glucagon and catecholamines in congestive heart failure and coronary shock. Circulation (Suppl. 3) 42: 82, 1970.

54. Sobel, B. E., Henry, P. D., Robison, A., Bloor, C., and Ross, J., Jr.: Depressed adenyl cyclase activity in the failing guinea pig heart. Circ. Res. 24: 507, 1971.

55. Boura, A. L. A., Green, A. F., McCoubrey, A., Laurence, D. R., Moulton, R., and Rosenbaum, M. L.: Darenthin: hypotensive agent of new type. Lancet 2: 17, 1959b.

56. Boura, A. L. A., Green, A. F.: The action of bretylium: adrenergic neurone blocking and other effects. Brit. J. Pharmacol. 14: 536, 1959.

57. Exley, K. A.: The persistence of adrenergic nerve conduction after TM or bretylium in the cat. In Vane, J. R., Wolstenholme, G. E. W., and O'Connor, M. (eds.): *Adrenergic Mechanisms.* J. & A. Churchill, Ltd., London, 1960, p. 158.

58. Kirpekar, S. M., and Furchgott, R. F.: The sympathomimetic action of bretylium on isolated atria and aortic smooth muscle. J. Pharmacol. Exp. Ther. 143: 64, 1964.

59. Cass, R., and Spriggs, T. L. B.: Tissue amine levels and sympathetic blockade after guanethidine and bretylium. Brit. J. Pharmacol. 17: 442, 1961.

60. Brodie, B. B., and Costa, E.: Role of norepinephrine in autonomic ganglia in

regulation of blood pressure. In Brest, A. N., and Moyer, J. H. (eds.): *Hypertension, Recent Advances*. Lea & Febiger, Philadelphia, 1961, p. 354.

61. Aviado, D. M., and Dil, A. H.: The effects of a new sympathetic blocking drug (Bretylium) on cardiovascular control. J. Pharmacol. Exp. Ther. 129: 328. 1960.

62. Boura, A. L. A., Copp, F. C., Duncombe, W. G., Green, A. F., and McCoubrey, A.: The selective accumulation of bretylium in sympathetic ganglia and their post ganglionic nerves. Brit. J. Pharmacol. 15: 265, 1960.

63. Gokhale, S. D., Gulati, O. D., and Kelkar, V. V.: Mechanism of initial adrenergic effects of bretylium. Brit. J. Pharmacol. 20: 362, 1963.

64. Siegel, J. H., and Gilmore, J. P.: Effect of bretylium tosylate on the myocardial release and extraction of catecholamine. Fed. Proc. 20: 126, 1961.

65. Herting, G., Oxelrod, J., and Patrick, R. W.: Actions of bretylium and guanethidine on the uptake and release of [^{3}H]-noradrenaline. Brit. J. Pharmacol. 18: 161, 1962.

66. Gaffney, T. E.: Effect of guanethidine and bretylium on the dog heart-lung preparation. Circ. Res. 9: 83, 1961.

67. Gaffney, T. E., Braunwald, E., and Cooper, T.: Analysis of the acute circulatory effects of guanethidine and bretylium. Circ. Res. 10: 83, 1962.

68. Bacaner, M. B.: Quantitative comparison of bretylium with other antifibrillatory drugs. Amer. J. Cardiol. 21: 504, 1968.

69. Amsterdam, E. A., Spann, J. F., Jr., Mason, D. T., and Zelis, R.: Characterization of the positive inotropic effects of bretylium tosylate: a unique property of an antiarrhythmic agent. Amer. J. Cardiol. 25: 81, 1970.

70. Markis, J. E., and Koch-Weser, J.: Characteristics and mechanism of inotropic and chronotropic actions of bretylium tosylate. J. Pharmacol. Exp. Ther. 178: 94, 1971.

71. Leveque, P. E.: Anti-arrhythmic action of bretylium. Nature 207: 203, 1965.

72. Bacaner, M.: Bretylium tosylate for suppression of induced ventricular fibrillation. Amer. J. Cardiol. 17: 528, 1966.

73. Bacaner, M., and Schrienemachers, D.: Bretylium tosylate for the suppression of ventricular fibrillation after experimental myocardial infarction. Nature 220: 494, 1968.

74. Wit, A. L., Steiner, C., and Damato, A. N.: Electrophysiologic effects of bretylium tosylate on single fibers of the canine specialized conduction system and ventricle. J. Pharmacol. Exp. Ther. 173: 344, 1970.

75. Bigger, J. T., and Jaffe, C. C.: The effect of bretylium tosylate on the electrophysiologic properties of ventricular muscle and Purkinje fibers. Amer. J. Cardiol. 27: 82, 1971.

76. Hoffman, B. F., and Bigger, J. T., Jr.: Antiarrhythmic drugs. In DiPalma, J. R. (ed.): *Drill's Pharmacology in Medicine*, Ed. 4, Chap. 40. McGraw-Hill Book Company, New York, 1971.

77. Bigger, J. T., Jr., Bassett, A. L., and Hoffman, B. F.: Electrophysiological effects of diphenylhydantoin on canine Purkinje fibers. Circ. Res. 22: 221, 1968.

78. Bigger, J. T., Jr., and Mandel, W. J.: Effect of lidocaine on the electrophysiological properties of ventricular muscle and Purkinje fibers. J. Clin. Invest. 49: 63, 1970.

79. Bigger, J. T., Jr., and Mandel, W. J.: Effect of lidocaine on conduction in canine Purkinje fibers and at the ventricular muscle-Purkinje fiber junction. J. Pharmacol. Exp. Ther. 172: 239, 1970.

80. Waxman, M. B., and Wallace, A. G.: The electrophysiologic effects of bretylium tosylate in the awake dog. Amer. J. Cardiol. 25: 135, 1970.

81. Watanabe, Y., Josipovic, V., and Dreifus, L. S.: Electrophysiological mechanisms of bretylium tosylate. Fed. Proc. 28: 270, 1969.

82. Pamintuan, J. C., Dreifus, L. S., and Watanabe, Y.: Comparative mechanisms of antiarrhythmic agents. Amer. J. Cardiol. 26: 512, 1970.

83. Weidman, S.: The effect of the cardiac membrane potential on the rapid availability of the sodium-carrying system. J. Physiol. 127: 213, 1955.

84. Singer, D. H., and Ten Eick, R. E.: Pharmacology of cardiac arrhythmias. Progr. Cardiovasc. Dis. 11: 488, 1969.

85. Hoffman, B. F.: The possible mode of action of antiarrhythmic agents. In Briller, S. A., and Conn, H. L., Jr. (eds.): *The Myocardial Cell.* University of Pennsylvania Press, Philadelphia, 1966, p. 251.

86. Bacaner, M. R.: Treatment of ventricular fibrillation and other acute arrhythmias with bretylium tosylate. Amer. J. Cardiol. 21: 530, 1968.

87. Day, H. W., and Bacaner, M. R.: Use of bretylium tosylate in the management of acute myocardial infarction. Amer. J. Cardiol. 27: 177, 1971.

88. Aravindakshan, V., Gettes, L. S., and Surawicz, R.: Use of bretylium tosylate in recurrent refractory arrhythmias. Circulation 41 and 42 (Suppl. 3): III–130, 1970.

89. Terry, G., Vellani, C. W., Higgins, M. R., and Doig, A.: Bretylium tosylate in treatment of refractory ventricular arrhythmias complicating myocardial infarction. Brit. Heart J. 32: 21, 1970.

90. Richards, A. M., and Jerde, O. M.: Bretylium tosylate and electroshock as combined therapy for intractable ventricular fibrillation and arrhythmias in myocardial infarction. Amer. J. Cardiol. 23: 13, 1969.

91. Krall, J. I., and Rakita, L.: Treatment of ventricular arrhythmias with bretylium tosylate. Amer. Heart J. 8: 288, 1971.

92. Macalpin, R. N., Zalis, E. G., and Kivowitz, C. F.: Prevention of recurrent ventricular tachycardia with oral bretylium tosylate. Ann. Intern. Med. 72: 909, 1970.

93. Saxton, S. H., Saxton, C., Davies, P. S., and Stoker, J. B.: Bretylium tosylate in prevention of cardiac dysrhythmias after myocardial infarction. Brit. Heart J. 32: 326, 1970.

94. Feldman, A. E., Hellerstein, H. K., Driscol. T. E., and Botti, R. E.: Repetitive ventricular fibrillation in myocardial infarction refractory to bretylium tosylate subsequently controlled by ventricular pacing. Amer. J. Cardiol. 27: 227, 1971.

95. Castenada, A. R., and Bacaner, M. B.: Effect of bretylium tosylate on the prevention and treatment of postoperative arrhythmias. Amer. J. Cardiol. 25: 461, 1970.

96. Mansour, E., Mason, D. T., Spann, J. F., Jr., Zelis, R., and Amsterdam, E. A.: Clinical evaluation of antiarrhythmic and hemodynamic properties of bretylium. Circulation 42 (Suppl. 3): 41, 1970.

21

Factors Affecting Myocardial Potassium Balance

TZU-WANG LANG, M.D., ELIOT CORDAY, M.D.,
HUGO CARRASCO, M.D., AND JOSE LOZANO, M.D.

Potassium efflux from the myocardium was first reported by Harris and his associates[1] in 1954 when they sampled the coronary sinus blood following coronary artery occlusion. They believed that the potassium released from the ischemic myocardium established an ectopic focus which produced ventricular tachycardia and fibrillation. This phenomenon was confirmed by many investigators,[2-6] but the recent study of Wexler and Patt[7] indicates that the relationship of intracellular potassium balance and arrhythmias might be a more complicated matter, because those animals with the greatest potassium efflux did not develop ventricular fibrillation. Thomas, Shulman and Opie[8] demonstrated that the changes in mean concentration of coronary sinus plasma potassium in the ischemic myocardium are not the major determinants of early arrhythmia after experimental coronary occlusion. They found that serious ventricular arrhythmias occurred frequently after occlusion of the left anterior descending artery or of its terminal branch but not after occlusion of anterolateral or apical branches. They hypothesized that anatomic factors appeared to be of greater importance than an increase in coronary venous potassium concentration in determining the onset of serious arrhythmias soon after coronary artery occlusion.

Evidence from our laboratory indicates that cardiac arrhythmias per se will cause a considerable net potassium loss from the myocardium;[9] ventricular tachycardia was produced by local application of aconite in 18 dogs. Elevation of the coronary sinus potassium started within 1 minute after the onset of the arrhythmia and increased progressively in all animals. The largest increases were from a control of 3.5 to 7.4 and from 2.6 to 6.5 mEq per liter. Potassium efflux from the myocardium of this magnitude would tend to perpetuate the arrhythmia, making it resistant to therapy, and could lead to fatal ventricular fibrillation. We believe this is the first study which demonstrates a large potassium loss from the myocardium during rapid ventricular tachycardia in the intact heart with normal coronary circulation and innervation.

Potassium is important for the normal repolarization of the cell and to extend the duration of the action potential. A loss of this cation, such as after coronary occlusion, would set the scene for the induction of an arrhythmia, which would cause a further loss of potassium and thus tend to perpetuate a more serious arrhythmia. Conversely, it would appear that, to correct a rapid cardiac arrhythmia, potassium must be actively returned back across the cell membrane so that normal activation processes and action potentials can be resumed.

ACTIVE IONIC TRANSPORT MECHANISMS

Mechanisms of ionic flux of the cations calcium-sodium-potassium across the myocardial cell membrane has shed considerable light on the cause of cardiac arrhythmias and their treatment.[10, 11] It is believed the current required for depolarization of the heart muscle cell is carried by positively charged sodium ions. Upon excitation, the permeability of the cell membrane suddenly changes to allow the rapid influx of sodium ions across the sarcolemma and the transverse tubular system. In the interval immediately following this sudden depolarization, sodium influx slows and potassium efflux subsequently supervenes. Depolarization of the cell also triggers the release of ionic calcium and causes it to enter the cell following the sodium influx.[10-12] As calcium influx ceases, potassium efflux increases to repolarize rapidly the cell and allow relaxation. During the period of repolarization, the sodium-calcium pump mechanisms become activated by high energy exchange systems which cause a net loss of sodium and a net gain of potassium. At the same time, calcium has to be stored in the cytoplasmic reticulum, and this is an energy-requiring process.

When potassium is lost from the cell in excessive quantities, the resting potential of the cell decreases toward positivity and reaches a point closer to the threshold for firing. Potassium loss also causes the action potential to shorten so that the absolute refractory period is reduced, and the non-refractory period during which the heart muscle cell can be excited is prolonged so that a small stimulus can have more chance to set up an arrhythmia. The shorter the distance between the resting potential and the depolarization threshold, the more irritable the cell. If a tachycardia supervenes, we believe that it will cause a further potassium egress, reducing the resting potential nearer the threshold level so that it requires only a small electrical excitation to cause depolarization, and also the duration of the action potential will continue to decrease. With still further potassium loss, the spike of the action potential becomes slowed and of low amplitude.

Thus the excitation process cannot become elicited, the cell becomes inexcitable, and cardiac standstill ensues which can give rise to ventricular fibrillation.

CAUSES FOR MYOCARDIAL POTASSIUM LOSS

Acute Cardiac Ischemia

Harris et al.[1] first demonstrated that coronary ligation could produce a net loss of potassium from the heart muscle and, because this was accompanied by arrhythmias, they suggested that potassium released from the ischemic myocardium might act as an excitatory factor at the boundary of the infarction to establish an ectopic focus leading to ventricular tachycardia and fibrillation. Cherbakoff et al.,[4] Cummings,[5] and Regan et al.[6] confirmed this phenomenon. However, Wexler and Patt[7] believe that potassium efflux is not the etiological agent which causes ventricular fibrillation following coronary artery occlusion because, in their study, only 33 per cent of the 69 dogs had an elevation of coronary sinus potassium. In 12 animals who developed ventricular fibrillation after coronary ligation, only 3 showed a significant elevation of coronary sinus plasma potassium concentration.

Thomas, Shulman, and Opie[8] recently demonstrated that when they ligated a coronary artery there was a marked rise in potassium concentration in the local vein draining the area of ischemia which persisted for a period of up to 40 minutes. Although as much as 20 per cent of the myocardium was involved in the ligation, the coronary sinus did not reflect a rise in the potassium content. This would suggest that the coronary sinus might not always reveal the serious local potassium egress from the myocardium.

Sarnoff et al.[13] demonstrated that a net myocardium potassium gain occurred when norepinephrine was administered, but when they constricted coronary flow to induce a myocardial ischemia, infusion of norepinephrine caused an increase in the coronary sinus potassium as a result of a loss of potassium from the heart muscle.

Glycosides

Glycosides can cause a serious intracellular myocardial potassium loss. This was first demonstrated by Calhoun and Harrison[14] in 1931 and confirmed by Wedd,[15] Wood and Moe,[16] Shatzman,[17] Hadju and Leonard,[18] Regan et al.,[6] Lown,[19] and Lown and Levine.[20] There are several theories which attempt to explain this potassium egress. Keynes and Lewis[21] suggested that digitalis attaches itself to a specific site on the external surface of the cell membrane that gives it the ability to inhibit the action of sodium-potassium-activated ATPase and thus interferes with potassium influx. Sarnoff *et al.*[13, 22] believed that the acutely induced loss of potassium resulting from the administration of acetyl strophanthidin is importantly related to increased myocardial contractility.

Electrical Shock

Childers *et al.*[23] and Regan *et al.*[24] demonstrated an increased coronary sinus potassium concentration immediately after electrical cardioversion. They also demonstrated that, when strophanthidin was administered intravenously in nontoxic doses, subsequent electrical countershock caused a still greater loss of potassium which extended over a longer period.[24] Cardiac arrhythmias often supervened and persisted for about 7 minutes. We believe that the arrhythmias which follow countershock are primarily due to the net myocardial potassium loss which disturbs normal resting and action potentials.

Acidemia

It has been suggested that an overall shift of potassium from the intracellular to the extracellular space occurs during acute metabolic acidosis and hypercapnia, which causes a progressive rise in plasma potassium level.[25] This might be a primary factor in the causation of cardiac arrhythmias and arrest during and after surgery.[26-28] During the immediate posthypercapnic recovery period, an additional sharp increase in the coronary sinus plasma potassium level accompanied by serious electrocardiographic and arrhythmic disturbances sometimes terminates in ventricular fibrillation or standstill.[29-31] Early administration of hypertonic glucose and saline solutions may reverse these electrocardiographic changes.[28] This has been explained by the fact that the increased heart rate increases metabolic activity and oxygen consumption, and this is accompanied by an increased CO_2 production and hydrogen ion concentration. Thus, the increase in the ratio of $H_i^+ : H_e^+$. (where H_e^+ is the extracellular hydrogen ion concentration and H_i is the intracellular hydrogen ion concentration) promotes a net loss of potassium from the cell.[13, 32, 33]

Increased Preload and Afterload

In isolated supported heart preparations, Gilmore and Gerlings[34] and Sarnoff *et al.*[13] noted that when contractility increased there was a net loss of potassium from the heart, and that when contractility decreased there was a net gain of potassium. The net loss of potassium appeared to vary with the observed increase in oxygen consumption.[35] They believed that a causal link existed between increased oxygen utilization and the net loss of potassium.

Arrhythmias

We have demonstrated that tachycardias caused a significant potassium egress from the intact heart in all 18 experiments, and this terminated in ventricular fibrillation.[9]

We note that Harris and his associates[1] obtained blood samples taken only at one time, that is, 7 minutes after coronary occlusion while ventricular tachycardia existed. Their figures display a simultaneous rise in potassium concentration in the local venous blood drained from the intact myocardium as well as from the coronary sinus. We demonstrated that ventricular tachycardia in itself will cause potassium egress from the intact heart, and we believe that this accentuates a further potassium loss from the ischemic as well as the normal myocardium. This might explain why Harris *et al.* noted a simultaneous rise in potassium level in coronary sinus blood drained from the myocardium which was ischemic, as well as from the normal myocardium. Probably the levels were much higher in the blood draining the ischemic zone because of an overlapping effect.

Although Regan *et al.*[6] and Cherbakoff *et al.*[4] confirmed that potassium loss following coronary ligation is the major cause of cardiac arrhythmia, none of them noted that ventricular tachyarrhythmias aggravated a further myocardial potassium efflux following coronary occlusion. However, when we reviewed their tracings, we noted that a secondary potassium loss in the myocardium often occurred following the onset of the ischemic or digitoxic arrhythmias. After countershock, the cardiac arrhythmias which supervened appear to have caused a further net potassium loss.[24]

Recent studies by Ebert[35] demonstrated that the potassium content of the atrial muscle was much lower in patients with chronic atrial fibrillation than in those with regular sinus rhythm. Parker and his associates[36] recently reported that cardiac pacing at rapid rates was associated with net myocardial potassium loss and that those losses were immediately restored during the postpacing period. Myocardial potassium loss was significantly greater in the group of patients with coronary artery disease, and this was closely associated with myocardial lactate production and reduction in coronary sinus blood pH.[36] In our study, we have also noted a myocardial potassium egress during aconite-induced ventricular tachycardia which was associated with excessive production of myocardial lactate and a reduction of pH in coronary sinus blood.

MECHANISM OF MYOCARDIAL POTASSIUM EGRESS DURING TACHYARRHYTHMIAS

The mechanism of myocardial potassium egress during tachycardia has not yet been elucidated. Sarnoff and his associates[13, 37] noted a relationship between increased contractility and the observed net potassium loss. The amount of the net potassium loss appeared to vary with the observed increase in oxygen consumption. They postulated that a causal link between the observed net loss of potassium and the increased contractile state as well as oxygen utilization is based on an increased metabolic activity and, thus, on an increased $H_i^+:H_e^+$ ratio.[13, 33] Gilmore and Gerlings[38] suggested that, when the heart rate is increased by stimulus, the duration of the interstimulus interval is a determinant of myocardial potassium balance. The interstimulus interval is greatly shortened in tachycardias, and this could account for the potassium loss. Langer *et al.*[10-12] postulated that the loss of potassium observed with increasing frequency of contraction is due to a sodium pump lag which allows for a transient net loss of potassium. They have shown that, as the rate is increased, the ATPase mechanism is stimulated by the net sodium gain inside the cell and this is associated with a potassium loss. Eventually, as the rate speeds up past a certain point, the ATPase mechanism reaches its maximal performance, and then a more progressive potassium loss results.[39, 40]

RATIONALE FOR TREATMENT OF RESISTANT TACHYARRHYTHMIAS

As a result of our studies, we conclude that one of the principles basic to the treatment of tachyarrhythmias should consider methods which restore myocardial potassium balance. Cherbakoff *et al.*[4] demonstrated that infusion of insulin-glucose and/or sodium bicarbonate solution into the coronary artery will reduce the coronary sinus potassium efflux following the coronary ligation, and that the cardiac rhythm will remain regular for a prolonged period of time. Sodi-Pallares *et al.*[41-43] and Maciel *et al.*[44] have observed that administration of potassium in the form of a polarizing solution (glucose, insulin, potassium chloride) prevents or diminishes the appearance of ectopic beats or rhythms following coronary occlusion in animals and in man with or without relation to digitalis administration. Regan *et al.*[6] demonstrated that, when the administration of glucose is combined with insulin, it restored the ionic potassium loss and this corrected the ischemic arrhythmias. They noted that procaine amide also restored potassium balance and converted ischemic arrhythmias. The administration of drugs such as diphenylhydantoin[45] and beta adrenergic blocking agents[46, 47] also is known to force potassium back across the cell membrane, and this restoration of intracellular potassium might explain some of their antiarrhythmic effects. These findings support our postulation that restoration of the myocardial potassium balance provides a new basis for the treatment of tachyarrhythmias.

REFERENCES

1. Harris, A. S., Bisteni, A., Russell, R. A., Brigham, J. C., and Firestone, J. E.: Excitatory factors in ventricular tachycardia resulting from myocardial ischemia. Potassium a major excitant. Science 119: 200, 1954.
2. Russell, R. A., Crafoord, J., and Harris, A. S.: Changes in myocardial composition after coronary artery ligation. Amer. J. Physiol. 200: 995, 1961.
3. Hano, J. E., and Harris, A. S.: Effects of histamine and potassium release agents on ventricular arrhythmias before and after coronary occlusion. Amer. Heart J. 65: 368, 1963.
4. Cherbakoff, A., Tozanna, S., and Hamilton, W. F.: Relation between coronary sinus plasma potassium and cardiac arrhythmias. Circ. Res. 4: 517, 1957.
5. Cummings, J. R.: Electrolyte changes in heart tissue and coronary arterial and venous plasma following coronary occlusion. Circ. Res. 8: 865, 1960.
6. Regan, T. J., Harman, M. H., Lehan, P. H., Burke, W. M., and Oldewurtel, H. A.: Ventricular arrhythmias and potassium transfer during myocardial ischemia and intervention with procain amide, insulin, or glucose solution. J. Clin. Invest. 46: 1657, 1967.
7. Wexler, J., and Patt, H. H.: Evidence that serum potassium is not the etiological agent in ventricular fibrillation following coronary artery occlusion. Amer. Heart J. 60: 618, 1960.
8. Thomas, M., Shulman, G., and Opie, L.: Arteriovenous potassium changes and ventricular arrhythmias after coronary artery occlusion. Cardiovasc. Res. 4: 327, 1970.
9. Lang, T. W., Corday, E., Lozano, J., Carrasco, H., and Meerbaum, S.: Dynamics of potassium flux in cardiac arrhythmias. Amer. J. Cardiol., (in press).
10. Langer, G. A.: Ion fluxes in cardiac excitation and contraction and their relation to myocardial contractility. Physiol. Rev. 68: 708, 1968.
11. Langer, G. A., and Serena, S. D.: Effects of strophanthidin upon conduction and ionic exchange in rabbit ventricular myocardium: relation to control of active state. J. Mol. Cell. Cardiol. 1: 65, 1970.
12. Langer, G. A., and Brady, A. J.: Potassium in dog ventricular muscle: kinetic studies of distribution and effect of varying frequency of contraction and potassium concentration of perfusate. Circ. Res. 18: 164, 1966.
13. Sarnoff, S. J., Gilmore, J. P., McDonald, R. H., Jr., Daggett, W. M., Weisfeldt, M. L., and Mansfield, P. B.: Relationship between myocardial potassium balance, oxygen consumption, and contractility. Amer. J. Physiol. 211: 361, 1966.
14. Calhoun, H. A., and Harrison, T. R.: Studies in congestive failure. IX. The effect of digitalis on potassium content of the cardiac muscle of dogs. J. Clin. Invest. 10: 13, 1931.
15. Wedd, A. M.: Influence of digoxin on the potassium content of heart muscle. J. Pharmacol. Exp. Ther. 65: 268, 1939.
16. Wood, E. H., and Moe, G. K.: Electrolyte and water content of the ventricular musculature of the heart-lung preparation with special reference to the effects of cardiac glycosides. Amer. J. Physiol. 136: 515, 1942.
17. Schatzman, H. J.: Herzglykoside als Hemmstoffe fur den aktiven Kalium-und-Natrimentransport durch die Erythroegtenmembran. Helv. Physiol. Pharmacol. Acta 11: 346, 1953.
18. Hadju, W. S., and Leonard E.: The cellular basis of cardiac glycoside action. Pharmacol. Rev. 11: 173, 1959.
19. Lown, B.: Digitalis and potassium. Advan. Intern. Med. 8: 125, 1956.

20. Lown, B., and Levine, S. A.: Current concepts in digitalis therapy. New Engl. J. Med. 250: 771, 1954.
21. Keynes, R. D., and Lewis, P. R.: Resting exchange of radioactive potassium in crab nerve. J. Physiol. 113: 73, 1951.
22. Sarnoff, S. J., Gilmore, J. P., Mitchell, J. H., and Remens-Nyder, J. P.: Potassium changes in the heart during hemeometric autoregulation and acetyl-strophanthidin. Amer. J. Med. 34: 440, 1963.
23. Childers, R. W., Rothbaum, D., and Arnsdorf, M. F.: Effect of direct current shock on the electrical properties of the heart. Circulation 35-36 (Suppl. 2): 85, 1967.
24. Regan, T. J., Markov, A., Oldewurtel, H. A., and Harman, M. A.: Myocardial potassium loss after countershock and the relation to ventricular arrhythmias after non-toxic doses of acetyl strophanthidin. Amer. Heart J. 77: 367, 1969.
25. Keating, R. E., Weichselbaum, T. E., Alanis, M., Margraf, H. W., and Elman, R.: The movement of potassium during experimental acidosis and alkalosis in the nephrectomized dog. Surg. Gynec. Obstet. 96: 323, 1953.
26. Young, W. G., Jr., Sealy, W. C., Harris, J. S., and Botwin, A.: The effects of hypercapnia and hypoxia on the response of the heart to vagal stimulation. Surg. Gynec. Obstet. 93: 51, 1951.
27. Johnstone, M.: Cyclopropane anesthesia and ventricular arrhythmias. Brit. Heart J. 12: 239, 1950.
28. Miller, F. A., Brown, E. B., Buckley, J. J., Van Bergen, F. H., and Vareo, R. L.: Respiratory acidosis: its relationship to cardiac function and other physiologic mechanisms. Surgery 32: 171, 1952.
29. Young, W. G., Jr. Sealy, W. C., and Harris, J. S.: The role of intracellular and extracellular electrolytes in the cardiac arrhythmias produced by prolonged hypercapnia. Surgery 36: 636, 1954.
30. Brown, E. B., Jr., and Mowlem, A.: Potassium loss from the heart during the immediate post-hypercapnic period. Amer. J. Physiol. 198: 962, 1960.
31. Lade, R. I., and Brown, E. B., Jr.: Movement of potassium between muscle and blood in response to respiratory acidosis. Amer. J. Physiol. 204: 761, 1963.
32. Brown, E. B., Jr., and Goutt, B.: Intracellular hydrogen ion changes and potassium movement. Amer. J. Physiol. 204: 765, 1963.
33. Clancy, R. L.: The effect of changes in intracellular pH on intracellular potassium in cardiac muscle (Ph.D. thesis). University of Kansas, Lawrence, Kansas, 1965.
34. Gilmore, J. P., and Gerlings, E. D.: Influence of developed tension on myocardial potassium balance in the dog heart. Circ. Res. 22: 769, 1968.
35. Ebert, P. A.: Relationship of myocardial potassium content and atrial fibrillation. Circulation 41-42 (Suppl. 2): 137, 1970.
36. Parker, J. O., Chiang, M. A., West, R. O., and Case, R. B.: The effect of ischemia and alterations of heart rate on myocardial potassium balance in man. Circulation 152: 205, 1970.
37. Sarnoff, S. J., Gilmore, J. P., Daggett, P. B., Mansfield, W. M., Weisfeldt, W. M., and McDonald, R. H., Jr.: Myocardial dynamics contractility, oxygen consumption, and potassium balance during paired stimulation. Amer. J. Physiol. 211: 376, 1966.
38. Gilmore, J. P., and Gerlings, E. D.: Influence of interstimulus interval on myocardial potassium balance. Amer. J. Physiol. 217: 136, 1969.
39. Langer, G. A.: The role of sodium ion in the regulation of myocardial contractility (editorial). J. Mol. Cell. Cardiol. 1: 203, 1970.

40. Blesa, E. S., Langer, G. A., Brady, A. J., and Serena, S. D.: Potassium exchange in rat ventricular myocardium. Its relation to rate of stimulation. Amer. J. Physiol. 219: 747, 1970.
41. Sodi-Pallares, D., Bisteni, A., Medrano, G. A., Testelli, M. R., and de Micheli, A.: The polarizing treatment of acute myocardial infarction. Possibility of its use in other cardiovascular conditions. Dis. Chest 43: 424, 1962.
42. Sodi-Pallares, D., de Micheli, A., Fishleder, B. L., Cisneros, F., Vizcaino, M., Bisteni, A., Medrano, G. A., Polanski, B. J., and Testelli, M. R.: Effets d'un régime hyposode hyperpotassique et riche en eau sur l'évolution clinique et électrocardiographique de certaines cardiopathies. Acta Cardiol. 16: 166, 1961.
43. Sodi-Pallares, D., and de Micheli, A.: Un tentativo di reintegrazione ionica cellulare in alenne malattie cardiovascular. Atti Accad. Med. Lombard. 17: 509, 1962.
44. Maciel, J. P., Mancini, D., Gemenez, H., and Etchegary, E.: Tratamiento de algunas cardiopatias con la terapentica polarizante. Prensa Med. Argent. 50: 2995, 1963.
45. Helfant, R. H., Riccinti, M. A., Scherlag, B. J., and Damato, A. N.: Effect of diphenylhydantoin sodium (Dilantin) on myocardial AO potassium differences. Amer. J. Pharmacol. 214: 880, 1968.
46. Lucchesi, B. R., Whitsitt, L. S., and Stickney, J. L.: Antiarrhythmic effects of beta-adrenergic blocking agents. Ann. N. Y. Acad. Sci., 139: 940, 1967.
47. El-Fiky, S. B. I., and Katzung, B. G.: Effect of hypothermia and pronethalol on ionic correlates of ouabain arrhythmias in dogs. Circ. Res. 24: 43, 1969.

22

Therapy of Power Failure of the Heart

TZU-WANG LANG, M.D., JOHN K. VYDEN, M.B.B.S.,
AND ELIOT CORDAY, M.D.

Effective management of patients with acute cardiac perfusion failure depends upon early recognition, ascertaining the degree of shock, and a thorough knowledge of pathophysiology and of the benefits, drawbacks, and limitations of therapeutic agents and other procedures. New concepts of the pathophysiology, diagnosis, and treatment of cardiogenic shock suggest, however, that we are approaching a new era during which the overwhelming mortality rate associated with this dreaded complication will be progressively reduced.

ACUTE CARDIAC PERFUSION FAILURE

Time of Onset

About one-third of patients develop shock within 6 hours after the onset of infarction, one-half within 24 hours, and two-thirds in 36 hours. About 13 per cent develop shock after 1 week.[1]

Recognition

The clinical manifestations of shock are cold, clammy skin, an altered level of consciousness with resultant confusion, agitation, and oliguria. The onset of oliguria and hypotension may occur in many other conditions such as those caused by hypotension due to opiates, the use of sedatives, and bacterial infection.

Inherent difficulties in the diagnosis and management of shock secondary to cardiac infarction are compounded when it is realized that a cuff blood pressure is often erroneous. Indeed, if the arterial pulse pressure is small or the patient is peripherally vasoconstricted, there may be a large discrepancy between the cuff pressure and the actual intra-arterial pressure.[2] Cohn has reported discrepancies of as much as 164 mm. Hg.[3] This discrepancy is greatest in patients receiving vasopressor drugs because their peripheral

245

vessels may constrict. Sometimes patients can become hypertensive during norepinephrine infusion, but the arm cuff pressure is either unobtainable or low. Many previously published studies comparing various agents used to treat patients in shock are invalid because their pressure measurements are unreliable. Because of the difficulty associated with the recognition and the setting of criteria for drug intervention in shock, the search for easily usable methods other than cuff pressure is continuing. The direct measurement of intra-arterial blood pressure is desirable for the management of shock.[4]

It is known that, when the cardiac output is markedly reduced, the speed of blood flow is correspondingly slowed. Hence, the appearance and mean transit time of indicator dye are correspondingly prolonged. Measurements of circulation time by the earpiece technique after injection of indocyanine green dye into a central venous catheter provides very useful information on the patient's hemodynamic status. Even under conditions of profound circulatory failure, when the earpiece dye curve is markedly distorted, changes in appearance time are indicative of improvement or deterioration in cardiovascular function.[5, 6] A recent study showed that simple measurement of the great toe temperature provides objective information on the severity of shock.[7]

It is essential that the physician rule out shock associated with a coincident illness. If the elderly patient with cardiac infarction needs bladder catheterization and he develops the shock syndrome on the 2nd or 3rd day of illness, it may be due to gram-negative bacteremia rather than cardiac infarction. Since urinary tract instrumentation in the elderly is associated with a high incidence of bacteremia, precipitation of bacteremic shock in acute cardiac infarction is probably common.

Pathophysiology

Cardiac output is normal in 70 per cent of patients with cardiac infarction. Extensive myocardial dysfunction pump failure is common after myocardial infarction and results in a drop of 30 to 50 per cent in the cardiac index.[5]

The fall in cardiac output may have as its cause a decrease in heart rate or stroke volume. Heart rate is generally increased in shock, and the fall in output is attributed to a reduction in stroke volume. Bradycardia often occurs as a result of excessive vagotonia and is associated with hypotension which is promptly corrected by administration of atropine. Stroke volume may in turn be caused either by a decrease in cardiac filling pressure resulting from impaired venous return or by a decrease in the strength of ventricular contraction. Weakness of ventricular contraction despite an adequate filling pressure or, in other words, "pump failure," is the source of the hemodynamic maladjustment. According to Starling's law of the heart, the energy of ventricular contraction is a function of the length of the muscle fiber, which in turn is a function of filling pressure. Filling pressure or central venous pressure may be decreased because of hypovolemia or because of an increased tone of capacitance vessels. Hypovolemia is often present in shock without overt evidence of external blood or fluid loss. It is due to seepage of fluid volume into the extravascular spaces and gut. Fluid replacement is now accepted as an essential part of the treatment in many instances.[8] Since patients with acute cardiac infarction almost always have severe coronary disease involving the vessels supplying the non-infarcted myocardium,[9] there will be other areas in which the coronary flow is pressure-dependent.[10] Hence, coronary circulation and its collateral flow will tend to fail if pressure drops.[11] Since hypoxia is a powerful stimulus to systemic vasodilatation,[12] the collateral vessels surrounding the area of infarction may be maximally vasodilated and, because of this, flow in these areas will also be pressure-dependent.

Feedback Mechanisms

An immediate adjustment to a fall in arterial blood pressure occurs through baroreceptor reflexes, causing a sympathoadrenal discharge and an elevation of blood levels of catecholamines which has both beneficial and deleterious effects. There are certain beneficial effects of these sympathoadrenal mechanisms such as a positive inotropic response, redistribution of organ blood flow, and coronary vasodilation.[13] Their deleterious effect is prolonged reduction of blood flow to the gut, kidneys, and musculoskeletal system. Reduction of blood flow in capillaries causes venous pooling, production of systemic acidosis because of lactic acid accumulation resulting from poor tissue perfusion, and reduction in peripheral blood flow at the microcirculatory levels, which encourages the formation of diffuse intravascular thrombosis. Acidosis and hypoxemia reduce contractility still further.

As arterial pressure falls, perfusion to the ischemic cardiac muscle decreases, and this may cause extension of the infarct. The progressive increase in the area of ischemia induced by hypotension explains the rapid clinical deterioration and also cardiac irritability.

Prognostic Indices

In assessing the prognosis of acute cardiac infarction and shock, individual measurements reflecting the stroke index or cardiac index are more reliable than measurements of blood pressure as indicators of survival. When sets of observations from survivors and from patients who failed to recover from shock are analyzed, then the measurement of stroke index and diastolic pressure can predict the outcome with an estimated accuracy of 95 per cent.[14]

A single great toe temperature measurement 3 hours after admission to the hospital correctly predicts the patient's outcome 67 per cent of the time.[7] Massive infarction is usually accompanied by a high risk of mortality. The size of the infarct can be evaluated by electrocardiographic, vectorcardiographic, and roentgenographic means.

We believe that monitoring of the central venous pressure is essential since a fluid challenge is often an essential part of treatment.[4, 8] The objection that, in a great number of patients, central venous pressure may be a poor reflection of left ventricular end diastolic pressure has been overcome with the advent of a new flow-directed catheter which can measure pulmonary artery and capillary wedge pressure simply and without the need for fluoroscopy.[15]

As outlined above, the techniques for evaluating exactly the functional state of a patient require a high level of sophistication. We believe that, ideally, the best interests of the patient are served by progressive serial measurements of cardiac index, direct intra-aortic blood pressure, and pulmonary wedge pressure. We chose these measurements because they act as a guide to functional change and effectiveness of therapy. We also know that direct intra-aortic diastolic blood pressure and cardiac index together provide, up to the present time, the optimal indices from which we can predict the outcome of a patient. We choose to measure pulmonary wedge pressure because the heart must be fully loaded with volume so as to make full use of the Starling mechanism of contraction of the left ventricle. In this situation, a wedge pressure of up to 25 mm. Hg is considered desirable. Under certain circumstances, for example, with pathology of the mitral valve, direct catheterization of the left ventricle is desirable so that left ventricular end diastolic pressure may be directly measured as a guide to volume loading. In addition to the above, the clinician must carefully watch clinical signs of shock such as cold limbs, confusion, sweating, etc. We do not believe that the religious measurement of urinary output is of great value because in shock the renal artery is vasoconstricted. Thus, when an agent such as norepinephrine, with its renal vasoconstrictive mechanism, is added to a treatment regime, the use of urine output as a major guide to status is often misleading.

THERAPEUTIC APPROACHES

Trendelenburg Position and External Warming

The once widely used head-down Trendelenburg position and the additional concern with conservation of body heat by the liberal use of blankets or even external warming devices have been discarded. These maneuvers nearly always decrease intra-arterial blood pressure and cardiac index, and the vasodilation induced by surface warming is likely only to intensify rather than minimize the circulatory deficit underlying shock.[16]

Relief of Anxiety and Pain

The relief of anxiety and pain in the patient is of major importance for several reasons: it reduces the pain stimulus which induces the shock state by excessive catecholamine production, it helps improve ventilation and reduce bronchospasm, and it reduces restlessness.[17]

New studies of the effect of single intravenous doses of morphine have disclosed that morphine tends to reduce the systemic vascular resistance and the blood pressure, as well as to depress the rate and depth of respiration with a reduction in pO_2 and a rise in pCO_2.[18, 19] If a hypotensive effect occurs, this often engenders an erroneous diagnosis of shock and a train of unwarranted aggressive therapy. Hypotension is sometimes magnified by concomitant sedatives. This may increase myocardial hypoxia and the tendency of the infarcted myocardium to develop ventricular fibrillation. Single doses of morphine may sometimes increase the heart rate and output and thus increase cardiac work. Also the vagotonic effect of morphine may result in bradycardia and this in turn causes secondary "escape" tachyarrhythmias.

Meperidine (Demerol), like morphine, may cause hypotension and respiratory depression, but it also has a favorable atropine-like effect. Pentazocine (Talwin) given intravenously in a dosage of 60 mg. seems preferable to morphine[19]; this drug does not produce the hypotension which is seen following morphine administration. It usually causes slight increases in blood pressure. Although, like morphine, it causes respiratory depression, it does not increase the ratio of physiological dead space to tidal volume and the pulmonary arterial-alveolar oxygen gradient, such as occurs with morphine, changes which are associated with an unfavorable prognosis.[19] However, further studies of the hemodynamic effects of pentazocine must be undertaken before it can be endorsed as preferable to agents such as morphine sulfate.

Eradication of Undesirable Cardiac Arrhythmias

Both supraventricular and ventricular arrhythmias usually cause a drop of one- to two-thirds in coronary artery blood flow and cardiac index.[20-22] Hence, their prompt eradication in the already hypotensive patient is essential.

However, consideration of the methods used is critical. Quinidine, procainamide, propranolol, and diphenylhydantoin take considerable vital time to correct the cardiac irritability. They are all potent myocardial depressants, and their long-term action is therefore often associated with undesirable side effects in shock.[23] Lidocaine is preferable because, when given intravenously, it has a very rapid antiarrhythmic action.[24-26]

If hypotension exists with the arrhythmias, the prompt administration of a vasopressor, such as norepinephrine, will often terminate the arrhythmia when pressure is restored.[11]

Electrical cardioversion will often revert an arrhythmia, but if concomitant hypoxia or metabolic acidosis are left untreated, the tachyarrhythmia will be resistant to electrical conversion. The tachyarrhythmia might best be managed by rapid atrial pacing (via a transvenous pacemaker in the right atrium), which can take over pacemaking from the abnormal focus.[27, 28] Then the pacemaker can gradually be slowed either until sinus rhythm again takes over or until the heart is paced at a more desirable heart rate.

Treatment of Concomitant Pulmonary Edema

Generally, if cardiac output improves with the treatment of shock, the signs of heart failure disappear. If essential, diuretics are preferred to glycosides in this situation, but they carry hazards of their own. Kirkendall and Wilson, for instance, showed that ethacrynic acid may cause an acute fall in systemic arterial blood pressure, mean right atrial pressure, cardiac index, and total peripheral resistance.[29]

Correction of Metabolic Acidosis

Periods of inadequate cardiac output result in inadequate tissue perfusion, which may lead to the development of excess lactate production and metabolic acidosis.[30] In humans, this metabolic acidosis reduces the sensitivity of the adrenergic receptor sites to the effect of catecholamines.[31] Since the sympathetic nervous system plays a major role in homeostasis and cardiac contractility, which are essential to combat acute shock, acidosis must be recognized and promptly treated.

Oxygen Therapy

In patients with cardiogenic shock, the arterial oxygen tension is greatly reduced and, although it can be elevated by breathing oxygen, it remains significantly below normal.[32] Oxygen administration diminishes cardiac output and increases total peripheral resistance. Deficiency in tissue oxygenation and a consequently anaerobic metabolism are recognized by elevation of arterial lactate concentration. If given in high concentration, oxygen lowers abnormally elevated arterial lactate levels, and it is often presumed that these metabolic advantages of oxygen therapy outweigh the consequences of its diminishing cardiac output and increasing vascular resistance. However, it has not been demonstrated that the benefits of conventional oxygen therapy have resulted in a reduction in mortality or even a diminution in the extent of myocardial necrosis.[33]

Although beneficial effects have been reported in isolated patients treated with hyperbaric oxygenation, the number of controlled studies to evaluate the results is inadequate.[33, 34]

Vagotonia

When a patient develops sudden arterial hypotension associated with a fall in central venous pressure and bradycardia, the apparent shock state may be due to vagotonia, and it should be promptly treated with intravenous atropine.

Volume Challenge

There is a high incidence of hypovolemia seen in the shock state because of fluid loss into the extravascular spaces which has been called "third spacing." An initial trial of volume loading is accepted as a rational approach when vasopressors fail.

All patients who meet the criteria of cardiogenic shock, showing no radiological signs of cardiac decompensation, and having a right atrial pressure of less than 10 cm. fluid should be challenged with a test volume load of 100 to 300 ml. of 5 per cent dextrose in water infused over a period of 5 to 15 minutes. If they respond with no rise, or only a slight rise in pulmonary wedge pressure, they should be treated with a further infusion of larger volumes of fluid, up to 120 to 300 ml. per hour, until the pressure is restored.[8, 35]

Pharmacological Intervention

Norepinephrine

If needed, norepinephrine should be given in amounts just sufficient to increase the intra-arterial pressure to about 100 mm. Hg systolic, since no further benefit is obtained with greater amounts.

Some clinicians formerly believed that norepinephrine had a deleterious effect because it caused a disproportionate increase of oxygen utilization in the myocardium. However, Sarnoff and his associates showed that this does not occur unless large unphysiological dosages are given.[36]

If vasopressors are to be used, it is essential that they be started promptly. It is known that, at 22 minutes after coronary occlusion, the first irreversibly damaged cells appear. After 45 minutes of total hypoxia, only 35 to 66 per cent of the cells remain viable.[37] Norepinephrine, however, reduces the size of cardiac infarction because it augments the collateral flow to the region of myocardial ischemia. This is the area which originally triggered the shock state.[38]

Few reliable survival statistics on the use of vasopressor drugs are available because in most studies implementation is delayed beyond the first few critical hours when viability of the myocardium might still be restored. Griffith et al.[39] showed that, when the pressure was restored within the first 3 hours of cardiogenic shock, the mortality was only 13 per cent. However, if this treatment was delayed beyond 3 hours, the mortality increased to 76 per cent. This emphasizes that, if vasopressors are to be of benefit, they must be instituted soon after the onset of the hypotensive state.

Norepinephrine cannot be endorsed as the perfect drug, for its prolonged use may compromise the splanchnic and renal circulations and damage the gastrointestinal tract and kidney.[40, 41]

3-Hydroxytyramine (Dopamine)

3-Hydroxytyramine (dopamine) may replace norepinephrine as the vasopressor of choice in treating cardiogenic shock. 3-Hydroxytyramine, which is the immediate biochemical precursor of norepinephrine, when given intravenously in doses of 2 to 8 μg. per kg. per min., increases mean blood pressure, mean cardiac output, mean coronary arterial blood flow and, at the same time, blood flow to the kidney and the gastrointestinal tract.[42] It appears to have an almost ideal proportion of alpha and beta adrenergic activity, enabling it to restore coronary and central hemodynamics without throttling the regional circulation of the kidney and gut as do most other vasopressors.[43]

L-Dopa

L-Dopa, which is a precursor of dopamine, has the properties of augmenting coronary flow, increasing left ventricular contractility, and reducing total peripheral vascular resistance.[44, 45] If eventually it is found that the increase in contractility is obtained without increasing the oxygen debt and that myocardial oxygen consumption is balanced by augmentation of coronary flow, L-dopa could prove to be a valuable drug.

Isoproterenol

After much controversy, it now appears that isoproterenol may be an unsatisfactory agent in the treatment of shock secondary to acute cardiac infarction because isoproterenol appears to increase myocardial oxygen requirements beyond the value gained by the concomitant increase in cardiac output.[4, 11, 46] Electrocardiographic changes reflecting myocardial ischemia are intensified when isoproterenol is given following coronary ligation in the experimental animal.[47] In addition, isoproterenol may cause a further reduction in pressure, resulting in marked generalized organ ischemia. Isoproterenol often increases the heart rate to augment cardiac work or causes serious cardiac irritability, effects which contraindicate its usage.[11]

Possibly, if isoproterenol has any place in treatment of shock secondary to cardiac infarction, then it is in the management of patients who exhibit the shock syndrome but maintain normal intra-arterial pressure. If isoproterenol reduces pressure, this signifies that vasodilation occurred and that the infusion should be accompanied by simultaneous plasma volume expansion.[4] Isuprel might be used in the short period between recognition of complete heart block and shock associated with acute cardiac infarction. If isoproterenol improves the shock state by increase in heart rate, the institution of electrical pacing is imperative.

Combined Vasopressor-Vasodilator Drug Therapy

The sympathoadrenal discharge which occurs in shock may be beneficial insofar as it increases cardiac output and redistributes blood flow to vital organs. The sustained and marked peripheral vasoconstriction which may occur has certain drawbacks because it increases cardiac work and causes complication such as renal shutdown,[40, 48] gastrointestinal ischemia and necrosis,[40, 49] failure of tissue perfusion with resulting acidosis, and also necrosis and intravascular thrombosis.[49] Excessive capillary filtrations resulting from a relatively greater increase in postcapillary than precapillary resistance are another deleterious effect of the adrenergic stimulus.

Alpha adrenergic receptor blockers such as phentolamine reduce the peripheral vasoconstriction effects without antagonizing the desirable beta-mediated inotropic response and coronary dilation. However attractive their use may appear on theoretical grounds, the clinical results of treatment with alpha blockade are disappointing.[50-52]

Hence, in treating shock, our attention should first be directed toward improving cardiac output by increasing filling pressure by volume challenge and then by the use of sympathetic amines with strong positive inotropic actions. If despite these measures and the concomitant treatment of acidosis, septicemia, and ventilation, there are signs indicating a continued state of inadequate perfusion and marked peripheral vasoconstriction, then an alpha blocker such as phentolamine should be added to the norepinephrine infusion. Such combined therapy appears promising but awaits more clinical evaluation.[53-55]

Digitalis

The specific indicator for digitalis therapy in the presence of overt heart failure or for the treatment of certain complicating arrhythmias is not questioned, but the value of digitalis in shock per se is considered controversial.

The glycosides increase the peripheral resistance and also the velocity and force of myocardial contraction, which augments myocardial oxygen consumption.[56-58] Therefore, it is postulated that glycosides increase relative myocardial ischemia and cause myocardial cells to suffer irreversible damage. Absolute scientific evidence proving that glycosides are beneficial or detrimental is not yet available.

If digitalis is used, it should be kept in mind that patients with acute cardiac infarctions are more sensitive to the cardiac glycosides, so that only 60 to 75 per cent of the amount normally utilized should be given.[59]

Glucagon[60-62]

While glucagon has been shown to increase cardiac output and stroke volume in patients undergoing routine diagnostic cardiac catheterization, when given as a bolus it produces inconsistent hemodynamic improvement and, when favorable changes occur, they are usually of small magnitude. When given as a continuous infusion in a dose range of 1 to 16 mg. per hour, it may improve blood pressure, decrease heart rate, and increase urine output. Occasional patients will respond dramatically to this drug when all else fails.

Corticosteroids

Although these agents may be efficacious in the management of other forms of shock,[63, 64] we do not believe that, used on their own, corticosteroids have any place in the management of shock secondary to cardiac infarction. Their exact role in an individual patient may become clearer as an increased knowledge of relative corticosteroid insufficiency in the pathogenesis of terminal shock is elucidated. Further studies evaluating massive doses of corticosteroids in cardiac infarction are underway at the present time.

Surgical Management of Shock

When all therapeutic maneuvers fail, one must ask the question, "Is there a surgically correctable lesion which might be operated upon?" Mechanical problems which cause myocardial dysfunction are now correctable, so that some patients may survive only with the help of successful cardiac surgery.[65]

Definitive treatment may take the form of surgical removal of infarcted or fibrosed ventricular muscle, correction of mitral insufficiency caused by papillary muscle dysfunction, closure of ruptures of the ventricular septum or free wall of the left ventricle, and direct myocardial revascularization procedures, depending on the location and extent of the pathology. Low cardiac output unresponsive to pharmacological treatment or suspicion of any of the above enumerated clinical complications are indications for emergency diagnostic procedures such as left ventricular angiography and/ or coronary angiography. Early infarctectomy and venous aorta-coronary artery jump grafts have been used by us successfully in some instances.[65-67]

Circulatory Assistance

Various modalities of circulatory assistance are now available which are becoming increasingly used in shock. While often successfully used late in shock when patients are terminal, these forms of treatment stand more chance for success if used earlier, before extensive necrosis and the secondary complications are allowed to develop.

Aortic balloon counterpulsation[68] and venoarterial pulsatile partial by-pass (VAPPB)[69, 70] might reverse the shock state both experimentally and clinically within a few hours. The present outlook for both of these devices in the coronary care setting offers much promise because they (1) improve cerebral and mesenteric circulations, (2) improve coronary perfusion and myocardial contractility, (3) correct hypoxemia and acidosis, (4) reduce ventricular end diastolic pressure and total peripheral vascular resistance, and (5) reduce systolic pressure and thus cardiac work and oxygen consumption.

A new simple practical form of temporary circulatory assist, ascending aorta synchronized pulsation (AASP),[71] appears most promising. It requires the insertion of only one single lumen cannula into the ascending aorta. With synchronized positive and negative pulsation of 3 to 10 ml. of blood, cardiac output and coronary flows improved markedly in experimental animals.

Another new concept in the treatment of shock secondary to cardiac infarction is coronary sinus perfusion with oxygenated blood.[72] Since the coronary sinus perfusion offers access to the myocardial capillaries as do the coronary arteries, the heart can be supported by their retrograde perfusion. In the experimental animal, this new technique is successful and is now undergoing extensive trials in patients with cardiac infarction and shock.

Cardiac Transplantation

Various temporary improvements can be achieved pharmacologically or with surgery and circulatory assist devices. It is axiomatic that there must be enough viable myocardium remaining to ensure long-term survival. Regrettably, in many patients most of the myocardium is lost.

If the involvement of other organ systems is minimal or seems reversible, then consideration of cardiac transplantation becomes tenable. Further study is needed, however, to conquer the problems of acute and late rejection.[73, 74] At present, cardiac transplantation must be considered an expensive and only temporary means of extending life for a few selected patients. It should become a practical technique, however, when medical science conquers the rejection phenomena.

Artificial Heart

It is reasonable to assume that within the next decade a completely implantable heart will be perfected which will provide life for the patient whose heart has been literally destroyed by myocardial infarction.[75]

REFERENCES

1. Scheidt, S., Aschem, R., and Killip, T., III: Shock after acute myocardial infarction. A clinical and hemodynamic profile. Amer. J. Cardiol. 26: 556, 1970.
2. Gunnar, R. M., Loeb, H. S., Pietras, R. J., and Tobin, J. R., Jr.: Hemodynamic measurements in a coronary care unit. Progr. Cardiovasc. Dis. 11: 29, 1968.
3. Cohn, J. N.: Blood pressure measurement in shock. J. A. M. A. 199: 972, 1967.
4. Gunnar, R. M., Loeb, H. S., Pietras, R. J., and Tobin, J. R., Jr.: Hemodynamic effects of myocardial infarction and results of therapy. Med. Clin. N. Amer. 54 (Suppl. 1): 235, 1970.
5. Weil, M. H., and Shubin, H.: Cardiogenic shock: pathogenesis and rationale of therapy. Coronary Heart Dis. 1 (Suppl. 2): 165, 1969.
6. Thomas, M., Malmcrona, R., and Shillingford, J.: The accuracy of the photoelectric earpiece technique in the treatment of cardiac output. Brit. Heart J. 27: 805, 1965.
7. Toby, H. R., and Weil, M. H.: Temperature of the great toe as an indication of the severity of shock. Circulation 39: 131, 1969.
8. Swan, H. J. C., Danzig, R., Sukumalchantra, Y., and Allen, H.: Current status of treatment of power failure of the heart in acute myocardial infarction with drugs and blood volume replacement. Circulation 39–40 (Suppl. 4): 277, 1969.
9. Blumgart, H. L., Schesinger, M. J., and Davis, D.: Studies in the relationship of the clinical manifestations of angina pectoris, coronary thrombosis, and myocardial infarction to pathologic findings. Amer. Heart J. 19: 1, 1940.
10. Moster, P., Ross, J., McFate, R. H., and Shaw, R. F.: Control of coronary blood flow by an autoregulatory mechanism. Circ. Res. 14: 250, 1964.
11. Corday, E., Vyden, J. K., Lang, T. W., Baszomenyi, E., Gold, H., Goldman, A., and Rosselot, E.: Re-evaluation of the treatment of shock secondary to cardiac infarction. Dis. Chest 56: 200, 1969.
12. Berne, R. M.: Regulation of coronary blood flow. Physiol. Rev. 44: 1, 1964.
13. Abboud, F. M.: The sympathetic nervous system and alpha adrenergic blocking agents in shock. Med. Clin. N. Amer. 52 (Suppl. 5): 1049, 1968.
14. Shubin, H., Afifi, A. A., Rand, W. M., and Weil, M. H.: Objective index of hemodynamic status for quantitation of severity and prognosis of shock complicating myocardial infarction. Cardiovasc. Res. 2 (Suppl. 4): 329, 1968.
15. Swan, H. J. C., Ganz, W., Forrester, J., Marcus, H., Diamond, G., and Chonette, D.: Catheterization of the heart in man with use of a flow-directed balloon-tipped catheter. New Engl. J. Med. 283: 447, 1970.
16. Taylor, J., and Weil, M. H.: Failure of the Trendelenburg position to improve circulation during clinical shock. Surg. Gynec. Obstet. 124: 1005, 1967.
17. Richardson, J. H.: Circulating levels of catecholamines in acute myocardial infarction and angina pectoris. Progr. Cardiovasc. Dis. 6: 56, 1963.

18. Thomas, M., Malmcrona, R., Fillmore, S., and Shillingford, J.: Hemodynamic effects of morphine in patients with acute myocardial infarction. Brit. Heart J. 27: 863, 1965.

19. Lal, S., Savidge, R. S., and Chabra, G. P.: Cardiovascular and respiratory effects of morphine and pentazocine in patients with myocardial infarction. Lancet 1: 379, 1969.

20. Corday, E., Gold, H., De Vera, L. B., Williams, J. H., and Fields, J.: Effect of cardiac arrhythmias on the coronary circulation. Ann. Intern. Med. 50: 535, 1959.

21. Corday, E., and Irving, D. W.: *Disturbances in Heart Rate, Rhythm and Conduction*. W. B. Saunders Company, Philadelphia, 1964, p. 306.

22. Corday, E., and Lang, T. W.: Hemodynamic consequences of cardiac arrhythmias. In *The Heart*, Ed. 2. New York, McGraw-Hill Book Company, 1970, p. 486.

23. Paulk, E. A., Jr., and Hurst, J. W.: Intractable heart failure and its management. Med. Clin. N. Amer. 54 (Suppl. 2): 309, 1970.

24. Lown, B., and Vassaux, C.: Lidocaine in acute myocardial infarction. Amer. Heart J. 76: 586, 1968.

25. Jewitt, D. E., Kishon, Y., and Thomas, M.: Lignocaine in the management of arrhythmias after acute myocardial infarction. Lancet 1: 266, 1968.

26. Harrison, D. C., Sprouse, J. H., and Morrow, A. G.: The antiarrhythmic properties of lidocaine and procaine amide. Circulation 28: 486, 1963.

27. Sowton, E., Leatham, H., and Carson, P.: The suppression of arrhythmias by artificial pacemaking. Lancet 2: 1098, 1964.

28. Beller, B. M., Kotler, M. N., and Collens, R.: The use of ventricular pacing for suppression of ectopic ventricular activity. Amer. J. Cardiol. 25: 467, 1970.

29. Kirkendall, W. M., and Wilson, C. B.: Treatment of the patient with refractory heart failute. Med. Clin. N. Amer. 52: 1157, 1968.

30. Scheurer, J.: Myocardial metabolism in cardiac hypoxia. Amer. J. Cardiol. 19: 385, 1967.

31. Zelis, R., Mason, D. T., and Braunwald, E.: A comparison of vasodilator stimuli peripheral resistance vessels in normal subjects in patients with congestive heart failure. J. Clin. Invest. 47: 960, 1968.

32. Mackenzie, G. J., Flenley, D. C., Taylor, S. H., McDonald, A. H., Staunton, H. P., and Donald, K. W.: Circulatory and respiratory studies in myocardial infarction and cardiogenic shock. Lancet 2: 825, 1964.

33. Camerson, A. J. V., Hutton, I., Kenmure, A. C. F., and Murdoch, W. R.: Hemodynamic and metabolic effects of hyperbaric oxygen in myocardial infarction. Lancet 2: 833, 1966.

34. Moon, A. J., Williams, K. G., and Hopkinson, W. I.: A patient with coronary thrombosis treated with hyperbaric oxygen. Lancet 1:18, 1964.

35. Allen, H. N., Danzig, R., and Swan, H. J. C.: Incidence and significance of relative hypovolemia as a cause of shock associated with acute myocardial infarction. Circulation 36 (Suppl. 2): 50, 1967.

36. Sarnoff, S. J., Gilmore, J. P., Weisfeldt, M. L., Daggett, W. M., and Mansfield, P. B.: Influence of norepinephrine on myocardial oxygen consumption under hemodynamic conditions. Amer. J. Cardiol. 16: 217, 1965.

37. Brachfield, N.: Maintenance of cell viability. Circulation 39–40 (Suppl. 4): 202, 1969.

38. Edlich, R. F., Burner, J., Quattlebaum, F. D. W., and Lillihei, C. W.: Limitation of size of myocardial infarction by administration of L-norepinephrine. Circulation 38 (Suppl. 6): 70, 1968.

39. Griffith, G. C., Wallace, W. B., Cochran, B., Nerlich, W. E., and Frasher, W. C.: Treatment of shock associated with myocardial infarction. Circulation 9: 527, 1954.
40. Corday, E., and Williams, J. H.: Effects of shock and of vasopressor drugs on the regional circulation of the brain, kidney and liver. Amer. J. Med. 29: 228, 1960.
41. Corday, E., Irving, D. W., Gold, H., Bernstein, H., and Skelton, R. B. T.: Mesenteric vascular insufficiency. Amer. J. Med. 33: 3, 1962.
42. Carvalho, M., Vyden, J. K., Bernstein, H., Gold, H., and Corday, E.: Hemodynamic effects of 3-hydroxytyramine (Dopamine) in experimentally induced shock. Amer. J. Cardiol. 23: 217, 1968.
43. Talley, R. C., Goldberg, L. I., Johnson, C. E., and McNay, J. L.: Hemodynamic comparison of dopamine and isoproterenol in patients in shock. Circulation 39: 361, 1969.
44. Carrasco, H. A., Lozano, J. R., Lang, T. W., and Corday, E.: Hemodynamic effects of L-Dopa. Geriatrics, in press.
45. Lozano, J. R., Carrasco, H. A., Lang, T. W., and Corday, E.: Pharmacodynamic application of L-Dopa for the treatment of experimental cardiogenic shock, in press.
46. Gunnar, R. M., Loeb, H. S., Pietra, R. J., and Tobin, J. R., Jr.: Ineffectiveness of isoproterenol in the treatment of shock due to acute myocardial infarction. J. A. M. A. 202: 1124, 1967.
47. Maroko, P. R., Kjekshus, J. K., Sobel, B. E., Watanabe, T., Covell, J. W., Ross, J., Jr., and Braunwald, E.: Factors influencing infarct size following experimental coronary artery occlusions. Circulation 43: 67, 1971.
48. Boughton, G. A., and Sommers, S. C.: Renal changes in shock treated with levarterenol. Amer. J. Clin. Pathol. 27: 29, 1957.
49. Brunson, Y. G., Eckman, P. L., and Campbell, Y. B.: The increasing incidence of unexplained liver necrosis. U. Minn. Med. Bull. 28: 197, 1957.
50. Riordan, J. F., and Walters, G.: Effects of phenoxybenzamine in shock due to myocardial infarction. Brit. Med. J. 1: 155, 1969.
51. Cowley, R. A.: Personal communication, January 21, 1966.
52. Goldberg, L. I.: The treatment of cardiogenic shock. VI. The search for an ideal drug. Amer. Heart J. 75: 416, 1968.
53. Gold, H., Baszomenyi, E., Lang, T. W., Enesen, V., Utsu, F., and Corday, E.: The augmentation of coronary flow in experimental cardiogenic shock with combined drug therapy. Acad. Med. N. J. Bull. 12: 180, 1966.
54. Wilson, R. F.: Combined use of norepinephrine and dibenzyline in clinical shock. Surg. Forum 15: 30, 1961.
55. Thal, A. P.: Panel discussion (F. A. Simeone, moderator). In Mills, L. C., and Moger, J. H. (eds): *Shock and Hypotension*. Grune & Stratton, New York, 1965, p. 421.
56. Wilson, R. F., Chiscano, A. D., and Quadros, E.: Some observations in 58 patients with cardiac shock. Anesth. Analg. 46: 764, 1967.
57. Sonnenblick, E. H., Williams, J. F., Jr., Glick, G., Mason, D. T., and Braunwald, E.: Studies on digitalis. XV. Effects of cardiac glycosides on myocardial force-velocity relations in the non-failing human heart. Circulation 34: 532, 1966.
58. Sonnenblick, E. H., Ross, J., Jr., Covell, J. W., Kaiser, G. A., and Braunwald, E.: Velocity of contraction as a determinant of myocardial oxygen consumption. Amer. J. Physiol. 209: 919, 1965.
59. Killip, T.: Management of the patient with acute myocardial infarction. Med. Clin. N. Amer. 52: 1061, 1968.

60. Parmley, W. W., Glick, G., and Sonnenblick, E. H.: Cardiovascular effects of glucagon in man. New Engl. J. Med. 279: 12, 1968.

61. Williams, J. F., Childress, R. H., Chip, J. N., and Border, J. F.: Hemodynamic effects of glucagon in patients with heart disease. Circulation 39: 38, 1969.

62. Linhart, J. W., Barold, S. S., Cohen, L. S., Hildner, F. J., and Samet, P.: Cardiovascular effects of glucagon in man. Amer. J. Cardiol. 22: 706, 1968.

63. Dietzman, R. H., and Lillehei, R. C.: The treatment of cardiogenic shock. V. The use of corticosteroids in the treatment of cardiogenic shock. Amer. Heart J. 75: 274, 1968.

64. Sambhi, M. P., Weil, M. H., and Udhoji, V. N.: Acute pharmacodynamic effects of glucocorticoids. Circulation 31: 523, 1965.

65. Lillehei, C. W., Jande, A. J., Rassman, W. R., Tanak, S., and Block, J. H.: Surgical management of myocardial infarction. Circulation 39–40 (Suppl. 4): 315, 1969.

66. Spencer, F. C.: Venous bypass grafts for occlusive disease of the coronary artery. Amer. Heart J. 79: 568, 1970.

67. Sabiston, D. C., Jr.: Direct revascularization procedure in the management of myocardial ischemia (editorial). Circulation 43: 175, 1971.

68. Krakauer, J. S., Rosenbaum, A., Freed, P. S., Jaron, D., and Kantrowitz, A.: Clinical management ancillary to phase-shift balloon pumping in cardiogenic shock. Preliminary comments. Amer. J. Cardiol. 27: 123, 1971.

69. Lang, T. W., Rosselot, E., Gold, H., Vyden, J. K., Goldman, A., Herrold, G., and Corday, E.: Effect of venoarterial pulsatile bypass on the coronary, renal and mesenteric circulations in cardiogenic shock. Amer. J. Cardiol. 27: 41, 1971.

70. Corday, E., Swan, H. J. C., Lang, T. W., Goldman, A., Matloff, J. M., Gold, H., and Meerbaum, S.: Physiologic principles in the application of circulatory assist for the failing heart. Amer. J. Cardiol. 26: 595, 1970.

71. Lang, T. W., Meerbaum, S., Lozano, J. R., Carrasco, H., and Corday, E.: Ascending aorta synchronized pulsation—AASP—a new temporary circulatory assist technique for the treatment of cardiogenic shock, in press.

72. Spann, J. F., Jr., Mason, D. T., Zelis, R. F., and Amsterdam, E. A.: A new concept in the treatment of shock in myocardial infarction. Coronary sinus perfusion with oxygenated blood at systemic pressure (abstract). Amer. J. Cardiol. 25: 129, 1970.

73. Terasaki, P. I., von Diepow, M., Davidson, C. J., and Mickey, M. R.: Serotyping for homotransplantation. XXIV. Heart transplantation. Amer. J. Cardiol. 24: 500, 1969.

74. Fernbach, D., Nora, J., and Cooley, D.: Prospective tissue typing for heart transplants. Lancet 1: 425, 1969.

75. De Bakey, M. E.: Left ventricular bypass pump for cardiac assistance. Clinical experience. Amer. J. Cardiol. 27: 3, 1971.

23

Maintenance of Cell Viability in Acute Myocardial Infarction

NORMAN BRACHFELD, M.D.

I have long been a fan of H. L. Mencken's and, as a third year medical student, I came across an essay of his entitled "Exeunt Omnes." It was written in 1919 as a commentary on a news story about Dr. George Crile, Sr., and it seems particularly apt and just as true 50 years later.

Mencken quotes Crile as saying:

". . . Death was acidosis—that it was caused by the failure of the organism to maintain the alkalinity necessary to its normal functioning. . . . [Mencken himself comments] I thus think of death as a sort of deleterious fermentation, like that which goes on in a bottle of Château Margaux when it becomes corked. Life is a struggle, not against sin, but against hydrogen ions. The healthy man is one in whom those ions, as they are dissociated by cellular activity, are immediately fixed by alkaline bases. The *sick* man is one in whom the process has begun to lag, with the hydrogen ions getting ahead. The *dying* man is one in whom it is all over save the charges of fraud."

Medicine could add little to the established concepts of religion and folklore in understanding the process of death until the middle of this century. Modern science has helped to extend the average life span by reducing the causes of infant mortality, infectious diseases, and other pathological processes, but it has had little or no impact on the built-in obsolescence of the human machine. The individual physiological life span remains fixed and apparently determined by a genetically programmed failure of the body's parts. After age 30, the probability of death doubles about every 8 years. Hayflick[1] points out that even if "heart disease, stroke, and cancer were eliminated, the average life expectancy would not be lengthened by much more than 10 years." Efforts to protect those 10 years against the common geriatric causes of death occupy a disproportionate amount of the clinician's time.

The feasibility of techniques for cardiopulmonary resuscitation and the

260

remarkable success of single and multiple organ transplants have not yet led to a sharpening of the inadequate, imprecise, and invariably confusing definitions of death given in contemporary lay and medical dictionaries. Death is variously defined as "suspension or cessation of vital processes of the body, as heart beat and respiration," [2] or "the ending of all vital function without possibility of recovery either in animals or plants or any parts of them: the end of life." [3] Legal definitions now current accept the concept of irreversibility which conceivably may lead to awkward medico-legal entanglements. Actually, the functional medical definition of death has been gradually changing. Until recently the physician was concerned primarily with gross evidence of the lack of viability; we now require a more qualitative definition of organ and cellular death. Classic definitions may leave those involved in transplantation programs in a dilemma. While hopefully extending the life of the recipient, transplantation requires that the functionally decerebrate "life" of the donor be shortened. Most authors stress the importance of establishing the "death" of the donor but urge that the decision be made on the state of cerebral function[4] and with a disregard for the viability of other organs and tissues. Some[5] urge that the decision be made in cases of brain injury on the basis of gross anatomic damage visible on physical examination, by craniotomy or by angiography. In the absence of universally acceptable, objective, early criteria, death must be operationally determined by when the doctor says it occurs.[6] Legal guidelines vary and most often are not available: thus shrouded in imprecision, this most critical diagnosis inevitably is left to the entirely subjective criteria established by physicians with widely divergent training and experience. With few exceptions, our medical schools have been unable to provide instruction in the prerequisites for a diagnosis of death, and they usually relegate this subject to brief consideration in a course on medical jurisprudence. The vagaries of current criteria also have led the most popular current textbooks on physical diagnosis either to ignore this area completely or to give it only token notice. One might well consider the definition of the death of the organism by first examining those factors that sustain cellular viability.

Therapy designed to prevent or diminish the severity of a pathological process requires control observations that will permit an evaluation of the response of the cell, tissue, or organ being studied. These remarks therefore first review briefly the histological, histochemical, and biochemical phenomena that occur when the cell is challenged by an ischemic insult. Since the theme of this presentation is the maintenance of cell viability in acute myocardial infarction, I shall focus on myocardial ischemia, although many of the changes described are quite nonspecific and occur as well in response to other types of cellular trauma. I hope to indicate those factors in the myocardial cellular environment which support viability and help maintain cellular homeostasis, and to suggest promising areas for future investigation into the pathogenesis of myocardial infarction and into improved methods of treatment.

The clinician's chief concern is whether or not the injury induced by coronary occlusion will cause temporary and reversible changes or permanent damage requiring *de novo* reparative tissue synthesis; *i.e.*, whether or not he is dealing with ischemia or cell necrosis (cell death). An early distinction between these two states is crucial to designing an effective program for treating coronary artery disease. Differentiation between the two also will help to define the permissible limits of nonperfusion of the arrested heart at surgery.

Open heart surgery has successfully challenged the dogma that the active aerobic metabolic activity of the myocardial cell limited to a few minutes the life span of the myocardium deprived of its circulation. Although electrocardiographic and biochemical changes were evident soon after surgically induced cessation of the coronary circulation, viability and the ability to return to adequate, if not optimal, functional activity were observed. At body temperatures, the nonperfused heart may be arrested for 25 to 30 minutes with the full expectation that it will return to normal function when the circulation has been re-established and defibrillation has been performed. If the temperature is lowered to 30°C. this period of nonperfused arrest can be extended to 1 hour. Andreev[7] reported resuscitation of the whole human heart as long as 43 hours after autopsy. Hearts were removed 60 to 90 minutes after autopsy, kept at 5 to 10°C., and perfused with Tyrode's solution. Once contraction had begun, they remained active for as long as perfusion was continued (up to 13 hours). Animal transplantation experiments are limited, but they have shown that the arrested heart can be removed and beating reinstituted as long as 72 hours later if the heart is stored at 3°C. and at from 3 to 7 atmospheres of O_2.[8] An initial 10-minute perfusion of the coronary vessels with lactated Ringer's solution to remove all blood permitted canine hearts to maintain viability without coronary circulation for up to 90 minutes at body temperature and to resume a resting cardiac work load when the circulation was restored.[9] Viability and return to normal function also have been observed in human cardiac transplants with as long as 2 hours of elapsed time between the removal and the completion of the transplant.

It is difficult to reconcile reports of survival after intentional whole heart cardiac arrest with the experience of laboratory investigators and clinicians that sudden occlusion of a segment of the coronary circulation can, and frequently does, lead to permanent, irreversible impairment of cardiac activity. The apparent paradox may be resolved by considering that ultimate vulnerability to myocardial ischemia is not a fixed phenomenon but is influenced by multiple factors. Models of myocardial ischemia must be precise in describing all parameters of energy production as well as the steady stage environment of the tissue so traumatized. We continue to be handicapped by the lack of adequate animal models of coronary artery disease, and extrapolation of information obtained from the experimental animal laboratory may be misleading. When the entire heart is subjected to surgical anoxic arrest, the presence or absence of concomitant perfusion, the pH, ionic composition and substrate composition of perfusing fluids (if used), the environmental temperature and the state of the coronary circulation before arrest all bear directly on its recovery of function when reperfused with well-oxygenated blood.

To the internist, anoxic arrest has a quite different meaning. It is never induced, is always an emergency, and frequently takes the life of the patient. If the insult does not cause arrest or ventricular fibrillation or if the patient survives this episode, one rarely sees a homogeneous, localized myocardial infarction. The result is more often a heterogeneous mixture[10] of progressively changing proportions of necrotic and living tissue determined by the location of the occlusion, the state of the collateral circulation, and the location of the infarct.

Under both circumstances, "surgical" and "medical," the ischemic state initially induces potentially reversible cellular changes. Under optimal surgical control of the arrested heart, all changes are reversed with the restitution of perfusion. Under "medical" conditions, total reversibility may occur, but here it is much less likely. More frequently, changes become fixed or progress to eventual necrosis and cell death. The severity of the response is determined by the state of the cell before the injury, the level of endogenous glycogen stores, and the condition of the arterial supply of the heart. There is a significant difference in cellular mortality, as well as in biochemical and histological changes, when the large infarct caused by occlusion of a component artery of a diffusely diseased system with a poor collateral circulation is compared with other areas of ischemic tissue which are supplied with a poor but potentially good collateral supply. In the former, the intrinsic glycogen store of the cell is the only possible substrate available; in the latter, a restricted circulation provides the opportunity for significant anaerobic metabolism, changes in pH, and variations in protein and lipid metabolism (discussed below). Viability also may be regulated in part by the rapidity with which blood supply to the ischemic area can be reestablished. Reversibly injured cells in an area distal to a coronary occlusion recover rapidly when circulation has been restored. Stainable glycogen is resynthesized, and contractile activity ensues. The need for a high level of efficient aerobic metabolic activity to meet the contractile demands made upon the injured tissue seriously compromises its potential for recovery and explains the differences in the rate of survival between anoxic arrest induced at surgery and that caused by coronary artery disease. The demands of muscle contraction help seal the fate of borderline ischemic cells, the infarct becomes sharply demarcated from adjacent normal myocardium, and contraction bands of normally functioning cells tend to distort the architecture of the zone of infarction. Caulfield and Klionsky[10] have shown that the actual disintegration of muscle fibers was dependent in part upon the activity of the muscle during the period of ischemia.

Finally, Bing et al.[11] have stressed the fact that survival of the major physiological and biochemical functions of the heart need not follow the same timetable. The factors that determine normal cardiac excitability are most vulnerable to anoxia or severe ischemia; those concerned with energy production and utilization survive for much longer periods. Thus loss of electrical potential may doom the cell at a time when other essential functions are viable and cell injury is potentially reversible.

HISTOLOGY AND HISTOCHEMISTRY OF MYOCARDIAL ISCHEMIA

The general pathologist is not chiefly concerned with the process of cell death. It is self-evident that routine histological preparations produce tissue sections in which all of the cells are dead and may have been for hours before fixation and staining. Observations made from these specimens often reflect secondary degenerative changes that actually occurred some time after cell death. Under the most favorable circumstances, human studies rarely can be performed until long after the actual process of cell death has been accomplished. Precision in timing the onset of the ischemic insult is not possible by available clinical or laboratory techniques so that the "evolution time"[12] of the lesion can be only roughly estimated. Despite the many problems presented by the use of laboratory models, the experimental pathologist can present a visual demonstration of the cellular changes which follow induced tissue ischemia. He can describe these changes in a more operational mode as a function of the time following induced occlusion. I hope to demonstrate that these observations can contribute to our understanding of the pathogenesis of a process which extends from an early period of potentially reversible alterations to ultimate irreversible cell death. Most studies have been performed upon the liver, kidney, and spleen; nevertheless, experiments with skeletal muscle and myocardium indicate qualitatively similar alterations for all nonconnective tissues. Slight tissue differences are due to variations in the type of cellular protein and the composition of existing enzyme systems.[13, 14]

The use of the phenothiazine dye methylene blue and other oxidation-reduction-sensitive color indicators permits gross identification of an ischemic zone within 10 to 15 seconds of inception. Although diagnostic changes are not apparent by light microscopy for from 1 to 2 hours after the onset of ischemia, histochemical changes become manifest in from 20 to 30 minutes. Fortunately, the electron microscope shortens this time considerably and can provide visual evidence of initial diagnostic alterations within 5 to 15 minutes. A review of the subsequent sequence of visible changes can help to establish the minimal period necessary to produce necrosis, to determine the point in time that separates reversible from irreversible injury, to describe the areas of greatest resistance to ischemia, and to provide anatomic correlation with electrocardiogram (ECG) and biochemical abnormalities. Examination of routine histological sections to determine the extent and severity of ischemic tissue damage is both difficult and misleading. Changes may be delayed or may be the result of the secondary causes described. Conversely, recent evidence indicates that drastic visual changes may be induced in cell constituents without causing or signifying permanent damage.[12] The loss of contractile activity and the relaxation of myofibers seen after the induction of ischemia are not necessarily permanent and tell little about ultimate disposition. Other reversible alterations include swelling of endothelia,[15] hyperemia of capillaries and venules,[16] margination of leukocytes,[17] an influx of fluid into the cell, leading to clear spaces and cellular swelling,[10] and marked reduction in adenosine triphosphate (ATP) concentration.[12] Glycogen depletion begins almost immediately, is evident by light microscopy within 5 minutes, and is accompanied by a decrease in, or marked loss of, phosphorylase activity. At 10 minutes, glycogen granules are difficult to locate, although they never disappear completely, which suggests a stable, bound pool of this compound unresponsive to the usual glycogenolytic stimuli.[10, 15, 16, 18] Marked clumping of nucleoplasm occurs early, before extensive cytoplasmic changes can be seen. Small neutral lipid droplets stainable with oil red O appear opposite the A bands of sarcomeres, at the poles of sarcolemmal nuclei, and between myofibrils adjacent to mitochondria.[17, 19] Mitochondrial swelling with enlargement, rounding of outer contour, pallor of matrix, and shrinkage of cristae are accompanied by swelling of the endoplasmic reticulum.[10, 15, 17, 20] There is disagreement as to the etiology of the mitochondrial changes. Some investigators feel that it reflects uncoupling of oxidative phosphorylation and can be reversed by the addition of ATP.[17] Others suggest that neither oxygen deficiency nor a rise in pCO_2 is solely responsible, but that mitochondrial abnormalities are due to intracellular ionic changes, particularly those involving calcium transport.[15]

Studies on hepatic parenchymal cells after the induction of hypoxia have resulted in noteworthy observations. Majno *et al.*[13] have demonstrated cellular protein denaturation within 30 minutes of interruption of the blood supply and at a stage when damage is still reversible. Although the denaturation is not reversible, the cell is not necessarily doomed. Glinsmann and Ericsson[20] have found that organelles, portions of cytoplasm, and mitochondria damaged by hypoxia are segregated within the ischemic cell and subsequently are digested within intracellular cytosegresomes through the action of lysosomal hydrolases (discussed below). The mechanism of these pathological changes in protein is not known, but they are accelerated in areas surrounded by normal tissue and are probably induced by the intra-cellular acidosis which accompanies anaerobic glycolysis. The alterations noted above may appear to be severe, but they are nevertheless potentially reversible. If blood flow to the ischemic tissue is re-established before irreversible changes are induced, recovery is rapid and cells return to full functional activity.

IRREVERSIBLE ISCHEMIC CELL DEATH

Rarely is there a sharp line of demarcation between reversible and irreversible ischemic damage. More frequently there is a gradual transition as more and more cells pass beyond the point of recovery. Jennings et al.[16] stress the fact that damaged cells do not die simultaneously. Death in the traumatized zone follows an exponential curve. At 22 minutes following occlusion, the first irreversibly damaged cells appear. Even after 45 minutes of total hypoxia, 35 to 66 per cent of the cells remain viable.

The ultimate fate of the cell is determined by multiple factors, some of which are described above. Critical are its relative ability to maintain energy production at a level sufficient to support essential cellular activity, the maintenance of a satisfactory ionic environment, the repair or replacement of damaged organelles, proteins, and enzymes which is undoubtedly dependent upon the preservation of nuclear function, and the activity of alternate enzymatic pathways. Many of these factors are so intricately interrelated that a significant deficiency in any one will generalize quickly to several others. The point of irreversible injury undoubtedly is controlled by the combined effects of metabolic breakdown, autolysis and protein denaturation of advanced degree, and an increased permeability of the sarcolemma that permits excessive loss of coenzymes, enzyme molecules, and electrolytes. Eventually the biochemical processes of energy production cannot maintain cellular integrity.[13, 16] Most investigators feel that this point in time is reached between 20 and 60 minutes after occlusion.[13, 16-19, 21]

It has been noted that the irreversibly injured cells that lie toward the center of the infarcted zone die almost unaltered, whereas those closest to the normally perfused areas, usually at the periphery of the infarct, develop marked changes characteristic of infarction. Similar observations have been made when irreversible alterations resulting from total occlusion have been compared to those caused by transient occlusion followed by restoration of normal circulation.[21-23] Sommers and Jennings have demonstrated severe histological changes, differing from those seen after permanent occlusion, which appear within 20 minutes of the return of blood supply.[22] This restoration permits the exchange of intermediary products of metabolism, fluid, and electrolytes between dead or injured cells and the general circulation. Intracellular structure is disrupted rapidly and extensively. Sommers and Jennings[22] and Caulfield and Klionsky[10] describe other changes in irreversibly injured tissue to which the circulation has been restored, *e.g.*, the appearance of inflammatory cells, calcium deposition, an increase in cellular fluid, sodium, chloride, and metabolites, mitochondrial degeneration, increased granularity and loss of respiratory enzymes (cytochrome oxidase and succinic dehydrogenase), and marked distortion and displacement of nuclei. Lysosomal hydrolases are released and appear free in the cell sap. The sarcolemmal membrane is stretched and functionally disrupted, and lactic acid, coenzymes, small molecular weight enzymes, potassium, magnesium, and nucleotides diffuse from the area of injury into the venous circulation, where they may be sampled by various diagnostic maneuvers.

Light and electron microscopy indicates that the endocardium is most resistant to ischemic damage. The anatomic integrity of the endocardial zone often is maintained despite surrounding areas of massive infarction; its Purkinje fibers retain viability, and glycogen stores are abundant. The survival of this zone has been attributed to nourishment via direct diffusion of nutrients from the cardiac chambers or via Thebesian veins.

BIOCHEMICAL ASPECTS OF MYOCARDIAL ISCHEMIA

Significant changes in carbohydrate, lipid, and protein metabolism and alterations in cytoplasmic, mitochondrial, and lysosomal enzyme systems have been described in reversibly injured ischemic cells. Despite extensive pharmacological and surgical studies of this problem, there are few methods that are capable of supporting these borderline ischemic cells, resolving their precarious state of balance, or maintaining functional viability. I should like to stress those factors that seem to have a direct bearing on maintenance of viability.

Glycolysis is normally an inefficient and quantitatively insignificant pathway for the production of energy by the heart. During severe ischemia, areas of irreversibly injured myocardium are incapable of maintaining adequate stores of ATP solely by glycolytic means. Neill *et al.*[24] have shown that under control conditions a nonoxidative energy source (?glycolysis) could account for approximately 15 per cent of total myocardial energy production. When oxidative phosphorylation was uncoupled by cyanide, work plus heat production was equal to more than four times the energy available from substrate oxidation. Nevertheless, such anaerobic energy production may make a critical contribution to the maintenance of cell viability, to the survival of excitability, and to the function of nodal and conducting tissue until a competent collateral circulation is established (physiologically

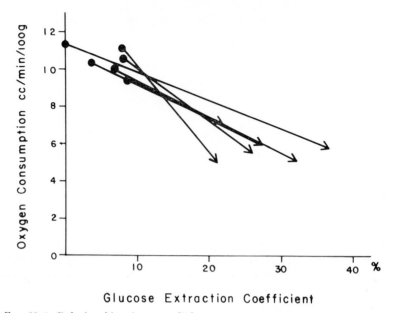

Glucose Extraction Coefficient

FIG. 23.1. Relationship of myocardial oxygen consumption to the percentage of glucose extracted (glucose extraction coefficient). Control determinations compared to a reduction in flow of 40 per cent.

or surgically) or until vasodilator tonus is induced. It may play an important role in promoting the recovery of the acutely anoxic heart.

Anoxic dependence on glycolysis implies an increase in glucose consumption for even marginal cellular function. We have shown that myocardial glucose extraction increases 504 per cent and glucose consumption increases 90 per cent when moderate, localized degrees of ischemia (flow reduced to 63 per cent of control) are induced in the dog heart *in vivo*.[25] In these studies, oxygen consumption and the glucose extraction coefficient showed a striking, fixed, inverse relationship (Fig. 23.1). Biochemical evidence for enhanced glycolysis also is indicated by changes in lactate metabolism and by an accumulation of glycolytic intermediates in the reduced oxidation-reduction state.

Increased concentrations of lactate may be found in coronary sinus samples within 6 seconds after ligation of a coronary artery. Biopsy of the resultant area of ischemia demonstrates an 1800 per cent increase in tissue lactate concentration and a 700 per cent increase in α-glycerophosphate concentration (Table 23.1). Coronary sinus pH may fall more than 0.4 pH unit within 2 minutes.

Other studies in our laboratory and that of Weissler *et al.*[26] of severe myocardial anoxia in the isolated perfused rat heart have supported these

Table 23.1. *Mean myocardial tissue, coronary sinus lactate and tissue α-glycerophosphate concentration and calculated "excess lactate" determined at rest and 5 minutes after ligation of anterior descending coronary artery of the dog*

	Tissue lactate		Tissue α-glycero-PO₄		Coronary sinus lactate		Myocardial excess lactate	
	Control	Ischemic	Control	Ischemic	Control	Ischemic	Control	Ischemic
	$\mu M/gm.$		$\mu M/gm.$		$\mu M/l.$		$\mu M/l.$	
Mean ($n = 10$)	1.8740	35.750	0.2254	1.7940	2.127	4.587	−0.204	2.076
S.D.	0.7502	3.683	0.0499	0.2624	0.221	0.392	0.655	0.306
P	<0.001		<0.001		<0.001		<0.05	
Change vs. Control	1808%		696%		116%		1118%	

findings and have demonstrated that the inclusion of glucose in circulating perfusate not only enhanced the electrical and mechanical performance of the heart during anoxia but also permitted more rapid recovery. Weissler and associates also demonstrated that the sarcotubular dilation seen in anoxic hearts in the absence of glucose was prevented by its presence in the perfusate. Such protection could not be demonstrated when we attempted to substitute free fatty acid (FFA) as the sole substrate during anoxic perfusion. Yang[27] reported that anoxic rabbit atria could maintain long periods of reduced activity only when glucose was provided as a substrate for glycolysis.

The biochemical mechanisms which facilitate the transport, phosphorylation, and oxidation of glucose and glycogen and support the production of glycolytic energy undoubtedly play a major role in the maintenance of cell viability.

EFFECTS OF MYOCARDIAL TISSUE ACIDOSIS

The fall in intracellular pH induced by glycolysis is critical in determining the eventual fate of ischemic tissue. Katz and Long[28] as well as others have emphasized how susceptible the heart is to the accumulation of hydrogen ions. The pH at which activity becomes impossible is significantly higher in the heart than in skeletal muscle. Myocardium also demonstrates a much poorer intrinsic buffering capacity, which enhances the degree of change in pH caused by production of lactic acid. Myocardial refractoriness to vasoactive and inotropic agents and an enhanced susceptibility to the onset and persistance of potentially lethal dysrhythmias during acidosis are well known and may be related to a marked decrement in cardiac pacemaker activity. Acidosis can also cause a sharp fall in left ventricular contractility, in the index of isovolumic work, and in coronary flow.[29] Regional acidification also may induce intracapillary coagulation of blood. This response to tissue acidosis often is successfully treated with alkalinizing agents which demonstrate multiple actions including the enhancement of glycolysis and inhibition of autolysis. It is noteworthy that myocardial vulnerability to ventricular fibrillation apparently is induced by metabolic acidosis alone and not by respiratory acidosis.[30]

True intracellular pH has proven extremely difficult to measure by available techniques. Robin *et al.*[31] have emphasized the importance of this problem by demonstrating that the pH gradient between intracellular and extracellular water is great enough to permit the hydrogen ion concentration of the former to be maintained at a level twice that of the latter. They also have reported that bicarbonate, the most important extracellular buffer and most commonly used alkalinizing agent, demonstrates a relatively poor ability to influence intracellular pH despite its effectiveness in extracellular sites. Enzyme systems responsible for the maintenance of all intracellular synthetic and energy-producing systems have pH optima within the normal physiological range and are quite sensitive to changes in ionic concentration. Bate-Smith and Bendall[32] have shown that ATP disappears most rapidly at a pH of 6.3, a level at which soluble ATPase shows maximal activity. The proteolytic enzymes normally confined to lysosomes all show acid pH optima approached only by an ischemic cellular environment conducive to intraorganelle physiological or generalized pathological autolysis.

FUNCTION OF MYOCARDIAL ACID HYDROLASES (LYSOSOMES) IN PATHOLOGICAL ISCHEMIC AUTOLYSIS

Viability and the maintenance of cellular integrity depend on the survival of essential synthetic enzyme systems as well as on the activation state of those systems regulating physiological and pathological autolysis. The relation between an increase in H^+ ion and the rate of formation of protein cleavage products in liver brei is almost stoichiometric.[14] Addition of alkali causes an inhibition of autolysis. Many early investigators[33] believed that tissue proteins at their isoelectric points were most liable to be digested by cathepsins (usually within the range of pH 5 to 7). They felt that there was little digestion at pH 7.5 because the enzyme had been inactivated or had been adsorbed by resistant base protein salts. By 1930, complete protease systems had been identified which consisted of cathepsin, carboxypolypeptidases, aminopolypeptidases, and dipeptidases. The systems appeared to be bound to and inactivated by insoluble tissue proteins. The mechanism of activation of such systems *in vivo* remains largely conjectural.

De Duve *et al.*[34, 35] and Weissmann[36] have described subcellular sac-like particles enclosed by a single unit lipoprotein membrane and containing enzymes that are uniquely concerned with the catabolic processes of hydrolysis. Cogent histological and biochemical evidence substantiates the existence of these particles as distinct, if not completely homogeneous, entities. De Duve hypothesizes that the primary role of the particles, termed lysosomes, in the normal cell is autophagic digestion. Such autophagic vacuoles appear and soon acquire a complement of acid hydrolases whenever the cell must sacrifice a portion of its own cytoplasm in response to fasting, anoxia, or active catabolism. The products of digestion diffuse through the lysosomal membrane into the cell sap; indigestible material accumulates within the vacuole until it is finally extruded through the cell membrane. Enzymes identified within the particle include acid phosphatase, β-glucuronidase, acid ribonuclease, acid deoxyribonuclease, phosphoprotein phosphotase, cathepsin, β-N-acetylglucosaminidase, β-galactosidase, α-mannosidase, therylsulphatases α and β, and others. Essential to the identity of the particle as a distinct structure is the observation that, when the enzymes are isolated and their membranes are ruptured, they all are released simultaneously. Individual enzymes may therefore be used as tracers for the entire particle. When so identified, they indicate loss of integrity of the lysosomal membrane. This group of enzymes is capable of digesting the most important constituents of the cell. Destruction of the lysosomal membrane permits enzyme release into the cell sap and may be the primary mechanism for pathological autolysis. De Duve has suggested that anoxia may stimulate the formation of autophagic vacuoles or that the lipoprotein membrane of pre-existing lysosomes may be labilized with release of lytic enzymes into the cytoplasm and digestion of susceptible substrate, in this case the cell contents themselves. Release *in vitro* follows incubation at an acid pH.

Lysosome-like particles have been identified by biochemical techniques in the liver, kidney, spleen, thyroid, leukocytes, brain and, recently, the heart.[37, 38]

The myocardium undoubtedly is more sensitive to the effects of ischemia than any other tissue in the body and therefore presents a favorable environment for hydrolase activity. Anaerobic production of excessive amounts of lactic acid may overcome the buffering capacity of the sarcoplasm and decrease cellular pH to a point within the range of enzyme activation. In addition, such a decrease in pH may in itself trigger a cyclic mechanism by inhibiting glycolysis, leading to a further decrease in ATP production and contractility, a fall in blood pressure and consequently in myocardial perfusion, and a further decrease in pO_2. Studies on ischemic rat liver[35] and on the pathogenesis of experimental shock[39] indicate that solubilization and activation of lysosomal enzymes may occur in response to the acidosis that accompanies a fall in pO_2, rather than in response to the anoxia itself. Such studies suggest that autolysis of anoxic cells may start

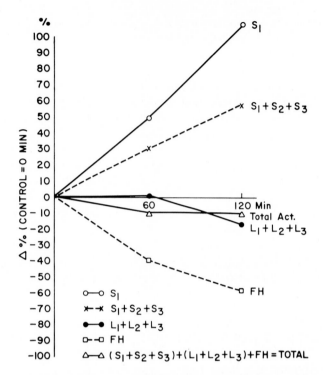

Myocardial Cathepsin Activity (time post-mortem)

Fɪɢ. 23.2. Redistribution of cathepsin enzyme activity from inactive sites within the lysosomal particle and bound to the final homogenate fraction. Assay was performed following cellular fractionation by preparative ultracentrifugation. Note progressive increase in "free" supernatant activity derived from the cell sap as a function of time post mortem. S_1, first supernatant extraction; $S_1 + S_2 + S_3 =$ total supernatant activity (three extractions); $L_1 + L_2 + L_3 =$ total large granule activity (bound); FH, final homogenate activity. Total cathepsin activity, which is represented by the sum of supernatant, large granule, and final homogenate assay, did not show a significant change.

with rupture of the lysosomal membrane. The process which renders the particles fragile is rapid and occurs early. As much as 80 per cent of the lysosomal enzymes may be released at a time when morphological and chemical cellular changes are still very discrete (Fig. 23.2).

A number of anti-inflammatory agents (cortisone, cortisol, prednisone, chloroquine, promethazine, etc.), stabilize the lysosomal membrane of non-cardiac tissue by direct interaction with surface lipid layers, thereby delaying or possibly preventing cellular autolysis. Low temperatures and maintenance of a neutral pH also appear to aid the preservation of lysosomal membrane integrity.

The full significance of these particle-bound enzymes in the myocardial response to ischemia is uncertain. The mechanism of their release and activation in the myocardium and techniques for neutralizing or inhibiting release are intriguing subjects for future research.

EFFECTS OF ISCHEMIA ON MYOCARDIAL LIPID METABOLISM

Myocardial lipid storage most commonly has been associated with acute infectious processes, poisoning, and malignancy, but there is significant histological evidence of lipid storage induced by myocardial ischemia in the experimental animal and man. In animals exposed to low atmospheric pressures or after ligation of the descending ramus of the left coronary artery, the heart shows cytoplasmic accumulation of fat droplets. Storage is temporary and lipids disappear completely after a competent collateral circulation to the ischemic area has been established.[19] Droplets are found only in living, actively metabolizing but ischemic tissue, which indicates that they are not an expression of autolytic degeneration. Cells that die rapidly do not accumulate neutral lipids. The myocardium of infants dying of hypoxia or related causes also shows a marked degree of lipid accumulation.[40] We have demonstrated that the availability of glucose markedly enhances the incorporation of palmitate into myocardial neutral lipids while simultaneously suppressing the oxidation of FFA[41] (Fig. 23.3). In the anoxic state, oxidation of extracted lipid decreases by more than 80 per cent, this fraction being recoverable in storage form as neutral lipid. In the absence of glucose, anoxia induced a similar decrease in oxidation of FFA, but such changes are associated with a decreased uptake of FFA and are not accompanied by the previously noted reciprocal increase in tissue neutral lipid. Thus, in contrast to glucose, cellular extraction of FFA appears to bear no fixed relation to the ability of the cell to oxidize this substrate. Uptake and storage occur under hypoxic conditions as long as sufficient glucose is available to support an actively glycolyzing system and despite the markedly reduced production of energy occurring under these conditions.

In the poorly perfused anoxic myocardium, unable to oxidize extracted and esterified FFAs, lipid stores may continue to accumulate and eventually may contribute to the decreased contractility associated with the ischemic myocardium. Maling and Highman[42] suggested that these accumulations may be toxic and reported myocardial fatty changes, stainable with oil red O, which persisted for 2 weeks after coronary artery ligation. It is clinically significant that the severity and duration of fatty changes parallel the severity and duration of the period of myocardial hyperirritability, which suggests that these changes may trigger fatal arrhythmias.[43]

α-Glycerophosphate is a most important precursor in triglyceride syn-

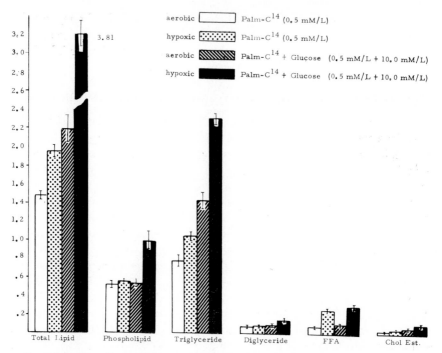

FIG. 23.3. The effects of glucose on the distribution of recoverable palmitate-C[14] (Palm-C[14]) activity following aerobic and hypoxic perfusion of the isolated rat heart preparation. Note that the increase in total lipid activity is expressed primarily in the phospholipid and triglyceride fractions and that this enhanced storage as neutral lipid is dependent upon the presence of glucose in the perfusate. FFA, free fatty acid; Chol Est., cholesterol esters.

thesis since it supplies the glycerol skeleton for esterification of FFA. It is an intermediary product of glycolysis and, when present in increased concentration, as noted during anaerobiosis, it may serve as a stimulus for FFA esterification. It is not unreasonable to speculate that, during all but the most severely ischemic states, anaerobic glycolysis may produce sufficient ATP for intracellular transport and for activation of extracted FFA, and that it concomitantly may enhance esterification of intracellular FFA by supplying high concentrations of the glycerophosphate required for glyceride synthesis (Tables 23.2 and 23.3). The increase in circulating arterial FFA concentration reported to exist in the post-myocardial infarction patient may enhance myocardial uptake and esterification and parallel a postulated increase in hepatic synthesis of very low density lipoproteins and glycerides in this state. Deposition of such neutral lipid in conduction pathways may well be related to subsequent dysrhythmias.

The foregoing observations permit us to hypothesize a sequence of events

Table 23.2. *Shifts in carbohydrate-lipid interrelationships following induction of hypoxia in the isolate perfused rat heart**

	Uptake		Lactate production	Recovery of C[14]		
	FFA	Glucose		As C[14]O$_2$	As total lipid	As nonlipid
	μM/gww		*μM glucose/gww*	*μM glucose/gww*		
Aerobic	6.036	26.8	24.2	2.52	0.378	3.238
	±0.336	±2.8	±5.0	±0.266	±0.027	±0.329
Hypoxic	6.351	119.3	111.6	1.69	0.643	2.195
	±0.940	±7.6	±5.4	±0.122	±0.035	±0.115
"T" test		0.001 > *p*	0.001 > *p*	0.02 > *p*	0.001 > *p*	0.02 > *p*
Change		+345%	+361%	−33%	+70%	−32%

Perfusate = KRB + glucose-C[14] (10.0 mM/l.) + palmitate (0.5 mM/l.) + albumin (0.1 mM/l.)

* Note the relatively fixed uptake of free fatty acid (FFA) and the marked increase in glucose uptake, balanced by an equivalent increase in lactate production. Glucose-C[14] oxidation to C[14]O$_2$ is depressed. Recovery of significant amounts of glucose-C[14] label is restricted to the total extractable tissue lipid fraction. Fractionation of this total activity is shown in Table 23.3. gww, grams wet weight; KRB, Krebs-Ringer-bicarbonate solution.

Table 23.3. *Determination of lipid fractional C[14] activity following aerobic and hypoxic perfusion with Krebs-Ringer-bicarbonate (KRB) solution containing glucose-C[14] and palmitate as substrate in the isolated perfused rat heart**

	Lipid fractionation				Localization of C[14] in TGFA	
	PL	TGFA	DG	FFA	Fatty acid	Glycerol
	μM/gww/30'				*μM/gww/30'*	
Aerobic	0.157	0.195	0.020	0.005	0.049	0.158
	±0.012	±0.018	±0.001	±0.0004	±0.01	±0.01
Hypoxic	0.142	0.466	0.025	0.010	0.053	0.411
	±0.009	±0.045	±0.002	±0.001	±0.01	±0.04
"T" Test		0.001 > *p*		0.01 > *p*		0.001 > *p*
Change		+139%		+100%		+160%

Perfusate = KRB + glucose-C[14] (10.0 mM/l.) + palmitate (0.5 mM/l.) + albumin (0.1 mM/l.)

* Note the significant quantitative recovery in the triglyceride (TGFA) fraction. The increase in free fatty acid (FFA) activity suggests enhanced synthesis but is quantitatively insignificant. Hydrolysis of the TGFA fraction demonstrates the glucose-derived C[14] activity to be confined to the glycerol portion of the molecule. PL, phospholipid; DG, diglyceride.

that ultimately lead to the death of the myocardial cell unless the process is halted before the changes have become irreversible. It is impossible to establish the exact relationship of these changes since many occur simultaneously. The outline presented here is abbreviated, and I have made no attempt to ascribe a cause and effect relationship to any but the major events.

The onset of cellular anoxia causes an immediate fall in creatine phosphate and ATP concentration and a rise in P_i, adenosine diphosphate, and adenosine monophosphate. There is an increase in anaerobic glycolysis which is supported by an increase in glucose consumption aided by enhanced cellular transport and phosphorylation. Glycogenolysis also is stimulated by an increase in phosphorylase a activity. The activity of phosphofructokinase increases many fold, and there is a shift of glycolytic intermediates to a reduced oxidation-reduction state. Lactate consumption falls and its production is enhanced, as is that of α-glycerophosphate. Esterification of FFA is enhanced by the increased concentration of α-glycerophosphate, and droplets of neutral lipid begin to accumulate in the perimitochondrial zone. Intracellular pH begins to fall as the capacity of intracellular buffer systems is gradually exceeded. The decrease in available energy permits ionic shifts, with loss of intracellular potassium and diffusion into the cell of sodium ions and extracellular fluid. Osmotic pressure within the cell gradually increases because of the autolytic breakdown of proteins, accumulation of free molecules, and shifts in electrolyte balance. Mitochondrial swelling and changes in endoplasmic reticulum now are visible histologically, as are the loss of glycogen and the appearance of clear fluid-filled, intracellular spaces. Cellular synthetic processes cease. Abnormal deflections in the ECG are induced by changes in membrane potential which reflect the failing function of the ionic pump. There is undoubtedly some protein denaturation at this stage and autophagic ingestion by increased numbers of lysosomal particles digesting portions of the living cell. The cell nucleus becomes slightly distorted.

Unless the circulation is restored, these reversible changes progress and become irremediable. The pH continues to fall, cathepsin and proteinase activators appear, the membrane of the lysosomal particle ruptures and releases acid hydrolases, which are activated rapidly: many now function at their pH optima. The combined damage of metabolic breakdown, autolysis, and protein denaturation destroys any potential for energy production, additional enzyme systems fail, the sarcolemma permits leakage of larger molecules, and the nucleus ceases to function. The cell is dead, it has lost its integrity as a functional unit, and a distinction between the internal and external environment ceases to exist. At this stage, the actual histological appearance is determined by the relative approximation of the dead tissue to an active circulation (as discussed).

When the area of totally infarcted myocardium is so extensive as to rupture or to interfere mechanically with the maintenance of perfusion pressure or cardiac output, the death of the entire organism results. Often, however, the outcome depends on the metabolic behavior of the reversibly injured cell. Clinical and experimental evidence indicates that severe, localized ischemia is an acute but temporary phenomenon which is soon resolved. It is induced by permanent coronary occlusion and also by periods of temporary occlusion both before and after the resumption of flow. The increase in circulating catecholamines accompanying coronary thrombosis indicates that adequate perfusion is prevented not only by the decrease in perfusion pressure and flow induced by obstruction of the large vessels but also by a temporary increase in peripheral myocardial vascular resistance caused by arteriolar vasoconstriction. Under optimal circumstances, collateral vascular channels open, blood is shunted from adequately perfused areas, and satisfactory aerobic metabolic activity can be reactivated. The treatment of coronary occlusion should be based on rapid revascularization of the myocardium or its equivalent before the persistent or progressive increase in ischemia leads to permanent and irreversible damage. Until such techniques become generally available, our knowledge of the alterations in metabolic and enzymatic pathways induced by myocardial ischemia suggests several areas for future investigation.

In addition to techniques that will permit a chronic reduction in cardiac work load without interfering with normal activity (hypotensive pharmacological agents, beta blockade, etc.) ,the most promising area for investigation may be the development of methods for prolonging the period of reversibility and encouraging the growth or function of a collateral circulation.

Surgical myocardial revascularization by implantation is apparently an effective technique, but its full effects may not be realized for many months. Recently, investigation has been aimed at the development of a method for "instant" revascularization. These venoarterial bypass procedures are being performed and their effects on hemodynamic, electrical and biochemical parameters are being actively evaluated in our institution and elsewhere. Although it is much too early to give definite answers, results thus far have been encouraging.

It has been demonstrated that intentional cardiac arrest can prolong viability significantly by reducing energy demands and preventing the electrical instability that may cause death in an otherwise not fatally damaged heart. Reduction in the temperature of the heart permits the stabilization of lysosomes, decreases the metabolic demands of the cell, helps to support the pH, and markedly retards protein denaturation. These observations encourage the development of mechanical devices that can assume the pumping function of the heart so that it may be shunted out of the circulation, kept at low temperatures, and perfused in the nonworking state with high oxygen mixtures until an adqeuate flow or other compensations have been established.

Little is known about methods for supporting anaerobic glycolysis, a process that has far-reaching effects in the metabolism of the ischemic myocardium. We all know that hypoglycemia is to be avoided. It would be useful to have a simple, reproducible, and efficient method to establish the degree of glycolytic activity and intramyocardial NADH:NAD ratios so that the determination of lactate and pyruvate balance, a gross and potentially misleading technique, may be replaced as a clinical diagnostic tool.

Routine determination of intracellular pH is not yet possible. Our inability to do so makes the evaluation of buffer agents difficult, despite the fact that the development of such agents to control intracellular acidosis is urgently required. Exhaustion of intracellular buffer capacity and the onset of significant acidosis signal a major step into the state of potential irreversibility. Cathepsins are activated, lysosomal enzymes are released, intracapillary thrombi are formed, and synthetic and energy-producing enzyme systems are inhibited or inactivated.

More information is required about the determinants of intracapillary thrombus formation and platelet adhesiveness in the post-occlusion period and about their role in the development of irreversible cellular changes, as well as about the true significance of the formation of intracellular neutral lipid. Finally, we all are handicapped by the lack of an adequate animal model that will permit study of this degenerative process under controlled laboratory conditions.

The research upon which this publication is based was performed pursuant to Contract Ph-43-67-1439 and Grant HE-06216 with the National Institutes of Health, Public Health Service, Department of Health, Education and Welfare. This study was also aided by support from the New York Heart Association and The Muscular Dystrophy Associations of America, Inc. Dr. Brachfeld is a Career Development Awardee of the National Heart Institute.

REFERENCES

1. Hayflick, L.: Human cells and aging. Sci. Amer. 218: 32, 1968.
2. *Dorland's Illustrated Medical Dictionary*, Ed. 24. W. B. Saunders Company, Philadelphia, 1965.
3. *Webster's New International Dictionary*, Ed. 3. G. and C. Merriam Company, Springfield, Mass., 1963.
4. A definition of irreversible coma. Report of the *Ad Hoc* Committee of the Harvard Medical School to examine the definition of brain death. J. A. M. A. 205: 337, 1968.
5. Moore, F. D.: Medical responsibility for the prolongation of life. J. A. M. A. 206: 384, 1968.
6. Arnold, J. D., Zimmerman, T. F., and Martin, D. C.: Public attitudes and the diagnosis of death. J. A. M. A. 206: 1949, 1968.
7. Andreev, S. V.: Resuscitation of cardiac activity in man after death. Medgiz, Moscow, 1955, as cited by Simonson, E.: Ann. Rev. Physiol. 20: 136, 1958.
8. Personal communication.
9. Webb, W. R., and Howard, H. S.: Extension of the limits of cardiac viability with total coronary occlusion. Surgery 42: 92, 1957.

10. Caulfield, J., and Klionsky, B.: Myocardial ischemia and early infarction. An electron microscopic study. Amer. J. Path. 35: 489, 1959.
11. Bing, R. J., Kardesch, M., Hogancamp, C. E., and Michal, G.: The survival of excitability, energy production and energy utilization of the heart. Trans. Ass. Amer. Physicians 71: 152, 1958.
12. Judah, J. D., Ahmed, K., and McLean, A. E.: Pathogenesis of cell necrosis. Fed. Proc. 24: 1217, 1965.
13. Majno, G., La Gattuta, M., and Thompson, T. E.: Cellular death and necrosis. Fed. Proc. 24: 1217, 1965.
14. Bradley, H. C.: Autolysis and atrophy. Physiol. Rev. 18: 173, 1938.
15. Meessen, H.: Ultrastructure of the myocardium. Its significance in myocardial disease. Amer. J. Cardiol. 22: 319, 1968.
16. Jennings, R. B., Kaltenbach, J. P., Sommers, H. M., Bahr, G. F., and Wartman, W. R.: Studies of the dying myocardial cell. In James, T. N., and Kayes, J. W. (eds.): *The Etiology of Myocardial Infarction*, Chap. 12. Little, Brown and Company, Boston, 1963.
17. Shnitka, T. K., and Nachlas, M. M.: Histochemical alterations in ischemic heart muscle and early myocardial infarction. Amer. J. Pathol. 42: 507, 1963.
18. Bajusz, E., and Jasmin, G.: Comparative morphogenesis and enzyme histogenesis of some occlusive and metabolic cardiac necroses. Rev. Can. Biol. 22: 181, 1963.
19. Wartman, W. B., Jennings, R. B., Yokoyama, H. O., and Clabaugh, G. F.: Fatty changes of the myocardium in early experimental infarction. Arch. Path. 62: 318, 1956.
20. Glinsmann, W. H., and Ericsson, J. L.: Observations on the subcellular organization of hepatic parenchymal cells. Evolution of reversible alterations induced by hypoxia. Lab. Invest. 15: 762, 1966.
21. Lowry, O. H., Gilligan, D. R., and Hastings, A. B.: Histochemical changes in the myocardium of dogs following experimental coronary arterial occlusion. Amer. J. Physiol. 136: 474, 1942.
22. Sommers, H., and Jennings, R. B.: Experimental acute myocardial infarction. Lab. Invest. 13: 1491, 1964.
23. Herson, P. B., Sommers, H. M., and Jennings, R. B.: A comparative study of the fine structure of normal and ischemic dog myocardium, with special reference to early changes following temporary occlusion of a coronary artery. Amer. J. Path. 46: 367, 1965.
24. Neill, W. A., Krasnow, N., Levine, H. J., and Gorlin, R.: Myocardial anaerobic metabolism in intact dogs. Amer. J. Path. 204: 427, 1963.
25. Brachfeld, N., and Scheuer, J.: Metabolism of glucose by the ischemic dog heart. Amer. J. Physiol. 212: 603, 1967.
26. Weissler, A. M., Kruger, F. A., Baba, N., Scarpelli, D. G., Leighton, R. F., and Gallimore, J. K.: Role of anaerobic metabolism in the preservation of functional capacity and structure of anoxic myocardium. J. Clin. Invest. 47: 403, 1968.
27. Yang, W. C.: Anaerobic functional activity of isolated rabbit atria. Amer. J. Physiol. 205: 781, 1963.
28. Katz, L. N., and Long, C. N.: Lactic acid in mammalian cardiac muscle. Proc. Roy. Soc. (London) Ser. B. 99: 8, 1926.
29. Opie, L. H.: Effect of extracellular pH on function and metabolism of isolated perfused rat heart. Amer. J. Physiol. 209: 1075, 1965.
30. Gerst, P. H., Fleming, W. H., and Malm, J. R.: Increased susceptibility of the heart to ventricular fibrillation during metabolic acidosis. Circ. Res. 19: 63, 1966.

31. Robin, E. D., Wilson, R. J., and Bromberg, P. A.: Intracellular acid-base relations and intracellular buffers. Ann. N. Y. Acad. Sci. 92: 539, 1961.
32. Bate-Smith, E. C., and Bendall, J. R.: Changes in muscle after death. Brit. Med. Bull. 12: 230, 1956.
33. Waldschmidt-Leitz, E.: The mode of action and differentiation of proteolytic enzymes. Physiol. Rev. 11: 358, 1931.
34. De Duve, C.: Lysosomes. A new group of cytoplasmic particles. In Hayashi, T. (ed.): *Subcellular Particles.* Ronald Press Company, New York, 1959.
35. De Duve, C., and Beaufay, H.: Tissue fractionation studies. Influence of ischemia on the state of some bound enzymes in rat liver. Biochem. J. 73: 610, 1959.
36. Weissman, G.: Medical progress. Lysosomes. New Engl. J. Med. 273: 1084, 1965.
37. Brachfeld, N., and Gemba, T.: Mechanisms of myocardial cell death. Release of lysosomal hydrolases after ischemia. Clin. Res. 13: 524, 1965.
38. Romeo, D., Scagni, N., Sottocasa, G. L., Pugliarello, M. C., DeBernard, B., and Vittur, F.: Lysosomes in heart tissue. Biochim. Biophys. Acta 130: 64, 1966.
39. Janoff, A., Weissmann, G., Zweifach, B. W., and Thomas, L.: Pathogenesis of experimental shock. J. Exp. Med. 116: 451, 1962.
40. Scott, J. M.: Fatty changes in the myocardium of the newborn. Brit. Med. J. 11: 1746, 1961.
41. Scheuer, J., and Brachfeld, N.: Myocardial uptake and fractional distribution of palmitate-1-C^{14} by the ischemic dog heart. Metabolism 15: 945, 1966.
42. Maling, H. M., and Highman, B.: Exaggerated ventricular arrhythmias and myocardial fatty changes after large doses of norepinephrine and epinephrine in unanesthetized dogs. Amer. J. Physiol. 194: 590, 1958.
43. Balsaver, A. M., Morales, A. R., and Whitehouse, F. W.: Fat infiltration of myocardium as a cause of cardiac conduction defect. Amer. J. Cardiol. 19: 261, 1967.

24

Changing Concepts in Mechanical Assistance and Surgical Excision

DWIGHT EMARY HARKEN, M.D.

INTRA-AORTIC BALLOON COUNTERPULSATION

Something over 10 years ago, the concept of assisted circulation by arterio-arterial counterpulsation was evolved in our laboratory and applied clinically.[1] By aspirating an aliquot of blood in synchrony with cardiac systole and returning that same aliquot of blood through the same cannula during diastole, the extravagant utilization of oxygen in myocardial pressure work was converted into more economical oxygen utilization of flow work. Furthermore, while the aortic valves were closed in diastole, there was increased diastolic pressure and therefore increased coronary flow. The favorable combination of reduced pressure work with increased coronary perfusion was attained. Credit for this ingenious synchronization with the electrocardiographic R wave must go to engineer Clifford Birtwell.

Adaptation of the Agress technique of microsphere embolization to the coronary arteries enables one to produce controlled coronary occlusion and infarction. It was also possible to establish a dose-related, standardized mortality of 85 per cent in dogs. This same 85 per cent mortality was converted to an 80 per cent survival by 2 hours of arterio-arterial counterpulsation. Sporadic efforts after cardiac arrest were made to utilize this technique of assisted circulation after patient demise. In order to test the system on a viable patient population and to assess the practicability in an organism with a cardiovascular system the size of an adult human, eight patients with intractable angina pectoris were counterpulsated from 1 to 2 hours. It was established by this mechanism that such arterio-arterial femoral counterpulsation was feasible in the unicameral aortic system from the heart, coronary arteries, aorta, iliac arteries, and femoral artery. Femoral counterpulsation effected a significant alteration in coronary flow. In these eight humans with intractable angina, the clinical relief was dramatic. However, as with all too many treatments for angina, clinical relief

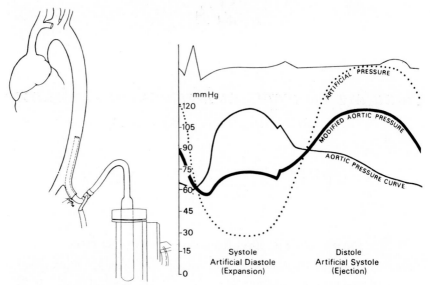

Fɪɢ. 24.1. Left, diagrammatic representation of relation of counterpulsation to circulation. Right, modification of aortic pressure curve by arterial counterpulsation.

is a poor assay. Objective studies of myocardial metabolism and coronary angiography were not feasible 8 years ago. This perhaps explains the fact that this work was not taken very seriously. However, it did seem logical because the remarkable laboratory salvage had been shown clearly to be due to the prompt establishment of intercoronary communicators. These extant but dormant communications were apparently opened in the microsphere-infarcted experimental animal by 2 hours of counterpulsation. The pattern of counterpulsation is shown in Figure 24.1. The ischemic coronary arterial tree, typical of a series of experiments with animals after death from microsphere occlusion, is shown in Figure 24.2 on the left. The opening of intercoronary communicators in animals electively sacrificed 2 hours after identical microsphere occlusion but undergoing 2 hours of counterpulsation is demonstrated on the right in Figure 24.2. This seems an adequate explanation of the 80 per cent survival after 2 hours of counterpulsation, as opposed to 85 per cent mortality without counterpulsation in an otherwise identical experimental preparation.[2]

At that time, Engineer Birtwell and Drs. Soroff, Jacobey, Taylor, and I felt that we should offer arterio-arterial counterpulsation to patients in cardiogenic shock. We outlined such a rigid protocol of cardiogenic shock that we all but eliminated patients with viable brains, livers, and gastro-intestinal tracts. The elimination of trial was further completed by randomization, wherein only five patients over a period of 18 months fell into

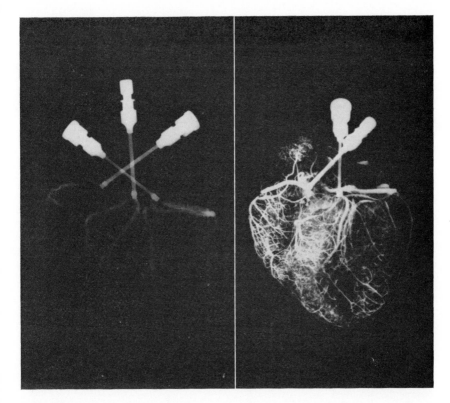

Fig. 24.2. Postmortem coronary arteriograms comparing two hearts studied 2 hours after acute coronary occlusion with the same dose of microspheres. The heart on the left shows multiple occlusions, predominantly in the secondary and tertiary branches. The heart on the right was counterpulsated for 2 hours. Note the marked increase in number and size of coronary collateral channels.

the protocol and all of those by randomization fell by chance into the control group. Thus the project never left the ground. Our patient selection would probably have defeated us in terms of salvage anyway, as we were allowing more than 2 hours of shock irreversible by a vigorous sequence of medical interventions. Again, at least the myocardium, brain, gastrointestinal tract, and kidneys would have almost certainly been beyond salvage, even though counterpulsation as a hemodynamic exercise might have restored heart action. In short, that phase of arterio-arterial counterpulsation had good laboratory basis and was feasible in humans as established by the surviving angina patients, but our "scientific study" had perhaps been inappropriately applied so that, with too little and too late, we offered nothing. This may well have been a continuing pattern in more recent experience.

At that time, Engineer Birtwell suggested an intra-aortic balloon similarly synchronized with aortic systole so that the balloon was collapsed in systole and inflated in diastole to reduce the myocardial pressure work of systole. While the aortic valve was closed, the balloon was to have been quickly inflated with helium through a catheter inserted through the femoral artery to augment diastolic pressure. This type of balloon was not developed. Dr. Adrian Kantrowitz did, however, develop just such a balloon and has accomplished effective counterpulsation. We have adopted his technique.

In preparation for this presentation today, Dr. Adrian Kantrowitz, pioneer of this form of assisted circulation and now of the Sinai Hospital in Detroit, has sent material derived from a combined study of some nine centers across the country. We are pleased to be participants in that study, which has had essential support from the John A. Hartford Foundation. Dr. Kantrowitz summarizes the intrathoracic balloon phase shift pumping or counterpulsation in medically refractory cardiogenic shock as of December 3, 1970 as follows.[3]

I. Early shock (onset less than 30 hours after acute myocardial infarction)
   A. Of 20 patients, 18 (90 per cent) recovered from shock during pumping.
   B. Five patients (25 per cent) died before circulatory stabilization was regained and pumping discontinued. Three of these deaths were due to procedure-related factors. Another of these deaths was due to a myocardial rupture.
   C. In the remaining 15 patients (75 per cent), shock was reversed and pumping was discontinued.
   D. Six patients (30 per cent) died 8 hours to 7 days after termination of pumping.
   E. Nine patients (45 per cent) recovered from their infarcts and were sent home. Three of them died—7, 19, and 24 months after pumping. The remaining six, so far as we know, are well 17 to 37 months after the procedure.
II. Delayed shock (onset more than 30 hours after acute myocardial infarction)
   A. Of 10 patients, seven (70 per cent) recovered from shock during pumping.
   B. Six patients (60 per cent) died during assistance, two as a result of procedure-related factors.
   C. Hemodynamic stabilization and termination of pumping were achieved in four patients (40 per cent), all of whom died within 10 days.
   D. Myocardial ruptures occurred in 6 patients (60 per cent).

Some of the experience has been very dramatic. One with which I am familiar might be mentioned. One of our hospital administrators suffered a massive coronary myocardial infarction from coronary occlusion and, after prolonged shock and repeated resuscitation, he was placed on balloon counterpulsation. He was unconscious and anuric, and his only blood pressure was being sustained by manual systole by the closed chest technique. While he received such manual assistance to circulation by chest compression, the transfemoral intra-aortic balloon was inserted. The counterpulsation was synchronized at first with manual circulatory assistance and then with restored heart action. After 7 days, he was able to sustain a good blood pressure and counterpulsation was discontinued. Some 57 hours later he had further infarction and shock returned. He was again placed on counterpulsation and he again became conscious with effective circulation, cerebrated, and resumed renal function. After 6 more days of counterpulsation, he was again taken off with an effective blood pressure, only subsequently to die of a massive gastrointestinal hemorrhage.

These clinical illustrations give some concept of the spectrum of problems that might benefit from this form of circulatory assistance. Furthermore, such counterpulsation can serve as a holding action until definition of the problem by coronary angiography can be followed by definitive surgery: either coronary bypass, myocardial resection, or combinations thereof. Success in each of these areas has now found its way into the medical literature. This all underscores the great potential of this little used modality. At the risk of extravagant speculation, I submit that we are on the verge of an exciting addition to our therapy for coronary artery disease. I hope that the use of counterpulsation will make even small infarcted zones smaller and make large and perhaps otherwise lethal infarcted zones consistent with survival or consistent with a holding action long enough for definitive combinations of bypass or excision.

It is even appropriate to hope that elective counterpulsation for severe coronary artery disease might expedite the development of protective intercoronary collateral communications.

NEW SURGICAL SYNDROMES: OCCULT VENTRICULAR ANEURYSM AND TACHYARRHYTHMIAS

The consequences of coronary artery disease with surgical consideration of various forms of surgery for various disease patterns constitute the substance of a panel in this symposium. There is specific surgery for various forms of coronary artery disease, and these patterns involve the following.

I. Central obstructive coronary artery disease by aortocoronary artery saphenous vein jump grafts.

II. Internal mammary artery implantation for diffuse disease. Here there is extending promise in the areas of "gas endarterectomy."

III. Localized excisional therapy for ventricular aneurysms producing intractable heart failure or embolic accidents.

IV. Valve replacement for papillary muscle rupture or dysfunction.

V. Excisional therapy with or without revascularization procedures as therapy for akinetic zones and with or without markedly dilated left ventricles.

VI. Repair of post-infarction septal defect.

VII. A remarkable variety of combinations of these specific surgical techniques.

The purpose of the second part of this presentation is to bring to your attention excisional therapy for two new syndromes that are receiving useful attention:

    I. Excisional therapy for occult aneurysm.
    II. Excisional therapy for intractable tachyarrhythmias.

Various studies by Burchell, Abrams, Hellerstein, and Gorlin place the incidence of post-infarction aneurysm of the left ventricle at 4 to 25 per cent. The record of clinically diagnosed and proven ventricular aneurysms before death is embarrassingly low as compared with the incidence of aneurysms found at autopsy. Perhaps the incidence of correct diagnosis is less than 20 per cent of those found at autopsy.

Gross aneurysms, as opposed to the occult aneurysms and tachyarrhythmias described here, represent areas in which aneurysmectomy is an established form of therapy. Patients succumb as a consequence of these gross aneurysms resulting from peripheral emboli in perhaps 10 per cent of cases, of congestive heart failure in something of the order of 50 per cent, and of reinfarction with or without rupture in something like 60 per cent. The combination of these three cardinal causes of death accounts for the tabulated excess of 100 per cent. It is not to this group of obvious and standard surgical indications that we address ourselves here. The foregoing statistics clarify the place for surgical excision in standard aneurysms. They also suggest that many patients die with unrecognized aneurysms. The further premise for this discussion of occult aneurysms submits, however, that unexplained refractory congestive failure following myocardial infarction deserves angiography. In some of these patients, aneurysms not otherwise detectable will be uncovered and can benefit from excisional therapy.

Note: To illustrate the occult aneurysm, roentgenograms were demonstrated of a man who had had previous coronary occlusion and who suffered from intractable congestive failure of progressive severity for some 7 months prior to review and hemodynamic evaluation by angiography. The angiograms showing a small antero-lateral dyskinetic zone were shown. Catheter figures of hemodynamics revealed a resting end diastolic pressure of 30 mm. Hg in the left ventricle. Minimal exercise produced pulmonary edema. This severe but small aneurysm was not recognizable in standard roentgenograms or standard fluoroscopic study. The patient was operated some 7 months previously, and that operation was presented to illustrate the technique of recognizing the dyskinetic zone of myocardium, its resection and repair. The patient has continued out of failure and has been rehabilitated since that surgery.

The second premise for discussion involves patients with uncontrollable post-infarction tachyarrhythmias. Occasionally patients totally refractory to all standard therapy may have the probable site of irritable focus demonstrated by angiography, again in the form of an occult aneurysm, and may respond to excisional therapy.

Note: A patient 56 years old, with a history of coronary occlusion 6 weeks previously, had had 71 episodes of resuscitation by manual systole and countershock. Unsuccessful attempts had been made to override this with an intravenous electrode to the pacemaker, and the standard and experimental forms of pharmaceutical control had also failed. Angiograms demonstrating a small zone of akinesis in the area of infarction led to surgical excision. The 80th resuscitation was performed on the operating table and documented in the moving picture. The operation was performed 5 months ago, the patient has been completely rehabilitated and has had no recurrence of his dangerous arrhythmias.

It is suggested that tachyarrhythmias unresponsive to electrical cardioversion, overriding pacing, or pharmacological control may have angiographic definition and surgical excision.

REFERENCES

1. Clauss, R. H., Birtwell, W. C., Albertal, G. A., Lunzer, S., Taylor, W. J., Fosberg, A. M., and Harken, D. E.: Assisted circulation. I. The arterial counterpulsator. J. Thor. Cardiovasc. Surg. 41: 447–458, 1961.
2. Jacobey, J. A., Taylor, W. J., Smith, G. T., Gorlin, R., and Harken, D. E.: A new therapeutic approach to acute coronary occlusion. I. Production of standardized coronary occlusion with microspheres. Amer. J. Cardiol. 9: 60–73, 1962.
3. Kantrowitz, A., Director of Surgery, Sinai Hospital, Detroit, Michigan: Personal communication derived from National Combined Study supported by John A. Hartford Foundation, Dec. 3, 1970.
4. Abelmann, W. H., Boston City Hospital: Personal communication, Jan. 1971.

25

Priorities in Cardiovascular Research

INTRODUCTION

THEODORE COOPER, M.D.

How did we, as scientists and physicians involved with the day-to-day care of sick patients, ever become involved with the question of priorities in cardiovascular research or the relative priority assessment of needs in cardiovascular research and care, as opposed to rehabilitation for alcoholics, problems of mental illness and pulmonary disorders, to name just a few? What should be our concern, if any, in the relative priorities of health as opposed to other national needs and goals? As I see it, we became involved and should be even more actively involved, because there is a finite limit to our resources: choices must be made as to where the available resources will be spent, and if we do not consider, advise, and advocate the cardiovascular medical priorities, then someone else with a great deal less knowledge and concern will, of necessity, make these decisions for us. This recognition that our resources are finite has forced us to believe that what René DuBois says is true: "The statement that we *must* do something because we *can* do it is operationally and ethically meaningless; it is tantamount to an intellectual abdication." Thus, there are a number of things we can do now in each of the fields to be considered, but the question really is what must we do, what should we do, now.

Such considerations are far from being intellectual exercises alone. Sometimes when the President's budget is presented to Congress and the nation, it appears as if there really were no choices, that life is quite simple, and that the priorities recommended are self-evident. No one in the Bureau of the Budget, or the Office of Management and Budget as it is now called, believes that these choices are easy or the options self-evident. But the officials responsible must present a budget which advocates the course recommended by the President, and hence the budget cannot emphasize the difficulty of the choices made. Seldom if ever does the budget document contain any mention of those contenders for adoption which were seriously considered but finally rejected. But it is important that these possibilities, these options, be discussed, debated, and presented so that the priorities which are finally chosen will in fact be the best ones for the greatest number of people.

Clearly, we are not about to enter into a discussion of the relative merits of health options as opposed to other social or national goals. Nor are we going to debate seriously the relative needs in cardiovascular diseases against those in other disease entities. For one thing, cardiovascular disease is the number one health problem by virtue of the death toll which it exacts from the total population and even by reason of the death toll which it takes among those in the prime of life. Furthermore, most of these deaths are due to myocardial infarction or coronary artery disease, and hence we are narrowing our considerations in this chapter to three specific aspects of myocardial infarction: the role of the hyperlipoproteinemias, the role of systemic hypertension, and the role of thrombosis. Each discussion is a thumbnail sketch of the present state of the art in each of these areas, including the opportunities to utilize present knowledge to effect prevention of disease or prevention of the expression of that disease in illness in the patient.

I hope that this discussion will not only highlight factual data which may be of immediate use, but that it will create a new awareness of the difficulties in establishing priorities and of the need for all of us who are involved in medical research and care to consider and weigh these priorities. From this base we may then more wisely seek effective means of either increasing our resources or rendering more efficient our present and planned activities so that, in fact, we can do more and better, even with less.

A.
TREATMENT OF THE HYPERLIPOPROTEINEMIAS

DONALD S. FREDRICKSON, M.D.

Recently Dr. Cooper and I heard the results of a private poll which, when combined with some public ones that we know about, leads me to believe that as many adult Americans are now worried about an increase in their cholesterol as are worried about the admission of Red China to the United Nations, or perhaps they are even more worried about it than they are about the decline in the purchasing power of the dollar.

People are more aware than we thought, and you can sense that, while there is only a very slight softening of our attitude toward Peking, there is very clearly a measurable softening of the adipose tissue reserves on a national level, because people are getting more unsaturated as they are changing their diets.

Now there is very much that I think is laudable in this. Many of us will even admit that it is probably a very sensible trend based on the now well-known risk factor analyses. But to a certain extent the nature of the movement is also a pity, because I suppose if one asked what is the most important question in terms of cardiovascular research related to the treatment of hyperlipoproteinemias, it is the question of whether we ought to treat them at all.

This is because we do not really know whether or not a lowering of the mean cholesterol of the population by 10 or 15 per cent will in fact lower the collective mortality or morbidity from coronary artery disease. We do not know whether a stringently low fat, low cholesterol diet is something for all people of all ages; we do not know, for example, whether one egg a day is one man's jeopardy but perhaps another's pleasure and, for a third, even a source of essential nutrients depending on what else he eats.

We do not know, and I wish we did, whether a lifetime diet containing 10 or 15 per cent of total calories as polyunsaturates is truly without other threats to health. And worst of all, I think there is a distinct possibility that, for lack of answers to these and similar questions, the present public mood may lose its momentum. The public may develop tachyphylaxis, because this is a social movement which is driven by social impulses alone, at the present, without the kind of incorporation of fact into statute or into public policy that a program can have when it is based on really firm facts.

Now faced with this uncertainty, we still have not reached agreement, all of us or any of us, about the options in terms of research on prophylaxis, a terribly important problem in this society. We do not all agree whether we ought now to strive for prophylaxis for all, or for all adults who are above 20 years of age, or only for some adults, particularly those who are most susceptible in relation to hyperlipidemia, or whether in fact we should try prophylaxis in anybody with our current state of knowledge.

Now I admit to a partiality toward emphasis on the susceptibles, because those of us who study mutants with severe hyperlipoproteinemia and a disproportionate share of coronary artery disease have recently inherited a particularly annoying dilemma, and this is the fact that we have now extremely encouraging success in the ability to lower blood lipids and lipoproteins in some of these more common disorders. As a result, we must cope with the question of whether it is really worthwhile to take the time and expense, that of the patient and that of the physician, to insist now that this be the lifetime mode for these many patients, some of whom we are beginning to detect and treat without delay in childhood.

The use of both diet and drugs imposes a very difficult regime; the physician can prescribe it, and the patient accept it, only when there is firm conviction that it is a healthy thing to do—and we still do not have positive proof that it is.

We just cannot indefinitely postpone convincing ourselves or patients on the basis of inadequate evidence. There are a number of prevention trials that are going on addressed to this question in this country and around the world. Just very briefly, let me remind you of the framework in which they lie. Some of them involve the general population. In these we have two different kinds of trials, one dealing with drugs and one dealing with diet.

With the exception of the British study of Atromid, none of the studies today, certainly not those with regard to diet, are of sufficient magnitude or proper design to give an answer to the question of prophylaxis for the general population. Consequently we must wait until a valid study is done; no such study is yet underway, particularly with regard to the question of diet.

The second major group of subjects who are now the objects of certain studies of prophylaxis are susceptibles. These may be grouped into two categories: (1) those who have already had an infarct, and (2) those identified as susceptible prior to infarction. In those who have already had an infarct, we have both good diet trials and good drug trials in progress, and these may give us some important answers to the question of prophylaxis. It is very interesting, however, that among the susceptibles there is no study in a group of patients before the infarct to determine whether or not our prophylactic measures are worth the candle. Now I have no doubt that, among the susceptibles, the patients with extreme elevations of low density lipoproteins, whether that be due to genetic or sporadic cause, are momentarily of the greatest interest to planners of intervention trials in susceptible individuals. The incidence of this disorder is rather high, although still not perfectly known. With regard to the familial extreme variety, as many as one in 200 Americans may have such a disorder.

Their atherosclerosis, to me at least, is simply an extreme exaggeration of that which occurs in the general population. This is not yet proved, but the studies so far show that the normal relatives of patients who have hyperbetalipoproteinemia, or Type 2 as we call it, seem to have no increase in incidence of coronary artery disease when compared with the general population.

Certainly now there is a striking ability to treat these hypercholesterolemic patients; between no treatment and maximal treatment, one can expect a 40 per cent difference in beta lipoprotein levels, and these levels can be held down for what looks like an indefinite period of time.

Thus there is a choice in these patients. For example, of two groups treated by diet, one may be given cholestyramine, the most effective agent for reducing the lipoprotein levels of these patients over long periods of time.

For proper control, there are potentials for double-blinding such a population, and certainly there are possibilities for randomization. There is always a question of end points. This is the major factor in delaying intervention trials across the broad spectrum of hyperlipidemia and coronary disease. In a selected population at extreme hazard, I think it is possible to consider end points other than mortality or morbidity, and this includes some maximal exercise tolerance or other noninvasive techniques; angiographic studies might also be indicated in appropriate subjects.

Thus, I would put the highest priority today on intervention trials in susceptibles. There are far fewer subjects who would be needed, there is the possibility of more extreme differences between the controls and the treated and, because of the increased severity of the problem, the increase in potential benefits to the individual patient could indeed be greater than in any other possible cohort. Moreover, some of the results of the first two considerations could be increased efficiency and decreased cost.

I certainly would not consider that any one trial in susceptibles will answer all of the questions relative to the general population, and more than one trial will undoubtedly have to be done, but I do believe, in summary, that this is a time of decision. As dietary trends are changing across the country, they may not in themselves effect a meaningful difference in coronary heart disease. I hope that they do, but such trends will make it increasingly difficult to compare a control and experimental population as each year goes on.

Finally, of course, if it does seem impossible for want of resources, for want of time, or for want of import to answer unequivocally the questions with which I began, then I think that those of us who are still on the fence had best come down and stand on one side or the other and go then about more important and productive activity.

B.
EFFECTIVE CONTROL OF ARTERIAL HYPERTENSION

RAY W. GIFFORD, JR., M.D.

The last 20 years of intensive research in the field of hypertension have yielded more answers with regard to epidemiology, natural history, and therapy than they have about the etiology and pathogenetic mechanisms of essential hypertension. At the present time, we must ask ourselves if we should redirect our efforts and our resources by realigning our priorities with respect to the conquest of hypertension. So long as human and economic resources are limited, the assignment of priorities is a necessary, albeit an unpopular and thankless, task.

Taking cognizance of data pertaining to the effectiveness of antihypertensive therapy in altering favorably the natural history of the disease[1-4] and believing that we all agree that the common goal is reduction of mortality and morbidity from the complications of hypertension, I would like to propose the following order of priorities for research in the effective control of hypertension in the 1970s.

I. Demonstration studies in representative communities to define the most effective, efficient, and economical methods to: (a) screen large populations for hypertension, (b) select and evaluate those who should be treated, (c) initiate and maintain therapeutic programs when indicated, and (d) evaluate appropriately the results and impact of such studies.

II. Controlled, double-blind trials to determine the efficacy of antihypertensive therapy for: (a) men and women with diastolic blood pressures between 90 and 105 mm. Hg, (b) young persons with labile hypertension, and (c) older patients (>60 years) with primarily systolic hypertension.

III. Longitudinal, prospective epidemiological studies designed to determine the precursors of hypertension in a representative population.

IV. Investigation of etiological factors and pathogenetic mechanisms in essential hypertension.

V. Development of simplified techniques for measuring cardiac output and plasma and extracellular fluid volumes as an approach to more rational antihypertensive therapy, at least from the hemodynamic standpoint.

VI. Development of new antihypertensive drugs and further identification of the clinical pharmacology and mechanisms of action of presently available drugs.

VII. Refinements in diagnostic and therapeutic procedures for identifying and managing patients with curable forms of hypertension (renal vascular disease, pheochromocytoma, primary aldosteronism, coarctation of the aorta, etc.).

I am neither a liberal, visionary social planner nor an opponent of basic research. I would hope that in the next 10 years there would be ample funds and personnel to pursue all of these research activities vigorously. I do feel, however, that there is a certain urgency about the practical application of the knowledge that we have already gained through research.

PRIORITY I: DEMONSTRATION STUDIES

The complications of coronary and cerebral atherosclerosis are the number one public health problem in the United States today, being responsible for nearly half of the deaths and for immeasurable disability and economic loss. I do not need to remind this audience that strokes, myocardial infarction, and sudden death due to coronary insufficiency are not confined to the elderly but are major menaces to the productivity, economic stability, and emotional tranquility of middle-aged persons. Prospective epidemiological studies have consistently identified hypertension as one of the most important antecedents or risk factors in both coronary and cerebral atherosclerosis. Until recently, however, good evidence was not available to support the intuition shared by many of us that effective treatment of even mild or moderate hypertension is beneficial.

Public health statistics have shown a progressive decline in the death rate from hypertensive heart disease and stroke during the last 20 years. Numerous studies have confirmed the lifesaving potential of blood pressure reduction for patients with malignant (group 4) and premalignant (group 3) hypertension.[1, 5-8]

More recently, the results of the Veterans Administration Cooperative Study[3, 4] have shown that, for men with diastolic blood pressures between 90 and 129 mm. Hg, antihypertensive therapy eliminated congestive heart failure secondary to hypertensive heart disease, prevented renal failure, cerebral hemorrhage, and acceleration of hypertension, and dramatically reduced the incidence of brain infarcts. The morbidity and mortality rates were significantly higher in the placebo group than in the treated group. The only complication of hypertension that was not appreciably affected by treatment was myocardial infarction, and this may be due to the fact that the average age of the men in this study was 50 years and it is likely that many of them already had significant coronary atherosclerosis before treatment was started.

From the 1962 National Health survey,[9] it can be estimated that at the present time there are approximately 20 million people in the United States with hypertension (>160/95 mm. Hg). Probably 40 per cent of these victims of hypertension do not even know that their blood pressure is elevated.[10] Of those who did know that they are hypertensive, only one-third were on antihypertensive therapy, according to the Baldwin County, Georgia survey, and only half of these have adequate control of their hypertension.[10] Thus, it can be calculated that, of 20 million hypertensive Americans, only 2 million are presently receiving the protection against complications and premature death that effective therapy can bestow.

To get the other 18 million under appropriate therapy and to keep them under observation is a herculean task that will require the ingenuity of social planners, educators, psychologists, behavioral scientists, public relations and media experts, legislators, governmental officials, social workers, ancillary health personnel, and nurses as well as physicians.

If this can be accomplished, the implications are so great in terms of conserving human life and preventing devastating complications that I have placed it as the number one priority.

Well-designed demonstration projects must be established in communities of various sizes to determine how best to identify the hypertensives and, once they are identified, how to evaluate them expeditiously, effectively, and economically. Because of the shortage of physicians, ancillary medical personnel must be trained in case finding and must assume a large role, under appropriate medical supervision, for evaluating, treating, and following the hypertensives identified.

A comprehensive lay and professional educational effort is mandatory to overcome physicians' apathy about antihypertensive therapy and to motivate the public to accept and seek screening and diagnostic procedures and to adhere to medical regimens which may produce side effects and which are necessarily lifelong. One of the major obstacles to successful medical therapy of hypertension is the failure of patients to take the medication.[11] Only if physicians and patients are convinced of the value and efficacy of drug therapy and are sufficiently concerned about the perils of untreated hypertension will the necessary cooperation be forthcoming. To accomplish this will be no minor feat, and it will require the combined efforts of the medical society, the mass media, educators, public relations consultants, and behavioral psychologists, to mention a few.

Attractive facilities for identification, evaluation, and treatment must be made available and convenient at no charge to the economically deprived and to the medically indigent. To overcome the superstitition and natural reluctance of the uneducated to participate in such a program will require specialized persuasive techniques, as well as attractive and readily available facilities.

Finally, each demonstration project must be evaluated, not only from the standpoint of lives saved and morbidity prevented but, just as importantly, from the aspects of feasibility, efficiency, cost analysis, patient and physician cooperation, and general applicability on a wide scale in other communities. It is not reasonable to expect that a prototype can be developed which can or will be adopted by every community. Therefore, multiple demonstration projects will be necessary in a variety of settings to explore ways in which this program can be integrated into existing facilities and can utilize existing resources.

While some may question whether this is a truly scientific endeavor, I submit that, if it is not designed, executed, and evaluated with all of the expertise that social and medical scientists can bring to bear, it will surely fail, and tens of thousands of Americans will pay with their lives for our failure.

PRIORITY II: CONTROLLED TREATMENT STUDIES

I have designated as the number two priority an extension of placebo controlled double-blind treatment studies to segments of the population not included in the Cooperative Study of the Veterans Administration.[3, 4] While the Veterans Administration Study did not include women, I feel that placebo controlled studies in women with diastolic blood pressures greater than 105 mm. Hg are unnecessary, unjustifiable, and unethical. On the other hand, Veterans Administration data for men with diastolic blood pressures between 90 and 105 mm. Hg are not as convincing as they are for men with higher pressures. Consequently, I would advocate a study to determine the effectiveness of therapy for both men and women at all ages with diastolic blood pressures between 90 and 105 mm. Hg.

Similar studies should also be undertaken to delineate the benefits to be derived from antihypertensive therapy for patients, especially young people, with labile hypertension, and for patients of all ages, including young people as well as the geriatric age group with only systolic hypertension. No information at all is available with regard to the efficacy of antihypertensive therapy in these groups.

However, I think that such controlled studies should not be given preference to the establishment of demonstration projects in representative communities for case finding and treatment. It may take years, for example, to determine whether the treatment of mild labile hypertension in adolescents and young adults will prevent coronary atherosclerosis. Even if it does not, there are enough other benefits to be derived from antihypertensive therapy to recommend its widespread use. If we wait until we have proof positive of the benefits of antihypertensive therapy for every age group, male or female, mild or severe, systolic or diastolic, before advocating community trials, we are jeopardizing the lives of thousands of people. We have enough information to proceed with case finding and treatment on a large scale of those with diastolic blood pressures of over 105 mm. Hg, while at the same time we can gather information in a well-controlled double-blind fashion about the value of treatment for other groups of hypertensive patients.

PRIORITY III: EPIDEMIOLOGICAL STUDIES

While prospective population studies have convincingly demonstrated that hypertension is a precursor of premature cardiovascular disease,[12, 13] they have yielded very little information about the precursors of hypertension itself, probably because children have not been included in the study populations. As a matter of fact, it may be necessary to start such a study with observations on the parents of the cohort and to record prenatal influences as well as data obtained at time of birth. When the study group on hypertension of the Inter-Society Commission on Heart Disease Resources considered the problem of primary prevention of hypertension, the gaps in our knowledge became appallingly apparent. Other than some vague references to genetic influences, which we probably could not control if we could identify, what could we say?

It is my opinion that a particularly hopeful approach to this problem might be the identification and prolonged observation of adolescents with labile, primarily systolic hypertension with high cardiac output to determine whether they will eventually develop sustained diastolic hypertension with normal cardiac output. If half were treated appropriately on a randomized basis, it would be possible to accomplish simultaneously one of the objectives already discussed in Priority II.

It is axiomatic in medicine that prevention is the best weapon against disease. Without more knowledge about the antecedents of hypertension, we have no hope of preventing it. This is why I placed it third in my list of priorities in research.

PRIORITY IV: INVESTIGATION INTO MECHANISMS AND ETIOLOGY OF ESSENTIAL HYPERTENSION

Acknowledging the fact that the cure for essential hypertension is not likely to be forthcoming until we have identified its etiology (or etiologies), I have still chosen to give this a relatively low priority. From my vantage point, investigation on this subject seems to offer little promise for reducing the morbidity and mortality from hypertension in the next 10 years, barring of course the elusive breakthrough. Few in the field believe that what we now call essential hypertension is a single entity with a common etiology. So complex is the problem that its ultimate solution seems years away. I hope that my pessimism proves to be unfounded, but in any event it should be our immediate concern to prolong the lives of thousands of victims of hypertension until such a time that they too can benefit from the discoveries that will be made in research laboratories around the world, ultimately leading to the cure of hypertension.

PRIORITY V: IMPROVED TECHNOLOGY

Hypertension may result from either increased cardiac output or increased peripheral resistance or both. Recently it has been shown that the relative contributions of these two factors in an individual patient vary from case to case.[14] Furthermore, some hypertensive patients have high, some have normal, and some have low plasma volumes.[15] The possible combinations of hemodynamic abnormalities are therefore rather considerable, and this is complicated even more by the fact that certain types of therapy can alter these derangements by normalizing one factor while permitting a previously normal factor to become abnormal. Reliable noninvasive techniques for measuring cardiac output and simpler methods for measuring plasma and extracellular fluid volumes would permit us to use the antihypertensive drugs at our disposal in a more rational manner to combat selectively the specific hemodynamic effect or effects identified. It is not beyond the realm of possibility that computers will be programmed to take into account the severity of hypertension, the complications of hypertension, and the hemodynamic and plasma volume aberrations as well as symptomatology so that they can select a rational regimen for that individual. At the moment, a well-trained, experienced, and knowledgeable physician is a satisfactory substitute for a computer in prescribing antihypertensive drugs, but with the proliferation of knowledge and drugs he may not remain so.

PRIORITY VI: NEW DRUGS

The low priority that I have given to the development of new drugs and to refinements in our knowledge about clinical pharmacology and the mechanisms of action of presently available drugs reflects my satisfaction with the current status. It is vastly more important to use the drugs we already have to treat the estimated 18 million untreated hypertensives than it is to develop new ones. A diuretic with antihypertensive potency comparable to the thiazides without hyperuricemic, hyperglycemic, and kaliuretic effects would be nice, but it is not essential. Already under investigation are new direct-acting vasodilators to reduce peripheral resistance, including diazoxide. The latter will offer advantages over conventional drugs in the management of hypertensive crises if and when it is approved by the Food and Drug Administration. Ultimately new pharmacological avenues should be explored such as those opened by renin inhibitors and cadmium chelators. In my opinion, the new sympathetic inhibiting drugs offer the least promising approach.

PRIORITY VII: DIAGNOSTIC AND THERAPEUTIC PROCEDURES FOR CURABLE HYPERTENSION

Fewer than 5 per cent of hypertensive patients have a potentially reversible surgical lesion (*e.g.*, pheochromocytoma, renal vascular disease, primary aldosteronism, etc.), yet it is apparent that these rare causes for hypertension receive an inordinate amount of attention at medical meetings and consume a disproportionate amount of the physician's time in clinical practice. While simplified, less expensive, and less time-consuming methods for identifying patients with these lesions would be welcome, they would not contribute materially to a reduction in overall morbidity and mortality from hypertension, simply because so few patients have surgically correctable lesions and most of those who do (with the exception of patients with pheochromocytoma and coarctation of the aorta) will respond satisfactorily to medical therapy.

While it is always possible that investigation into the mechanisms of these rare forms of hypertension may shed light on the bigger problem of essential hypertension, it is more likely, in my opinion, that research directed at essential hypertension will identify other, as yet unrecognized, curable forms.

For reasons that I have outlined in detail elsewhere,[16] the tremendous cost in time and money of evaluating hypertensive patients to identify or exclude curable causes should not be a deterrent to mass screening because more good than harm would result if mass diagnostic investigation had to be minimized and all patients with secondary hypertension were treated as if they had essential hypertension.

SUMMARY

As much as we need better understanding of the pathogenetic mechanisms and etiological factors in essential hypertension, as much as we need more information about the precursors and prevention of hypertension, as much as we need controlled long-term studies to evaluate the efficacy of treatment in certain groups of hypertensives, our most urgent need is to devise methods of identifying and treating an estimated 18 million hypertensive Americans who are presently receiving inadequate treatment or none at all. This should remain our number one research priority until the majority of our fellow countrymen who are victims of this disease are enjoying the fruits of our research. The fact that we have drugs that can substantially reduce morbidity and mortality from one of the most prevalent diseases in this nation should be disquieting to us so long as cardiovascular disease remains our number one public health problem.

Today's youth have accused our generation, perhaps with justification, of being irrelevant and of having misdirected, inappropriate, and at times ambivalent priorities. I am suggesting that in the field of research in hypertension we redefine our goals and realign our priorities to make them relevant to the goals we seek, namely, the prolongation of useful life for millions of hypertensive patients in this country.

REFERENCES

1. Perry, H., Jr., Schroeder, H. A., Cantanzaro, F. J., Moore-Jones, D., and Camel, G. H.: Studies on the control of hypertension. 8. Mortality, morbidity, and remissions during twelve years of intensive therapy. Circulation 33: 958–972, 1966.
2. Mathisen, H. S., Loken, H., Brox, D., and Stenbaek, O.: The prognosis in long-term treated and "untreated" essential hypertension. Acta Med. Scand. 185: 253–258, 1969.
3. Veterans Administration Cooperative Study Group: Effects of treatment on morbidity in hypertension. I. Results in patients with diastolic blood pressures averaging 115 through 129 mm Hg. J. A. M. A. 202: 1028–1034, 1967.

4. Veterans Administration Cooperative Study Group: Effects of treatment on morbidity in hypertension. II. Results in patients with diastolic blood pressure averaging 90 through 114 mm Hg. J. A. M. A. 213: 1143–1152, 1970.
5. Bjork, S., Sannerstedt, R., Angervall, G., and Hood, B.: Treatment and prognosis in malignant hypertension: clinical follow-up study of 93 patients on modern medical treatment. Acta Med. Scand. 166: 175–187, 1960.
6. Dustan, H. P., Schneckloth, R. E., Corcoran, A. C., and Page, I. H.: The effectiveness of long-term treatment of malignant hypertension. Circulation 18: 644–651, 1958.
7. Harington, M., Kincaid-Smith, P., and McMichael, J.: Results of treatment in malignant hypertension; a seven-year experience in 94 cases. Brit. Med. J. 2: 969–980, 1959.
8. Farmer, R. G., Gifford, R. W., Jr., and Hines, E. A., Jr.: Effect of medical treatment of severe hypertension; a follow-up study of 161 patients with group 3 and group 4 hypertension. Arch. Intern. Med. 112: 118–128, 1963.
9. Hypertension and Hypertensive Heart Disease in Adults: United States 1960–1962 (data from the National Health Survey), Public Health Service Publication 1000, Series 11–13, 1966, p. 5.
10. Wilber, J. A.: Detection and control of hypertensive disease in Georgia, U.S.A. In *Epidemiology of Hypertension*. Grune & Stratton, Inc., New York, 1967, pp. 439–448.
11. Wilber, J. A., and Barrow, J. G.: Reducing elevated blood pressure; experience found in a community. Minnesota Med. 52: 1303–1305, 1969.
12. Kannel, W. B., Schwartz, M. J., and McNamara, P. M.: Blood pressure and risk of coronary heart disease: the Framingham Study. Dis. Chest 56: 43–52, 1969.
13. Kannel, W. B., Wolf, P. A., Verter, J., and McNamara, P. M.: Epidemiologic assessment of the role of blood pressure in stroke; the Framingham Study. J. A. M. A. 214: 301–310, 1970.
14. Frohlich, E. D., Tarazi, R. C., and Dustan, H. P.: Re-examination of the hemodynamics of hypertension. Amer. J. Med. Sci. 257: 9–23, 1969.
15. Tarazi, R. C., Dustan, H. P., Frohlich, E. D., Gifford, R. W., Jr., and Hoffman, G. C.: Plasma volume and chronic hypertension: relationship to arterial pressure levels in different hypertensive diseases. Arch. Intern. Med. 125: 835–842, 1970.
16. Gifford, R. W., Jr.: Evaluation of the hypertensive patient with emphasis on detecting curable causes. Milbank Mem. Fund Quart. 57: 170–186, 1969.

C.
PREVENTION OF CORONARY ARTERY THROMBOSIS

SOL SHERRY, M.D.

Currently, occlusive disease of the vessels is the primary health hazard facing the aging population of the Western world. Since arterial occlusive disease is most often related to atheromatous involvement of the vessel, the increasing concern over atherosclerotic disease of the arteries is both justifiable and reasonable; the control and prevention of this lesion are likely to have a far-reaching impact on morbidity, mortality, and longevity. Most important in this regard is the prevention of acute myocardial infarction since it is estimated that this complication alone will afflict more than 1 million individuals in the United States during 1970.[1]

In general, extensive occlusive disease of the arteries is a mixture of atherosclerosis and thrombosis; while the relative contribution of each and the relationship between the two remain unsettled, most pathologists agree that the decisive acute occlusive event which precipitates major pathological sequelae is usually thromboembolic in nature. Therefore it is quite surprising that, in the problem of acute myocardial infarction, the prevention of coronary artery thrombosis has not received the attention it deserves.

Lack of interest in the prevention of coronary artery thrombosis probably reflects a changing attitude concerning the importance of thrombosis in the pathogenesis of acute myocardial infarction. Two decades ago, the term acute coronary thrombosis was used almost synonymously with acute myocardial infarction; today the terms are used independently, and rarely does the physician attempt to identify the proximate event leading to the infarction and, when he does, thrombosis no longer appears to have the prominence it once enjoyed. Undoubtedly this changing attitude is based both on pathological observations which indicate that acute thrombi are infrequently found in patients dying suddenly of a "heart attack," [2] and on the argument that, when thrombi are found in patients with proven myocardial infarction, they represent an effect of the infarct rather than its cause. Let us analyze these aspects further.

INCIDENCE OF CORONARY ARTERY THROMBOSIS IN ACUTE MYOCARDIAL INFARCTION

Most of the confusion over incidence arises from difficulties in case selection and in the methods of pathological examination. In many of the studies, all cases dying acutely of a "heart attack" have been considered as having a myocardial infarction, and when the vessels were examined, they were either cut longitudinally, which is an excellent method for dislodging thrombi, or sectioned horizontally at several sites but far enough apart to overlook small thrombi.

Recent observations on sudden death (*i.e.*, death within 1 hour of the onset of symptoms) indicate that most patients probably die from an acute arrhythmia, not from a myocardial infarction, *i.e.*, the latter is not the usual cause of sudden death. Therefore, it is not surprising that the incidence of demonstrable coronary thrombosis is low in this group. When cases of sudden death are eliminated and examination of the coronary vessels is (a) restricted to patients who die with well-documented clinical and pathological evidence of recent infarction, and (b) carried out with serial sections made every 2 to 3 mm. (with heavily calcified vessels, the vessel should be removed first, fixed, and decalcified before sectioning) then each of the three most recent studies[3-5] has demonstrated an incidence of thrombi of over 90 per cent. The thrombi usually occurred at sites of narrowing of the vessel consequent to an underlying atheromatous plaque, and most often they were less than 5 mm. long, although some extended for several centimeters. The left anterior descending branch was most frequently involved (50 to 60 per cent of cases), followed by the right coronary artery (25 to 35 per cent) and the left circumflex branch (10 to 20 per cent). Interestingly, thrombi in the left anterior descending branch usually were found within the first 2 cm. of origin (50 per cent were within the first centimeter), while thrombi in the right coronary artery demonstrated no predilection as to site, with some thrombi found as far as 10 cm. from the origin of the vessel.

SIGNIFICANCE OF CORONARY ARTERY THROMBOSIS IN PATHOGENESIS OF ACUTE MYOCARDIAL INFARCTION

The high incidence of coronary artery thrombosis in patients with unequivocal evidence of acute myocardial infarction does not establish a pathogenetic role for this event, particularly as the suggestion has been made that the thrombosis is a consequence of the tissue necrosis.[2] The latter view is difficult to reconcile with the more detailed histological studies of Constantinides,[6] confirmed by Harland and Holburn[3] as well as others. These investigations established clearly that almost all thrombi were superimposed on and associated with breaks, *i.e.*, fissures, cracks, or ulcers, in the intima of atheromatous or fibrosed arterial walls. This has led to the inescapable conclusion that thrombosis in the major arteries of the heart is initiated in most cases by the breaks in the vessel wall, although admittedly the rate of growth, ultimate size, and fate of the thrombus are dependent on other factors, *e.g.*, platelets, fibrin formation, fibrinolysis, and vascular flow. Most convincing in establishing the primacy of the intimal interruption in initiating the thrombosis is the fact that the breaks are covered and filled by platelet masses, and fragments of the atherosclerotic wall, including shreds of collagen, are often buried in the thrombi.

PATHOGENESIS OF ACUTE CORONARY THROMBOSIS

Consequently, although many of the details remain to be elaborated, a useful outline has emerged for the pathogenesis of acute coronary thrombosis. For one or more reasons (aging and hardening, trauma from vascular flow or a microhemorrhage in the vascular wall), a plaque or fibrosed vessel fissures, cracks, or ulcerates, exposing the subendothelial microfibrils and collagen of the subintimal tissue; the latter trigger the sticking, aggregation, and formation of a platelet mass; this is followed by the release of platelet factors, which results in the deposition of fibrin sufficient to stabilize the platelet mass and to initiate the development of a superimposed fibrin-red cell coagulum. The end result is a typical arterial thrombus which occludes the vessel and leads to severe ischemia, myocardial necrosis, and infarction.

Acceptance of this view, which best fits the information available at present, re-establishes the primacy of acute coronary thrombosis as the immediate cause of most cases of acute myocardial infarction and stresses the importance of thrombus prevention as an immediate goal for strikingly influencing the incidence of acute myocardial infarction. Since thrombus prevention may be more readily achieved than the control of atherosclerosis, it is essential that it be given a very high priority for cardiovascular research in the 1970s.

PROSPECTS FOR PREVENTION OF CORONARY ARTERY THROMBOSIS

Current forms of anticoagulant (heparin and coumarin) therapy are not designed to have a major impact on the problem under discussion. In acute myocardial infarction, their value is restricted to thrombus growth in the coronary vessels and to the prevention of venous thrombosis and pulmonary embolism and of mural thrombus formation and systemic embolization. The former is not an important consideration, and the latter complications account for approximately only 6 per cent of the deaths. Although intensive conventional anticoagulant therapy is probably capable of eliminating half of these (3 per cent), this gain represents only a small fraction of the problem of survival following an acute infarct. More appropriate for the treatment of acute myocardial infarction is the use of thrombolytic or clot-dissolving agents, for the rapid restoration of blood flow could improve myocardial function and diminish irritability. The prospects in this area are good, but this is not the problem under discussion.

From a public health standpoint, the goal is the prevention of coronary artery thrombosis. Here, relatively little can be expected from the long-term use of coumarin compounds; these agents do not significantly affect platelet sticking and aggregation to the site of the vascular lesion, and it is the platelet mass which must be prevented if we are to inhibit the formation of a coronary thrombus. Thus the immediate objective is well defined, *i.e.*, to develop agents capable of inhibiting platelet sticking and/or aggregation at the site of vascular lesions in man.

The investigation and development of platelet antiaggregants has been underway for some time; the prospects look bright for the future, although admittedly much remains to be done. There are many pharmacologically active antiaggregating agents, but three have come to the fore (aspirin,[7] sulfinpyrazone,[8] and dipyridamole[9]); all have demonstrated an effect *in vitro* and in experimental animal models, and currently all are in various stages of clinical investigation. Considering that the effects *in vivo* of these agents in preventing arterial thrombus formation in man may not correlate too closely with observations on inhibition of platelet aggregation *in vitro* or on thrombus prevention in experimental animal models, it would be most helpful if we had available a human disease state in which the pharmacological effects of the antiaggregating agents could be screened quickly and under controlled conditions. This information would be most useful before embarking on major clinical trials, for such trials will require large numbers of patients and will extend over several years. From a practical standpoint, the most useful model for obtaining quick answers to the efficacy *in vivo* of an antithrombotic agent would be in the prevention of thrombosis in the deep veins of the lower extremity, particularly if this could be combined with a sensitive technique, *e.g.*, I^{125} scanning, for demonstrating early or incipient thrombosis. The lesion in this instance is a venous thrombus, however, and platelet mass formation may not be involved in its initiation. More appropriate would be an arterial lesion, and here the two most attractive areas for study are embolization from valvular prostheses and transient cerebral ischemic attacks; although either would be a good model, surgical developments are limiting their usefulness. New types of artificial valves are being introduced frequently (hopefully to circumvent the thromboembolic and other complications), while for transient ischemic attacks, surgical endarterectomy is being performed to an ever increasing extent, particularly when significant carotid vascular lesions are demonstrated by angiography. However, it is encouraging to note that plans are being formulated to test the effect of aspirin in reducing the frequency of transient ischemic attacks; this study could provide important information before the institution of a major clinical trial in the prevention of coronary thrombosis. Ultimately, and not in the too distant future, such a trial will have to be undertaken; one hopes that sufficient information will be at hand to make wise decisions as to the best agent and dosage to employ.

While platelet antiaggregants show promise in becoming the primary agents of choice in the prevention of coronary thrombosis, their efficacy in thrombus formation may prove to be synergistic when combined with agents capable of inducing a hypocoagulable state, *e.g.*, the coumarins, or with orally administered compounds which enhance circulating fibrinolytic activity. Such developments must await some proof of efficacy of the platelet antiaggregants alone.

In summary, this report (1) re-emphasizes the incidence and importance of coronary thrombosis in acute myocardial infarction, (2) stresses the need for the prevention of coronary thrombosis in strikingly reducing the morbidity and mortality from this disorder, and (3) cites the direction of current research in achieving this objective.

REFERENCES

1. Ibrahim, M. A., Sacket, D. L., and Winkelstein, W., Jr.: Acute myocardial infarction: magnitude of the problem. In Sherry, S., Genton, E., Brinkhous, K. M., and Stengle, J. M. (eds.): *Thrombosis*. National Academy of Sciences, Washington, D. C., pp. 106–114.
2. Spain, D. M., and Bradess, V. A.: The relationship of coronary thrombosis to coronary atherosclerosis and heart disease (a necropsy study covering a period of 25 years). Amer. J. Med. Sci. 240: 701, 1960.
3. Harland, W. A., and Holburn, M. A.: Coronary thrombosis and myocardial infarction. Lancet 2: 1158, 1966.
4. Mitchell, J. R. A.: The role of thrombosis in myocardial infarction. In Sherry, S., Genton, E., Brinkhous, K. M., and Stengle, J. M. (eds.): *Thrombosis*. National Academy of Sciences, Washington, D. C., pp. 117–125.
5. Davis, N. A.: Incidence of thrombosis in myocardial infarction. Aust. Ann. Intern. Med. 19 (Suppl. 1): 60, 1970.
6. Constantinides, P.: Plaque fissures in human coronary thrombosis. J. Atheroscler. Res. 6: 1, 1966.
7. O'Brien, J. R.: Effects of salicylates on blood platelets. Lancet 1: 779, 1968.
8. Packham, M. A., Warrior, M. F., Glynn, M. F., Senyi, A. S., and Mustard, J. F.. Alteration of the response of platelets to surface stimuli by pyrazole compounds: J. Exp. Med. 126: 171, 1967.
9. Emmons, P. R., Harrison, M. J. G., Honour, A. J., and Mitchell, J. R. A.: Effect of dipyridamole on human platelet behavior. Lancet 2: 603, 1965.

26

Stress Testing in Evaluating Cardiac Performance

LENORE R. ZOHMAN, M.D.

Those of us who choose to prescribe exercise training for our cardiac patients must answer one very important question. What dose of exercise do we prescribe for a patient which will be strenuous enough to result in physical fitness and not strenuous enough to impose detrimentally on his cardiovascular capacity? The ensuing discussion is oriented toward the use of exercise stress testing to provide information about the patient on which to base the prescription of exercise, rather than toward the use of such testing for the diagnosis of coronary disease. Chapter 27 explains the rationale and methods of translating the stress test results into a physical training program.

The Master two-step test and nonstandardized exercise tests have been accepted as useful in the diagnosis of coronary heart disease. Doyle and Kinch[1] have screened over 2,000 men (carrying out more than 20,000 tests since 1953) using exercise stress tests diagnostically and prognostically in identifying clinically silent coronary heart disease. In the known cardiac patient, however, exercise stress tests are also useful in determining the capacity for occupational work or exercise. When the patient's cardiovascular capacity is known, exercise may be prescribed relative to his capacity, the results of his participation in an exercise training program may be assessed, and in some cases the effectiveness of drug therapy in improving his performance may be determined.

STRESS TESTING METHODS

Exercise testing may be carried out, using step tests with various climbing rates on steps of various heights, treadmill tests at various grades and speeds, ergometer tests at various pedaling rates and against various resistances for variable periods of time, and even cranking tests involving upper extremity work, which sometimes is also combined with lower extremity work. Each method has its own rationale and its advantages and disadvantages, many of which are succinctly described in the work of Bruce *et al.*,[2] Haskell and Fox,[3] and Shephard *et al.*,[4] among others. In choosing the type of stress test, three decisions must be made by the physician: (1) whether to use a single stage or a multistage test, (2) whether to carry out a continuous or an intermittent test, and (3) whether a submaximal or a maximal performance test is preferred.

Single versus Multistage Testing

The single stage test may also be called a single load or a single level test. The single load may either demand the same oxygen consumption (and energy cost) of each individual, or it may impose a single external work load without respect to body size. The Master two-step test, for example, ostensibly demands the same amount of work of each subject by adjusting the number of trips over the steps according to age, sex, and weight of the subject. Ford and Hellerstein[5] have determined that this amount of work has an energy cost of 8.5 calories per minute for each subject. Single stage tests can also be carried out on treadmills[6] or on the bicycle[7] as well as on steps. In single load tests when one uses a fixed amount of external work, it is understood that a small man may be working at a larger percentage of his capacity than a large man. However, if both men can perform this work load without electrocardiographic (ECG) evidence of myocardial ischemia, then either man is capable of carrying out occupational work requiring this degree of performance. Thus, single load exercise testing of the fixed load type may be particularly useful to the industrial physician who knows the requirements of specific jobs and must match men to jobs.[8]

The multistage test presents a series of gradually heavier work loads to the patient with or without rest pauses in between the work periods (Fig. 26.1). The discontinuous series with rest pauses may also be called ntermittent. The continuous series of increasing loads without rest pauses

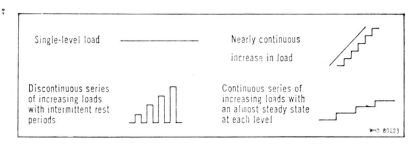

Fig. 26.1. Types of load used in exercise tests. Each of these types of load may be applied in any of the following types of exercise: steps or bench, upright bicycle, supine bicycle, and treadmill. (From Shephard, R. J., et al.[4])

may progress in a series of small steps of short duration or in fewer steps of a duration long enough to permit the attainment of a steady state at each work level before progressing to the next level. Multistage tests may be done on the bicycle as reported by Hellerstein[9] or on the treadmill according to Astrand[10] or even on steps as carried out by Sheffield *et al.*[11]

For example, in a continuous test, the grade on the treadmill may be increased in 1 per cent steps, or small increases in resistance may be imposed when small work increments are required on the bicycle ergometer. Those tests using large work increments allow the patient to exercise at the same work level for 3 to 5 minutes to achieve a balance between oxygen consumption and oxygen supply, and then alter the work load.[2, 12]

The multistage tests have the advantage of starting the patient slowly, permitting the observation of this performance at gradually increasing levels of stress as he approaches his maximal performance capacity. The early low work levels serve as a "warm-up" period, as well as allowing gradual adjustment of the circulation to the exercise. The single stage test permits no warm-up and, if done only once, generally does not provide information about maximal performance. Single stage tests with increasing intensities of effort may be repeated on subsequent days, however, and in this way they might yield the same information as the multistage tests. Whether done on treadmill, bicycle, or steps, on 1 day or several, multilevel testing takes time.

Continuous versus Intermittent Testing

Continuous testing is one method of decreasing the testing time of a multistage procedure since no rest pauses are required. Increasing the work load before the attainment of steady state at each level, that is, at intervals of less than 3 to 4 minutes, further decreases the testing time. Such tests may be continued until the patient reaches maximal performance. This type of testing is done easily with a treadmill or it can be done with a bicycle ergometer, but it is more difficult when it is necessary for a patient to increase his rate of stepping in order to increase the work load.

Kellerman *et al.*[13] Bonjer,[14] and Shephard *et al.*[4] compared the intermittent and continuous patterns of exercise loading and found little difference in physiological response at submaximal work loads or in predictions of maximal performance from the data obtained on normal subjects by either method. The maximal oxygen intake value derived from the test results was approximately the same whether the subject was tested in a continuous or an intermittent fashion.

There may be some disadvantages in patient testing by the continuous method, however. Significant electrocardiographic abnormalities have first appeared in one-eighth to one-sixth of cases as late as the 6th minute of the recovery period[15]; conceivably these abnormalities might have been avoided by observing their genesis during rest pauses. Conversely, some observers feel that these abnormalities are more frequent if rest pauses are permitted than if a continuous test is carried out. In our own laboratory, we are more comfortable with the opportunity to observe whatever electrocardiographic abnormalities might occur during the rest pauses rather than being surprised by their occurrence at the termination of the procedure. Patients exercising on a bicycle are also more comfortable when permitted to rest their leg muscles, shift position on the bicycle seat, and remove the mouthpiece during the rest period. Yet, in our experience, treadmill as contrasted to bicycle exercise is easier to carry out in a continuous rather than a discontinuous sequence.

Submaximal versus Maximal Exercise

Submaximal exercise is not strenuous enough to push the patient to exhaustion or to his physiological limits to performance, whereas maximal exercise is sufficiently strenuous. The maximal oxygen intake has been called "the international reference standard of cardiorespiratory fitness." [16] This point is reached when, with further increase of the work load, the oxygen consumption levels off, that is, it increases by less than 2 ml. per kg. of body weight per minute. At this point, the respiratory quotient $(CO_2$ produced$)/(O_2$ consumed$)$ reaches a value of 1.0, barring artifacts. The "respiratory equivalent" is usually 26 to 30, that is 26 to 30 ml. of air must be ventilated for each milliliter of oxygen consumed at maximal oxygen intake. This value is considerably lower at submaximal work loads.[17] Usually the blood lactate concentration at maximal aerobic capacity is close to 90 to 100 mg. %. Maximal heart rate and maximal oxygen consumption need not be attained simultaneously. Heart rate may continue to rise with increases in work load for a short time at maximal oxygen intake. Since the maximal pulse rate which can be attained decreases with advancing years, pulse rate at maximal performance is related to age[15] (Fig. 26.2). At maximal oxygen intake, the pulse rate is usually within 2 standard deviations of the expected maximal value for an individual of that age. This is the point of exhaustion. At exhaustion during treadmill exercise, the subject may complain of nausea (probably indicating gastrointestinal ischemia) or chest pain indicating myocardial ischemia, or an ataxic gait may be noted, resulting from cerebral ischemia. In exhaustion generated by bicycle exercise, the main problem is quadriceps muscle fatigue. Stepping exercise may generate any of the described symptoms at exhaustion. Patients with coronary heart disease are generally limited by symptoms or signs in advance of obtaining these high levels of performance. Moderately severe angina and ventricular arrhythmias indicate a "clinical maximum."

Certainly the most reliable method of determining maximal performance

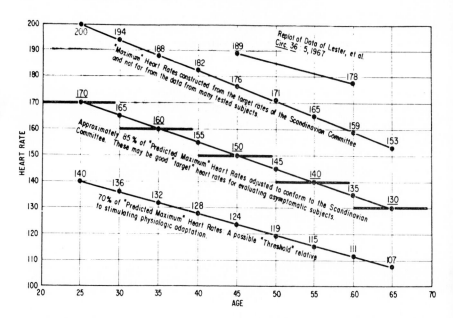

Fig. 26.2. The decline of "maximal" heart rate with age possible applications to exercise testing and training. (From Fox, S. M., and Haskell, W. L.[15])

is to stress each patient in a multistage test to maximal oxygen intake. This procedure leaves no doubt about whether that patient is capable of transferring oxygen from room air to the tissues effectively. The strenuousness of the procedure and the imperfections inherent in translating stress test results into an exercise prescription for the gymnasium make some of us feel that, for clinical purposes, maximal testing may not be indicated. Alternatively, submaximal testing at several progressively harder work loads can be used and the maximum can be calculated rather than measured. A line can be fitted to points on the plot of heart rate versus oxygen consumption derived from the submaximal tests and then extrapolated to maximal heart rate for age. The maximal oxygen consumption can be read off at that age-adjusted maximal heart rate (Fig. 26.3). Obviously the more points available (the more submaximal work loads carried out) the more exact the line. There are at least four methods of making this extrapolation, based primarily on the number of points available (Astrand and Ryhming nomogram,[18] formula of Von Dobeln et al.,[19] nomogram of Margaria et al.,[20] and extrapolation of Maritz et al.[21]). Extrapolations to maximal from submaximal test results for subjects unfamiliar with the procedure usually provide values from 5 to 10 per cent lower than measured maximal oxygen uptake values. There is also the possibility that a particular patient will not have the average maximal heart rate for someone his

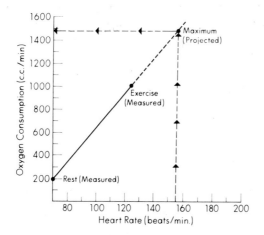

	Oxygen Consumption (c.c./min)	Heart Rate (beats/min)
Rest	200	70
Exercise	1000	120
Maximum predicted from age nomogram....................155		
Maximum oxygen consumption by extrapolation at heart rate 155 ∴1475 c.c./min. (Low)		

Fig. 26.3. Predicting maximal aerobic capacity from measurements made during submaximal work. (From Zohman, L., and Tobis, J. S.: *Cardiac Rehabilitation.* Grune & Stratton, Inc., New York, 1970, p. 158.)

age, so that these inaccuracies must be weighed against the value of strictly correct data from a maximal test. Haskell and Fox[3] point out that, if the distribution of maximal heart rates is reasonably normal, approximately 16 per cent of individuals will have a maximal heart rate below the mean value for age, *i.e.*, if the maximum for age is 190 beats per minute, 16 per cent will have a maximum of 178, so that testing at 85 per cent of maximal heart rate might actually be testing at 91 per cent of maximum for this group because maximum is lower than average. The same reasoning shows us that 16 per cent of subjects might be tested at 81 per cent rather than 85 per cent of maximum.

MEASUREMENTS DURING EXERCISE STRESS TESTING

Although more complicated measurements are done occasionally, the following five noninvasive measurements are frequent: (1) work load expressed as (a) speed and grade of the treadmill or (b) kilopond meters (kpm) of bicycle resistance, of (c) body weight multiplied by the distance the body is raised in climbing steps, (2) blood pressure, (3) oxygen consumption, and both (4) heart rate and (5) ECG configuration from the electrocardiogram. The work load is predetermined by the conditions of the test. Blood pressure is usually measured by cuff. The diastolic pressure is at times very difficult to measure during exercise, particularly at high work capacities. On occasion, a sound may continue to be heard at very low or even zero cuff pressures. Oxygen consumption measurement is usually carried out by collecting expired air in Douglas bags or weather balloons, with subsequent analysis by chemical methods or meters for carbon dioxide, oxygen, and volume. Alternatively, the composition and volume of expired air, values required for the oxygen consumption calculation, are obtained by on-line gas analysis, and a computer print-out completes such an automated system.

The electrocardiogram is often telemetered, displayed on an oscilloscope, and recorded on a paper strip chart. Sophisticated tachometers, pulse totalizers, and arrhythmia detectors are used in some laboratories.

The use of the electrocardiogram is of particular interest to the cardiologist. The electrical properties of the equipment, as well as the ease of use of various types of electrodes, the placement of electrodes, and the use of systems sensitive enough to detect significant ST changes, present monitoring problems somewhat different from those of the more familiar coronary care unit. Even small amounts of perspiration from the exercising subject, for example, may permit voltages to be generated between the subject and the telemetry transmitter or electrodes which can obscure the ECG signal.[22] This cannot be avoided during exercise except by placing the transmitter in a plastic bag, but it may be avoided in the coronary care unit by meticulous nursing care. Quantitation of ST displacement during ECG telemetry during exercise also seems more important than its immediate quantitation in the coronary care unit.

Reasonably, electrode placement should exclude as much noise as possible that might result from movement during exercise. To do this, some monitoring systems (*e.g.*, ear-ensiform-precordial) yield resulting ECG configurations which may be somewhat unfamiliar.

The choice of the location most likely to show ECG changes has been studied by many in depth.[23] Since Lachman *et al.*[24] have reported postural alterations which may be confused with ischemic changes in bipolar leads used on exercise, our own preference in exercise stress testing has been to use the **unipolar precordial lead** with the tallest R wave, or the one that we feel is most likely to show ischemia because of its relationship to previous infarction. However, Blackburn[23] finds the transthoracic bipolar lead useful (C-C5) or the manubrium-C5 lead (CM5) since there is no movement of the electrode over the manubrium. Irma Astrand also prefers bipolar leads (CR leads) since, among other advantages, they display 25 to 30 per cent greater amplitude and thus may reveal ST changes more readily than the V leads.[25]

If the volume of testing performed is sufficiently great to preclude manual totalization of pulse rates at various work loads from the ECG tracings, then the use of tachometers and pulse totalizers imposes still other restrictions on the monitoring lead chosen. To prevent double triggering and double counting by the pulse counters because of the near-equal size of the R and T waves (particularly on exercise when the T wave may increase in amplitude), there must be a sufficient difference in amplitude between these waves to permit the counter to discriminate and to count only the R wave; and lead choice may thus be influenced.

SIMPLIFIED PROCEDURES FOR THE OFFICE

The complicated and expensive instrumentation described above is certainly not feasible for an office or field testing station. Stepping platforms, a blood pressure cuff and an electrocardiograph machine can suffice in the office, however. Stepping platforms are available which permit adjustment of the height of the step, allowing the patient to be stressed at various multiples of his basal metabolic level (1 met). Raising the stepping platform 4.5 cm. every 2 minutes without interrupting the stepping rate permits stressing the patient in multiples of his resting oxygen consumption (Fig. 26.4). The stepping rate in this multistage test is maintained at 33 per minute or modified to 22 per minute at times.[26] A single Master two-step test is approximately 3 to 4 times basal and a double Master is approximately 7 to 8 mets. An office test may be monitored continuously by electrocardiogram using the ECG cable and by blood pressure measurements in rest breaks or at the termination of a continuous test. Using the traditional Master two-step apparatus, a multistage test can also be performed in the office. Master and Rosenfeld are now developing standards for imposing

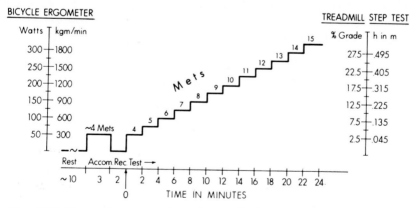

FIG. 26.4. Standard test procedures for treadmill, bicycle, and stepping ergometer. (From Balke, B.[26])

a 15 per cent increase in work load if the patient completes the double two-step satisfactorily.[27] Sheffield *et al.*[11] do a single Master, follow this by a rest period, and then carry out a double Master, followed by a recovery period. The third level is that amount of two-step activity which will elevate the heart rate to 85 per cent of maximum for age. Data are thus obtained at three submaximal work loads. Maximal oxygen consumption values, which can be obtained from tables for known work loads if heart rates are measured at these work levels,[28] may be extrapolated to maximum for indirect determination of maximal oxygen intake.

Submaximal office testing should be stopped in our opinion for any of the following reasons: (1) any clinical symptom which is obviously cardiac; (2) other symptoms which seem to be noncardiac such as claudication or eructation; (3) cerebral symptoms such as ataxia, dizziness, or slight confusion; (4) significant electrocardiographic abnormalities such as the appearance of successive or multifocal ventricular premature beats, tachyarrhythmia, more than 2 mm. of ST depression on the monitoring precordial lead, and T or U wave inversions; (5) inordinate rise in blood pressure (detected during rest periods or immediately after exercise) to greater than 250/125–130 mm. Hg; and (6) declining pulse pressure or failure of the blood pressure to rise on moderate exercise. Systolic blood pressures normally may increase from 10 to 40 mm. Hg on exercise. Conversely, a continuously rising diastolic pressure at increasing work intensities may warn of impending cardiovascular decompensation.[26] These guidelines are obviously not applicable in the presence of certain cardiac drugs which alter the exercise ECG shape or rate response. In the absence of limiting factors, testing may proceed to 85 per cent of maximal age-related heart rate, or until limited by local muscle fatigue.

Those individuals who cannot complete the submaximal performance test at several levels in the office because of muscle fatigue without cardiovascular limitations at this level or those patients on whom direct oxygen consumption measurements are desired might be referred to hospital-based testing stations.

MEDICOLEGAL CONSIDERATIONS

When high level performance evaluation or the testing of seriously ill patients is contemplated, in our opinion it is advisable to have a functioning defibrillator and know how to use it. Cardiac arrest has been reported following a negative maximal exercise stress test while the patient showered.[29] On the other hand, custom has not dictated that physicians carrying out the Master two-step or exercise tests below this level have a defibrillator, even though at times the Master test may elicit a heart rate which is 85 per cent of maximum or greater, without an antecedent warm-up period, and without knowledge of electrocardiographic changes until the exercise has been completed.

Information should be given to the patient about the test procedure, its benefits, and its risks. Obtaining the patient's informed consent for this type of test is important. The risk of a serious cardiac event (syncope, cardiac arrest, ventricular fibrillation) in testing a healthy middle-aged subject to maximal performance is "probably less than one in ten thousand." [30] Apparently untoward events can happen during inactivity following the test or as the result of superimposed stress, such as the heat of showering, and can be avoided by quiet, level walking or having the patient sit with the legs elevated for 15 minutes before taking a lukewarm shower. McDonough and Bruce compared the incidence of serious complications in maximal and submaximal testing.[31] In 102,000 submaximal tests, there were 7 myocardial infarctions and 4 deaths, compared to 2 infarctions (precipitated by hot showers) and no deaths among 6,000 maximal performance tests. The physician should be present during maximal testing but "may not be a requirement for submaximal tests of normal subjects."

DIFFERENCES BETWEEN THE DIAGNOSTIC AND PRETRAINING USE OF EXERCISE STRESS TESTS

Our orientation as physicians has in the past directed our use of exercise stress tests toward the diagnosis of coronary heart disease. In expanding their use to provide us with information helpful in prescribing exercise we must borrow concepts from the fields of rehabilitation medicine and physicial education, among others. Five examples of this difference in thinking are cited below. These may be summarized as differences in sensitivity, specificity, frequency, intensity, and duration (Fig. 26.5).

Sensitivity

None of our diagnostic methods for coronary heart disease is sufficiently sensitive nor sufficiently reliable in 100 per cent of cases; *e.g.*, in the clinical diagnosis of angina pectoris, the patient's subjective response and the physician's correct interpretation of these responses have a marked influence. There are problems in obtaining reliable results and making the correct interpretation of the exercise stress test results. The extent of pathology required to elicit an abnormal exercise stress test has not been precisely determined. And with cinearteriograms, lesions are demonstrated more easily than is disturbed flow. The size of the vessel involved also influences the usefulness of cineangiograms as the final arbiter of coronary heart disease.

However, precise correlation between the exercise stress test results,

	Diagnostic	Pre-Training
Sensitivity	Combination of tests preferred	Exercise stress test sufficient
Specificity	Other tests available	Must use exercise stress test
Frequency	Usually once; Soon if > once	At regular intervals
Intensity	Standardized	Variable
Duration	To symptoms/ECG changes, etc.	May "walk through"

FIG. 26.5. Differences in use of the exercise stress test.

the clinical picture, and the cineangiogram findings is not of major importance if the stress test is to be used as the basis for exercise prescription, whereas it may be of utmost significance in diagnosing myocardial ischemia. As Mason *et al.* state, "the majority of patients with positive ECG tests have clinical angina pectoris and severe disease by arteriogram, but not all of them. The majority of patients with severe arteriographic lesions have a positive ECG response to exercise and clinical angina pectoris but not all of them." [32] In prescribing exercise, cardiovascular function is of more importance than coronary anatomy. Regardless of the visualized lesions, "how much exercise is the patient capable of performing before the appearance of symptoms or physiological limitations" is the question to be asked in prescribing exercise. If the angiogram is negative and the patient has symptoms and a positive exercise stress test, exercise can be prescribed using these guidelines. If the angiogram is positive, the exercise can still be prescribed in the same way: based on demonstrated performance in the stress test and generation of symptoms. The sensitivity of various methods for *diagnosing* coronary heart disease is of lesser significance in using stress tests for "pretraining" evaluation.

Specificity

Another difference in thinking concerns the availability of alternate methods for diagnosis of coronary heart disease but not for exercise prescription. Hypoxia tests,[33] pacing tests to the point of angina,[34] and arteriograms are available for the diagnosis of coronary artery disease, in addition to the exericse stress test. For the prescription of exercise, however, these other methods have not been used. Exercise is prescribed on the basis of an exercise stress test, not on the arteriogram or hypoxia test.

Frequency

The frequency of follow-up testing may be different when the test is used diagnostically rather than for exercise prescription. Diagnostically, one exercise stress test may suffice, although at times this is insufficient and several tests may be needed, using different exercise modalities such as bicycles and treadmills or different work intensities or different lead placements. If more than one test is needed, it is usually carried out within days of the previous tests. Stress tests prescribed in exercise training programs are carried out usually at intervals of 6 to 12 weeks or longer, sometimes over periods of months to years. They are usually repeated in the original testing pattern in order to be useful for assessing the patient's response to the exercise regime by comparison with previous stress test results.

Intensity

Another difference between diagnostic and pre-exercise stress tests is the level or work load at which the patient must be tested. The physician may choose to test the patient only up to but not beyond the level of the exercise activity in which the patient wishes to participate, and this may be a level insufficient to detect myocardial ischemia—hence nondiagnostic.

Duration

Last, the length of the two types of test procedures may vary. The diagnostic test is generally terminated at the appearance of symptoms or significant ECG abnormality. In some cases, the pretraining or training reevaluation test is not terminated at this point. Kattus *et al.* test "cardiovascular adaptation" by permitting their patients to continue walking through their 3+ angina in the presence of electrocardiographic abnormalities of certain types in order to assess their potential for improvement on an exercise training program; those who can "walk through" generally are good candidates for such a program.[12]

SUMMARY

Exercise stress testing is important in evaluating the patient with coronary heart disease for whom exercise is to be prescribed. The physician may choose among treadmill, bicycle, or step tests, single level or multilevel, continuous or intermittent tests, and submaximal tests or those continued to maximal oxygen intake, to obtain the desired information. Measurements of work load, oxygen consumption, blood pressure, heart rate, and electrocardiographic configuration are conveniently made in the laboratory. Simpler tests on steps or stationary bicycle with measurements of blood pressure, heart rate, and ECG configuration can be carried out in the office to provide similarly useful information upon which to base an exercise prescription. Differences in concepts concerning sensitivity, specificity, frequency, intensity, and duration of exercise stress tests are discussed, relating these factors to whether the test is to be used diagnostically or in prescribing exercise therapy in coronary heart disease.

This work was supported by Grants RD1994-M from the Social and Rehabilitation Service of the United States Department of Health, Education and Welfare, and HD 00599 from the National Institute of Child Health and Human Development.

REFERENCES

1. Doyle, J. T., and Kinch, S. H.: The prognosis of an abnormal electrocardiographic stress test. Circulation 41: 545, 1970.
2. Bruce, R. A., Rowell, L. B., Blackmon, J. R., and Doan, A.: Cardiovascular function tests. Heart Bull. 14: 9, 1965.
3. Haskell, W. L., and Fox, S. M., III: Some factors to consider when selecting an exercise stress testing procedure for the detection of myocardial ischemia. Mal. Cardiovasc. 10: 189, 1969.
4. Shephard, R. J., Allen, C., Benade, A. J. S., Davies, C. T. M., DiPrampero, P. E., Hedman, R., Merriman, J. E., Myhre, K., and Simmons, R.: Standardization of submaximal exercise tests. Bull. W. H. O. 38: 765, 1968.
5. Ford, A. B., and Hellerstein, H. K.: Energy cost of the Master two-step test. J. A. M. A. 164: 1868, 1957.
6. Simonson, E.: Use of the electrocardiogram in exercise tests. Amer. Heart J. 66: 552, 1966.
7. Tornvall, G.: Assessment of physical capabilities. Acta Physiol. Scand. 58 (Suppl.): 201, 1963.
8. Taylor, H. L., Haskell, W., Fox, S. M., III, and Blackburn, H.: Exercise tests: a summary of procedures and concepts of stress testing for cardiovascular diagnosis and function evaluation. In Blackburn, H. (ed.): *Measurement in Exercise Electrocardiography*, Chap. 18. Charles C Thomas, Publisher, Springfield, Ill., 1969, p. 265.
9. Hellerstein, H. K.: Exercise therapy in coronary disease. Bull. N. Y. Acad. Med. 44: 1028, 1968.
10. Astrand, I.: Aerobic capacity in men and women with special reference to age. Acta Physiol. Scand. 169 (Suppl.): 47, 1960.
11. Sheffield, L. T., Holt, J. H., and Reeves, T. J.: Exercise graded by heart rate in electrocardiographic testing for angina pectoris. Circulation 32: 622, 1965.
12. Kattus, A. A., Alvaro, A., and MacAlpin, R. N.: Treadmill exercise tests for capacity and adaptation in angina pectoris. J. Occup. Med. 10: 627, 1968.
13. Kellerman, J. J., and Karniv, I.: *Rehabilitation of Coronary Patients*. Cardiac Evaluation and Rehabilitation Institute, Tel Hashomer Government Hospital, Tel Hashomer, Israel, 1970.
14. Bonjer, F. H.: Measurement of working capacity by assessment of the aerobic capacity in a single session. Fed. Proc. 2: 1363, 1966.
15. Fox, S. M., III, and Haskell, W. L.: The exercise stress test: needs for standardization. In Eliakion, M., and Newfeld, H. (eds.): *Cardiology: Current Topics and Progress.* Academic Press, New York, 1970, pp. 149–154.
16. Shephard, R. J., Allen, C., Benade, A. J. S., Davies, C. T. M., DiPrampero, P. E., Hedman, R., Merriman, J. E., Myhre, K., and Simmons, R.: The maximum oxygen intake. Bull. W. H. O. 38: 757, 1968.

17. Stoboy, H.: Physical fitness testing methods and criteria. Trans. N. Y. Acad. Sci. 30: 483, 1968.

18. Astrand, P. O., and Ryhming, I.: A nomogram for calculation of aerobic capacity (physical fitness) from pulse rate during submaximal work. J. Appl. Physiol. 7: 218, 1954.

19. Von Dobeln, W., Astrand, I., and Bergstrom, A.: An analysis of age and other factors related to maximal oxygen uptake. J. Appl. Physiol. 22: 934, 1967.

20. Margaria, R., Aghermo, P., and Rovelli, E.: Indirect determination of maximal O_2 consumption in man. J. Appl. Physiol. 20: 1070, 1965.

21. Maritz, J. S., Morrison, J. R., Peters, J., Strydom, N. B., and Wyndham, C.: A practical method of estimating an individual's maximum oxygen intake. Ergonomics 4: 97, 1961.

22. Hurzeler, P.: Practical considerations concerning exercise ECG telemetry equipment. In *Medical Research Engineering*, in press.

23. Blackburn, H.: The exercise electrocardiogram. Technological, procedural and conceptual developments. In *Measurement in Exercise Electrocardiography*, Chap. 17. Charles C Thomas, Publisher, Springfield, Ill., 1969, p. 220.

24. Lachman, A. B., Semler, H. J., and Gustafson, R. H.: Postural ST-T wave changes in the radioelectrocardiogram simulating myocardial ischemia. Circulation 31: 557, 1965.

25. Astrand, I.: Electrocardiographic changes in relation to the type of exercise, the work load, age and sex. In *Measurement in Exercise Electrocardiography*, Chap. 19. Charles C Thomas, Publisher, Springfield, Ill., 1969, p. 318.

26. Balke, B.: Report of the Committee on Physiological Measurements and Indices. In Atha, J. (ed.): *Proceedings of the International Committee on the Standardization of Physical Fitness Tests*. Magglingen, Switzerland, 1967.

27. Master, A., and Rosenfeld, I.: Augmented two-step test. In Master, A. M.: *Transactions of the Association of Life Insurance Medical Directors of America*, vol. 54, pp. 42–59, 1970.

28. Astrand, P. O., and Rodahl, K.: Evaluation of physical work capacity on the basis of tests. In *Textbook of Work Physiology*, Chap. 11. McGraw-Hill Book Company, New York, 1970, p. 341.

29. Bruce, R. A., Hornsten, T. R., and Blackmon, J. R.: Myocardial infarction after normal responses to exercise. Circulation 38: 552, 1968.

30. American Heart Association Statement for Physicians on Exercise Testing and Training of Apparently Healthy Persons, 8/26/70 (draft).

31. McDonough, J. R., and Bruce, R. A.: Maximal exercise testing in assessing cardiovascular function. J. S. Carolina Med. Ass. 65: 26, 1969.

32. Mason, R. E., Likar, I., Biern, R. O., and Ross, R. S.: Correlation of graded exercise electrocardiographic response with clinical and coronary cinearteriographic findings. In *Measurement in Exercise Electrocardiography*, Chap. 25. Charles C Thomas, Publisher, Springfield, Ill., 1969, p. 454.

33. Kimura, E., Ushiyama, K., Kojima, N., Hayakawa, H., Kanie, T., and Yoshida, K.: Exercise test and anoxia test in the diagnosis of angina pectoris: a comparative study. Jap. Heart J. 4: 313, 1963.

34. Balcon, R., Maloy, W. C., and Sowton, E.: Clinical use of atrial pacing test in angina pectoris. Brit. Med. J. 3: 208, 1968.

27

Transition from Exercise Stress Test to Physical Training Prescription

WILLIAM S. GUALTIERE, Ph.D.

The desirability of a scientific rationale for prescribing physical exercise programs has long been acknowledged by exercise physiologists and physical educators. With the recent addition of physical exercise to the therapeutic regime of selected heart disease patients, this objective has taken on greater significance. Although research has not provided answers to many of the questions which have been raised, there is available sufficient information to improve upon the intuitive nature of many of the physical training prescription practices in common use today.

The ensuing discussion reviews the physical training prescription process, specifically for patients with ischemic heart disease, using our clinical and research program in the Department of Rehabilitation Medicine at Montefiore Hospital to illustrate current thinking in this area. An overview of this process is given in Figure 27.1. Steps 1 and 2, dealing with the evaluation of the patient's capacity for physical training, are discussed in Chapter 26. Steps 3 and 4 comprise the subject of this discussion: the transition from exercise stress test to physical training prescription. The transition process presupposes that two conditions are satisfied: (1) that the necessary training stimulus (intensity, duration, and frequency) to elicit an improvement in cardiorespiratory capacity is known, and (2) that an objective assessment of the patient's tolerance level (clinical maximum) for physical training has been accomplished in terms of electrocardiogram (ECG) configuration, signs and/or symptoms, heart rate, and oxygen consumption. Both of these conditions can be adequately satisfied.

IMPROVEMENT OF CARDIORESPIRATORY CAPACITY: WHAT DOES RESEARCH SAY?

Cardiorespiratory capacity, aerobic capacity, and maximal oxygen intake are synonymous terms which refer to the functional capacity of the

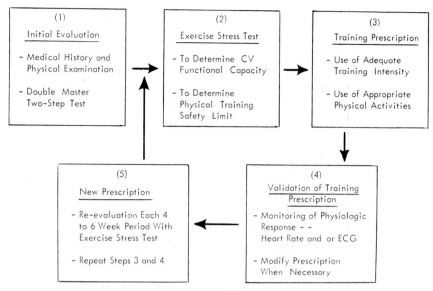

FIG. 27.1. Physical training prescription process.

body to take in, transport, and use oxygen in the working muscles. It is this capacity which is largely reflected in a person's ability to perform hard muscular work for long periods of time. The improvement of this capacity is the primary objective of physical training programs for both normal adults and cardiac patients.

Normal Adults (Table 27.1)

A significant cardiorespiratory training response can be demonstrated in normal male adults (>30 years) when training is undertaken 3 days per week for 30 to 45 minutes per session over a 5-month period. Training is usually adjusted every 1- or 2-month period by changing the intensity (*i.e.,* exercise rate and/or work load) and/or duration (time per session). The required training intensity appears to approximate a demand of 60 to 85 per cent of an individual's maximal oxygen intake for 10 to 20 minutes of a 30- to 45-minute session.

The popular training activities include calisthenics, walking, and running or jogging. These activities are sometimes carried out with intermittent periods of work and rest (interval training) or for 5- to 20-minute periods with no rest (continuous training). Both methods have been successfully employed with no significant advantage offered by either method. The usual changes indicating a favorable training effect are a decrease in heart rate for a fixed (standard) submaximal work load, an increase in the maximal oxygen intake, and a decrease in the time required to run a fixed distance of 1 or 2 miles.

Table 27.1. *Description of selected training programs used with normal middle-aged adults*

Study	Subject sample description					Training program			
	no.	age	sex	clinical impression	mo.	days/week	min./day	intensity	activities
Skinner et al.[1]	15	41.7*	M	13 normals 2 CV disease†	6	6 (minimum of 3)	30–45	Light to near exercise tolerance	Calisthenics, walking, running, IT, CT‡
Hanson et al.[2]	7	48.9*	M	7 normals	7	3	60–90	Self-imposed limit	Calisthenics, team sports, running
Mann et al.[3]	105	38*	M	105 normals	6	5	60	Three groups: 300, 400 and 500 kcal./hr., heart rate 160–190 beats per min.	Calisthenics, walking, running, IT, CT
Pollock et al.[4]	19	28–39	M	19 normals	5	2 groups (1) 2 (2) 4	~30	kcal./min. (1) 215–355 (2) 215–367	Calisthenics, walking, running, IT
Ribisl[5]	15	40.2*	M	15 normals	5	3	35	300 kcal./min. 1st mo. to 750 kcal./min. 5th mo.	Calisthenics, walking, running, IT, CT

* Mean.
† CV, cardiovascular.
‡ IT, internal training; CT, continuous training.

Cardiac Patients (Table 27.2)

There are at least three ways in which cardiac patients are trained differently from normal adults: intensity of training stimulus, training modality, and training method. Whereas a training stimulus of 60 to 85 per cent of maximal oxygen intake is used for normals, cardiacs frequently are symptom-limited even at intensities below 60 per cent of their projected maximal oxygen intake (their clinical maximum) so that it is not feasible to train them at the same stimulus level. For example, a patient with angina pectoris is generally permitted to exercise at an intensity which occasionally elicits mild to moderate pain during a training session. The onset of mild pain in this patient may correspond to 40 per cent of his projected maximal oxygen intake. A second patient with a known clinical maximum of 4-mm. ST depression trains at an intensity which produces an ST depression no greater than 2 mm. In this case, the training may require an oxygen demand equal to 55 per cent of the patient's projected oxygen intake capacity.

A second difference concerns the training modality. Cycling on a stationary bicycle is used more frequently for training cardiacs than normals because of the rigid control it apparently affords over the regulation of the training prescription. The use of a metronome for controlling cycling rate and the mechanical setting of a predetermined work resistance assure that the patient is consistently working within his safety limit. This feature may be of great importance for some cardiacs, especially those who are symptom-free but who have ventricular arrhythmias at clinical maximum.

The third difference is the strong preference for use of the interval training method with cardiacs. Usually the bouts of work in interval training are from 1 to 4 minutes and the rest periods take approximately one-half of that time. This principle of repeated bouts of exercise with intervening rest periods affords the deconditioned cardiac at least two advantages over the continuous training method: (1) a lower heart rate is incurred for the same amount of mechanical work, which permits the patient to exercise for a longer period of time; and (2) improvement in skeletal muscular efficiency or muscular endurance is facilitated because more time is spent per session in exercising rather than resting. This latter point is not necessarily applicable to the normal individual who may have a sufficient cardiac and skeletal muscular capacity to enable him to engage in continuous training for the greater part of an exercise session.

The cardiac's improvement in cardiorespiratory capacity to training is similar to that of the normal. The major difference in the response of these two populations is in the greater improvement in normal subjects. The lesser gains in cardiacs may possibly be related to the lower training intensity which of necessity must be used in cardiacs: below clinical maximum for the cardiac and 60 to 85 per cent of maximal oxygen intake for the normal. Moreover, it must be acknowledged here that some cardiacs

Table 27.2. *Description of selected training programs used with heart-disease patients*

Study	Patient sample description			cardiac problem			duration			Training program	
	no.	age	sex	MI*	an-gina	other	no.	days/week	min./day	maximal intensity	activities†
Mazzarella and Jordan[6]	4	41–69	M			X	2–2.5	3	20	73% max. $\dot{V}O_2$ (64–86%)	Treadmill, walking
Sloman et al.[7]	13	16–54	5 M, 8 F	X	X	X	3	7	15 + ?	Royal Canadian Air Force, 5 and 10 BX	Calisthenics, walking
Barry et al.[8]	6	36–49	M	X	X		1.5–13	?	?	Heart rate >130 beats/min. and/or below ECG criteria (?)	Cycling (upright), IT
Hellerstein et al.[9]	189	Middle-age	M	X	X	X	6–84	3	30–60	400 kcal./hr. in trained state	Calisthenics, walking, running, IT, recreation
Rechnitzer et al.[10]	8	45‡	M	X			5–6	2	30 + ?	?	Calisthenics, walking, jogging, running, swimming
Zohman and Tobis[11]	18	41–75	17 M, 1 F	X	X		1.5	3	5	Immediately below pain	Cycling (supine), CT
Frick and Katila[12]	7	37–55	M	X	X		1–2	3	25–30	Onset of chest pain or heart rate of 150 beats/min.	Cycling (upright), CT, IT
Clausen et al.[13]	9	52‡	M	X			1–1.5	5	20–30	Below pain, initial heart rate 120–158, final heart rate 129–157	Cycling (upright), IT

Kasch and Boyer[14]	11	50‡	M	X	X	6	4	45–60	Heart rate = ST depression of 2 mm. or more	Running, IT
Heller[15]	22	38–59	M	X	X	18–42	3–5	?	Level below symptoms	Calisthenics, walking, running, CT, IT
Gualtiere et al.[16]	8	36–61	M	X	X	6–9	3	20–50	65–95% of clinical max. VO_2	Cycling (upright), IT

* Myocardial infarction.
† IT, interval training; CT, continuous training.
‡ Mean.

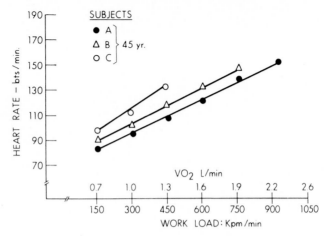

F$_{IG}$. 27.2. Stress test: heart rate and VO_2 response of three ischemic heart disease patients.

fail to show a favorable response to physical training. The lack of improvement may be related to the extent and type of pathology. Drs. MacAlpin and Kattus have described patients with "strategically placed, proximal stenotic lesions in major coronary vessels without frank collaterals" who appear to be poor candidates for deriving benefit from physical training.[17]

TRANSITION FROM EXERCISE STRESS TEST RESULTS TO PHYSICAL TRAINING PRESCRIPTION

Having reviewed research information regarding the cardiorespiratory adaptation to training and methods of training cardiacs, the case material which follows uses hypothetical although typical ischemic heart disease cases to explain how some of these research data may be applied.

Figure 27.2 gives the exercise stress test plot for heart rate and oxygen consumption from three male patients with documented ischemic heart disease. The performance was terminated in each case at a heart rate level below the predicted maximum for this age group (approximately 175 beats per minute). Patient A was able to work to the desired predetermined end point of 85 per cent of maximal predicted heart rate, while Patients B and C were stopped short of this level because of angina and/or ECG changes (clinical maxima) which contraindicated additional exercise stress (Table 27.3). Thus, each patient's safety limit for physical exercise has been objectively determined. Expressed in terms of heart rate, oxygen consumption, and caloric expenditure,* these limits are: 150 beats per minute and 2.2 liters of VO_2 (11.0 kcal. per minute); 140 beats per minute and 1.9

---

* One liter of oxygen equals approximately 5 kcal.

Table 27.3. *Stress test: end point summary data of three ischemic heart disease patients*

Stress test parameter	Subjects*		
	A (45 yr.)	B (45 yr.)	C (45 yr.)
Work load (Kpm†)	900 (85% max. HR)	750 (clinical max.)	450 (clinical max.)
Heart rate (beats/min.)	150	140	132
Oxygen consumption (l./min.)	2.2	1.9	1.3
Blood pressure (mm. Hg)	170/72	162/76	160/78
Angina	No	Mild	Severe
Electrocardiogram			
ST depression (mm.)	1.0	1.5	3.5
Extrasystoles	3 PACs, 1 PVC	Multifocal PVCs	1 PAC

* HR, heart rate; PAC, premature atrial contraction; PVC, premature ventricular contraction.

† Kpm, kilopond meters per minute.

liters of VO_2 (9.5 kcal. per minute); and 132 beats per minute and 1.3 liters of VO_2 (6.5 kcal. per minute) for Patients A, B, and C, respectively.

The transition from exercise stress test to the development of a physical training prescription is influenced by whether the stress test and the training will be conducted using the same exercise modality, *e.g.*, the use of cycling in the test and in the training prescription, in which case the **transition is direct.** If cycling is used for testing and the patient is trained on a walking program the **transition is indirect.** Since both mechanisms are used routinely in the prescription process, both are considered here in the development of the same prescription; that is, with regard to the peak energy demand required for the execution of the training prescription. This is carried out for Patient C only.

Patient C

Table 27.4 contains Patient C's physical training prescription. In this case, the exercise stress test and prescription used the same exercise modality, cycling on a stationary bicycle. Thus, a direct transition was possible. Note that the prescription has three distinct periods; warm-up, cardiorespiratory, and cool-down. The prescription requires a peak oxygen demand of approximately 1.0 liter per minute or 5 kcal. during the cardiorespiratory conditioning period (stimulus period). Note in Table 27.3 that the exercise stress is below the patient's clinical maximum of 1.3 liters per minute of oxygen (6.5 kcal. per minute).

The indirect transition of this same prescription is given in Table 27.5. This procedure involves the use of caloric expenditure values for many of

Table 27.4. *Physical training prescription**

Name: Patient C   Frequency: Mon. Wed. Fri.

Warm-up period		Cardiorespiratory conditioning period		Cool-down period	
time	event	time	event	time	event
min.		*min.*		*min.*	
0–3	0 Kpm		300 Kpm for 4 min., followed by	38–42	150 Kpm
3–5	150 Kpm	10–38	2 min. rest; repeat 4 times	42–45	0 Kpm
5–6	Rest				
6–9	150 Kpm				
9–10	Rest				

* Direct transition from stress test data to physical training prescription.

Table 27.5. *Physical training prescription**

Name: Patient C   Frequency: Mon. Wed. Fri.

Warm-up period		Cardiorespiratory conditioning period		Cool-down period	
time	event	time	event	time	event
min.		*min.*		*min.*	
0–3	Walking 2½ mph		Walking 3½ mph for 4 min., followed by 2-	38–42	Walking 3 mph
3–5	Walking 3 mph	10–38	min. rest; repeat 4	42–45	Walking 2½ mph
5–6	Rest		times		
6–9	Walking 3 mph				
9–10	Rest				

* Indirect transition from stress test data to physical training prescription.

the popular physical activities. Here the objective is to match the oxygen consumption and/or equivalent caloric expenditure data obtained from the stress test (cycling) to the caloric expenditure required to perform other physical activities. In this case, the activity selected involves walking at different speeds. By using the caloric expenditure values appearing in Table 27.6 for different walking speeds, a prescription was developed which closely approximates the same peak energy expenditure required for the prescription given in Table 27.4. It can be observed that walking at 3½ miles per hour and cycling at 300 Kpm per minute each requires an expenditure of 5 kcal. per minute.

The "equicaloric" matching principle can also be utilized in the prescription process without actually measuring the patient's oxygen consumption as he performs the exercise stress test. In this situation, an estimate of his oxygen consumption for the work done is obtained from existing tables which give values for the commonly used stress test modalities of cycling, walking, running, and bench-stepping at various work inten-

Table 27.6. *Caloric expenditure of physical activities*

Activity	Cal./min.
Walking 2 mph	2.8*
Walking 2½ mph	3.8*
Walking 3 mph	4.4*
Walking 3½ mph	5.0*
Walking 4 mph	5.8*
Swimming, breaststroke, 1 mph	6.8†
Swimming, crawl, 1 mph	7.0†
Swimming, backstroke, 1 mph	8.3†
Swimming, sidestroke, 1 mph	9.2†
Running (horizontal) 5⁷⁄₁₀ mph	12.0†
Running (horizontal) 7 mph	14.5†
Running (horizontal) 11²⁄₅ mph	21.0†

* Passmore and Durnin.[18]
† Morehouse and Miller.[19]

sities.[20-30] With this information in hand, the transition is made as described above.

The relative accuracy of exercise prescription from stress test results using these methods may be ranked in descending order as follows: the direct transition from test to training modality using measured oxygen consumption values is the most accurate; next is the indirect transition from one type of stress testing modality to another physical training modality also using measured oxygen consumption values, and least accurate is direct or indirect transition from work load and table values for oxygen consumption.

The next step in the prescription process concerns the validation of the physical training prescription. Ideally, the patient should be monitored in the same manner as during the exercise stress test. This may be neither practical nor administratively feasible. An alternative procedure is to have the patient monitor his heart rate at designated time periods, usually for 15 seconds immediately following the peak stress activities (cardiorespiratory conditioning period). The heart rate values are then compared to those obtained from the stress test, permitting an estimate of the energy demand of the activity from the linear relationship between heart rate and oxygen consumption previously determined for that individual. Prescriptions can thus be adjusted if the matching by oxygen consumption results in different heart rates than expected.

In addition to the sources of error inherent in the transition process, there are other factors which would invalidate the prescription developed for certain ischemic heart disease patients. Table 27.7 contains a list of some of these factors as well as the directional change which they usually

Table 27.7. *Modification of PTRx* intensity: influencing factors*

Factor	Directional change of PTRx intensity
Exercise environment	
hot climate	Decrease
cold climate	Decrease
competitive activities	Decrease
Drugs	
propranolol	Increase
procainamide, quinidine	Increase
isosorbide dinitrate, nitroglycerin	Increase
digitalis	Increase

* Physical training prescription (References 31 to 41).

necessitate in the intensity of the prescription. These factors are grouped into two categories, exercise environment and drugs. An increase in myocardial oxygen consumption for the same amount of work results from both hot (increased heart rate) and cold (increased systolic pressure via increased peripheral resistance) exposure. The addition of competition to the exercise environment (emotional factor) has a similar effect, particularly if the prescription is of a low intensity. Drugs are not discussed here as this topic is covered extensively in Chapter 28.

SUMMARY

A rational approach to the problem of converting a patient's exercise stress test data to a physical training prescription is discussed. To conduct this transition, two conditions must be satisfied: the necessary training stimulus (intensity, duration, and frequency of training) to elicit an improvement in cardiorespiratory capacity must be known, and an objective assessment of the patient's exercise tolerance (clinical maximum) must have been determined. Sample prescriptions are presented as established, using the same exercise for stress testing and physical training (direct transition) and different exercises for testing and physical training (indirect transition). A method for validating the prescription is also suggested.

This work was supported by Grants RD1994-M from the Social and Rehabilitation Service of the United States Department of Health, Education and Welfare, and HD 00599 from the National Institute of Child Health and Human Development.

REFERENCES

1. Skinner, J. S., Holloszy, J. O., and Cureton, T. K.: Effects of a program of exercise on physical work. Capacity and anthropometric measurements of fifteen middle-aged men. Amer. J. Cardiol. 14: 747–752, 1964.
2. Hanson, J. S., Tabakin, B. S., Levy, A. M., and Nedde, W.: Long-term physical

training and cardiovascular dynamics in middle-aged men. Circulation 38: 783–799, 1968.

3. Mann, G. V., Garrett, H. L., Farhi, J. A., Murray, H., Billings, T., Shute, E., and Schwarten, S. E.: Exercise to prevent coronary heart disease. Amer. J. Med. 46: 12–25, 1969.

4. Pollock, M. L., Cureton, T. K., and Greninger, L.: Effects of frequency of training on working capacity, cardiovascular function, and body composition of adult men. Med. Sci. Sports 1: 70–74, 1969.

5. Ribisl, P. M.: Effects of training upon the maximal oxygen uptake of middle-aged men. Int. Z. Angew. Physiol. 27: 154–160, 1969.

6. Mazzarella, J. A., and Jordan, J. W.: Effects of physical training on exertional myocardial ischemia in middle-aged men. Circulation (Suppl. 2, abstracts) 32: 147–148, 1965.

7. Sloman, G., Pitt, A., Hirsch, E. Z., and Donaldson, A.: The effect of a graded physical training programme on the physical working capacity of patients with heart disease. Med. J. Aust. 1: 4–7, 1965.

8. Barry, A., Baily, J. W., Pruett, E. D. R., Steinmetz, J. R., Birkhead, N. C., and Rodahl, K.: Effects of physical training in patients who have had myocardial infarction. Amer. J. Cardiol. 17: 1–8, 1966.

9. Hellerstein, H. K., Hornsten, T. R., Goldbarg, A. N., Burlando, A. G., Friedman, E. H., Hirsch, E. Z., and Marik, S.: The influence of active conditioning upon subjects with coronary artery disease. In Physical Activity and Cardiovascular Health, Can. Med. Ass. J. 96: 901–903, 1967.

10. Rechnitzer, P. A., Yuhasz, M. S., Paivo, A., Pickard, H. A., and Lefcoe, N.: Effects of a 24-week exercise programme on normal adults and patients with previous myocardial infarction. Brit. Med. J. 1: 734–735, 1967.

11. Zohman, L. R., and Tobis, J. S.: The effects of exercise training on patients with angina pectoris. Arch. Phys. Med. 48: 525–532, 1967.

12. Frick, M. H., and Katila, M.: Hemodynamic consequences of physical training after myocardial infarction. Circulation 35: 192–202, 1968.

13. Clausen, J. P., Larsen, O. A., and Trap-Jensen, J.: Physical training in the management of coronary artery disease. Circulation 40: 143–154, 1969.

14. Kasch, F. W., and Boyer, J. L.: Changes in maximum work capacity resulting from six months training in patients with ischemic heart disease. Med. Sci. Sports 1: 156–159, 1969.

15. Heller, E. M.: Practical graded exercise program after myocardial infarction. Arch. Phys. Med. 50: 655–662, 1969.

16. Gualtiere, W. S., Zohman, L. R., Lopez, R. H., and Flores, A. M.: Effects of physical training on the cardio-respiratory functional capacity of ischemic heart disease patients. In preparation.

17. MacAlpin, R. N., and Kattus, A. A.: Adaptation to exercise in angina pectoris. Circulation 33: 183–201, 1966.

18. Passmore, R., and Durnin, J. V. G. A.: Human energy expenditure. Physiol. Rev. 35: 801–840, 1955.

19. Morehouse, L. E., and Miller, A. T.: *Physiology of Exercise.* The C. V. Mosby Company, St. Louis, 1967, pp. 190–191.

20. Astrand, I.: Aerobic work capacity in men and women with special reference to age. Acta Physiol. Scand. (Suppl. 169): 49, 1960.

21. Astrand, P.: Human physical fitness with special reference to sex and age. Physiol. Rev. 36: 307–335, 1956.

22. Bobbert, A. C.: Physiological comparison of three types of ergometry. J. Appl. Physiol. 15: 1007–1014, 1960.

23. Bobbert, A. C.: Energy expenditure in level and grade walking. J. Appl. Physiol. 15: 1015–1021, 1960.

24. Dill, D. B.: Oxygen uses in horizontal and grade walking and running on the treadmill. J. Appl. Physiol. 20: 19–22, 1965.

25. Glassford, R. G., Baycroft, G. H. Y., Sedgwick, A. W., and MacNab, R. B. J.: Comparison of maximal oxygen uptake values determined by predicted and actual methods. J. Appl. Physiol. 20: 509–513, 1965.

26. Grimby, G., and Soderholm, B.: Energy expenditure of men in different age groups during level walking and bicycle ergometry. Scand. J. Clin. Lab. Invest. 14: 321–328, 1962.

27. Hellerstein, H. K.: Techniques of exercise prescription and evaluation. J. S. Carolina Med. Ass. 65 (suppl.): 46–56, 1969.

28. Nagle, F. J., Balke, B., and Naughton, J. P.: Gradational step tests for assessing work capacity. J. Appl. Physiol. 20: 745–748, 1965.

29. Shephard, R. J.: The relative merits of the step test, bicycle ergometer, and treadmill in assessment of cardio-respiratory fitness. Int. Z. Angew. Physiol. 23: 219–230, 1966.

30. Workman, J. M., and Armstrong, B. W.: A nomogram for predicting treadmill-walking oxygen consumption. J. Appl. Physiol. 19: 150–151, 1964.

31. Brouha, L., Maxfield, M. E., Smith, P. E., and Stopps, G. J.: Discrepancy between heart rate and oxygen consumption during work in the warmth. J. Appl. Physiol. 18: 1095–1098, 1964.

32. Dagenais, G. R., Pitt, B., Mason, R. E., Friesinger, G. C., and Ross, R. S.: Evaluation of long-acting nitrates and beta-adrenergic blocking agents in angina pectoris. Amer. J. Cardiol. (abstract) 25: 90, 1970.

33. Detry, J.-M. R., and Bruce, R. A.: Effects of nitroglycerin on "maximal" oxygen intake in coronary heart disease. Circulation (Suppl. 3, abstract) 41: 96, 1970.

34. Epstein, S. F., Robinson, B. F., Kahler, R. L., and Braunwald, E.: Effects of beta-adrenergic blockade on the cardiac response to maximal and submaximal exercise in man. J. Clin. Invest. 44: 1745–1753, 1965.

35. Epstein, S. E., Stampfer, M., Beiser, G. D., Goldstein, R. E., and Braunwald, E.: Effects of a reduction in environmental temperature on the circulatory response to exercise in man. New Engl. J. Med. 280: 7–11, 1969.

36. MacAlpin, R. N., Kattus, A. A., and Winfield, M. E.: The effect of a beta-adrenergic-blocking agent (nethalide) and nitroglycerin on exercise tolerance in angina pectoris. Circulation 31: 869–875, 1965.

37. Najmi, M., Griggs, D. M., Kasparian, H., and Novack, P.: Effects of nitroglycerin on hemodynamics during rest and exercise in patients with coronary insufficiency. Circulation 35: 46–54, 1967.

38. Parker, J. O., West, R. O., Ledwich, J. R., and DiGiorgi, S.: The effect of acute digitalization on the hemodynamic response to exercise in coronary artery disease. Circulation 40: 453–462, 1969.

39. Pirnay, F., Deroanne, R., and Petit, J. M.: Maximal oxygen consumption in a hot environment. J. Appl. Physiol. 218 (Suppl. 5): 642–645, 1970.

40. Pitt, B., and Ross, R. S.: Beta-adrenergic blockade in cardiovascular therapy. Mod. Concepts Cardiovasc. Dis. 37: 47–54, 1969.

41. Wolfson, S., and Gorlin, R.: Cardiovascular pharmacology of propranolol in man. Circulation 40: 501–511, 1969.

28

Interaction of Drugs and Exercise Training for Cardiacs

ABNER J. DELMAN, M.D.

Alteration of the hemodynamic response to exercise by a physical conditioning program has been well documented in patients with coronary artery disease. The exercise response may also be changed by the intervention of numerous cardiac drugs. Although there has been considerable experience accumulated in the use of either physical training or drug therapy in the management of patients with angina pectoris, there have been few reported observations on the possible interactions of these two modalities of treatment. This chapter discusses some of the hemodynamic alterations that may occur with training and with vasoactive drugs and considers their potential interactions.

The traditional approach to angina pectoris has focused attention on changes in coronary blood flow.[1, 2] Even with nitroglycerin, however, a consistent increase in myocardial blood flow has not been demonstrated.[3, 4] The pain of myocardial ischemia is related to an imbalance between myocardial oxygen needs and the availability of oxygen to the heart through a faulty delivery system of diseased coronary vessels.[5] The potential cardiac benefits of either drugs or training in patients with angina pectoris, then, must be considered in terms of whether they can diminish myocardial oxygen consumption, as well as any possible improvement in coronary blood flow. In this context, I would like to review briefly present concepts of the major determinants of myocardial oxygen consumption. The three most important factors are intramyocardial tension, heart rate, and the contractile state of the left ventricle[5, 6] (Table 28.1). Intramyocardial tension is related to the product of the transmural ventricular systolic pressure and the radius of the ventricle divided by its wall thickness. Ventricular systolic pressure is controlled by peripheral systolic pressure, and ventricular radius is related to ventricular volume. Therefore, an increase of peripheral systolic pressure or ventricular volume at rest or during exercise will

Table 28.1. *Major determinants of myocardial oxygen requirements*

Intramyocardial tension T = Pr/2h $\dfrac{\text{Tension} = \text{pressure} \times \text{radius}}{2 \times \text{wall thickness}}$

    ventricular systolic pressure
    intraventricular volume
    myocardial mass
Heart rate: activation per minute
    pressure-time per minute
    tension-time per minute
Contractile state of left ventricle
    force-velocity relationship
    V_{max} (maximal contraction velocity)
    LV dp/dt (maximal rate of rise of left ventricle pressure)

---

increase myocardial oxygen needs. A decrease in either of these factors will reduce oxygen requirements.[6] The second important oxygen determinant is the heart rate. Obviously, the myocardial tension per minute is controlled by the product of the tension per beat and the heart rate or beats per minute. This has been called the pressure-time index or the tension-time index, a major determinant of the heart's oxygen requirements.[7] The third factor is the contractile state of the ventricle as measured by the force-velocity relationship of the myocardium. This may be determined by obtaining the V_{max} (maximal contraction velocity), or the LV dp/dt (maximal rate of rise of the left ventricular pressure), which is a somewhat less accurate measure of contractility but relatively easy to obtain during hemodynamic studies. Increases or decreases in the contractile state will increase or decrease myocardial oxygen consumption, respectively.[8]

I would like now to discuss some aspects of the exercise response in patients with coronary artery disease. Patients with angina pectoris have more than a defect in oxygen delivery to the myocardium. They usually have abnormal hemodynamic responses to exertion that may play an important role in causing their ischemic pain (Table 28.2). During exercise, these patients usually have an abnormal elevation of the left ventricular end diastolic pressure and the mean pulmonary artery pressure as mani-

Table 28.2. *Abnormal exercise response in coronary artery disease*

    Abnormal increase in left ventricular end diastolic pressure
    Abnormal increase in mean pulmonary artery pressure
    Exaggerated increase in peripheral systolic pressure (variable)
    Exaggerated increase in heart rate (variable)
    Abnormal ventricular volume change
    Anginal pain at constant pressure-time index
    Decreased exercise performance
    Ischemic electrocardiographic changes

---

festations of a decrease in left ventricular function.[9, 10] In addition, many of these patients have an exaggerated elevation of peripheral systolic pressure and heart rate during exercise, with the occurrence of anginal pain at a relatively constant rate-pressure product, individualized for each patient.[11] These hemodynamic alterations are an important determinant of the decreased exercise performance and "ischemic" electrocardiographic (ECG) changes that occur during the exercise state.[11] Elevations of the left ventricular end diastolic pressure, pulmonary artery pressure, peripheral systolic pressure, and heart rate will all significantly increase myocardial tension per minute and myocardial oxygen requirements.

Whether physical conditioning improves ventricular function or increases coronary blood flow through stimulation of coronary vessel collaterals in humans with coronary artery disease is still to be determined. Alteration of the exercise response after physical training, however, has been well documented in such patients (Table 28.3). These changes may include a significant decrease in heart rate and systolic blood pressure during equal work loads, with a resultant decrease in the pressure-time and, probably, the tension-time per minute.[12-14] Cardiac output is unchanged or may decrease,[12, 13, 15] and stroke volume increases with no apparent change in ventricular volume.[13] Whether these alterations result from improved ventricular function, resetting of the "neurovegetative" system with changed catecholamine response, or differences in peripheral blood flow, the end result is a myocardial oxygen-sparing effect secondary to a reduction in myocardial tension per minute.[12-15] Thus, the concomitant improvement in exercise performance and ischemic electrocardiographic changes can be explained on a logical and physiological basis.

Let us now consider some of the actions of the vasoactive drugs during the exercise state in patients with coronary artery disease. The beneficial effects of the nitrites in angina pectoris is unquestioned. These drugs do not, however, consistently increase coronary blood flow in patients with coronary arterial disease.[4] These drugs, as exemplified by nitroglycerin, do alter the vascular dynamics in a number of ways. Nitroglycerin reduces venous tone, causing pooling of blood in the peripheral veins, and dilates the arterioles, with a subsequent fall in vascular resistance and a decline

Table 28.3. *Altered exercise response after physical training*

Decreased heart rate
Decreased systolic blood pressure
Decreased pressure-time per minute
No significant cardiac output change or decrease
Increased stroke volume with no apparent ventricular volume change
Improved exercise performance
Decreased ischemic electrocardiographic changes

DRUG	ALTERED EXERCISE RESPONSE WITH DRUGS (Cor. Art. Dis.)							
	PAP ↑	LVEDP ↑	SYST. BP	HR	PTI	LVV	dp/dt	CI
Nitroglycerin	↓	↓	↓	↑	↓	↓	↑	↑
Propranolol	→	→	↓	↓	↓	↑	↓	↓
Combined N-P	↓	↓	↓	↓	↓	→	↓	↓
Digitalis	↓	↓	→	↓	↓	↓→	↑	↑→
	Improved Exercise Performance Decreased Anginal Pain Decreased "Ischemic" EKG Changes							

Fig. 28.1. Alterations of pulmonary artery pressure (PAP), left ventricular end diastolic pressure (LVEDP), systemic blood pressure (Syst. BP), heart rate (HR), pressure-time index (PTI), left ventricular volume (LVV), rate of rise of left ventricular pressure (dp/dt), and cardiac index (CI) during exercise with cardiac drugs in patients with coronary artery disease. ↑, increase; ↓, decrease; →, no change.

in systemic arterial pressure. These changes result in decreased end diastolic and end systolic dimensions of the heart, reduced systolic intraventricular pressure and resistance to ventricular ejection, and a fall in the abnormally elevated left ventricular end diastolic pressure, with a resultant lowering in ventricular preload and afterload.[5, 16] The sum of these changes can be seen during exercise (Fig. 28.1). There is a significant decrease in the abnormal elevations of the pulmonary artery and left ventricular end diastolic pressures, a fall of systemic blood pressure, a decrease in left ventricular volume and a resultant significant diminution of the pressure-time and tension-time indices.[5, 17, 18] These oxygen-sparing effects dominate over the increased heart rate, dp/dt, and output responses that may be seen after administration of nitroglycerin in exercising patients with coronary artery disease, resulting in improved exercise performance, decreased anginal pain, and decreased ischemic electrocardiographic changes.

Beta adrenergic receptor-blocking agents, as exemplified by propranolol, reduce myocardial oxygen requirements during exercise by blocking the stimulation of the cardiac sympathetic nerves during exertion. The mechanism of action is considerably different from that of nitroglycerin (Fig. 28.1). The primary effects are a reduction in heart rate and blood pressure with resultant decrease in pressure-time per minute, a decrease in contractility, and a fall in cardiac output.[5, 18, 19] However, propranolol will not diminish the abnormal elevation in pulmonary artery and left ventricular end diastolic pressures during exercise, and it will result in an increase in ventricular dimensions-actions that tend to augment the oxygen requirements of the heart.[5, 18] The sum of these effects is usually a reduction of myocardial oxygen needs, with again a resultant improvement in exercise performance and a decrease in both anginal pain and electrocardiographic changes with exertion.

Since propranolol and nitroglycerin work by different mechanisms, a combination of these agents would appear to have significant advantages over the administration of either drug alone.[5, 18] These advantages have been demonstrated in hemodynamic studies. Combined nitroglycerin-propranolol will cause a fall in almost all of the measured parameters during exercise in patients with coronary artery disease, with a greater oxygen-sparing effect than is produced by either agent alone.[18] Recent studies have suggested an additive effect between isosorbide dinitrate and propranolol, with improved exercise performance.[19, 20]

The effect of digitalization on exercise performance in patients with coronary artery disease in the absence of congestive heart failure is not as clear-cut as that of nitroglycerin or propranolol. Administration of cardiac glycosides will not consistently reduce exertional angina or improve exercise tolerance.[21, 22] The inotropic effect of digitalis may increase myocardial oxygen consumption by its direct increase in myocardial contractility and velocity of contraction.[8, 23] On the other hand, digitalis will improve ventricular function and reduce the abnormal elevation of left ventricular end diastolic pressure during exercise in patients with angina pectoris,[21, 22] and it may reduce the heart rate. In the presence of cardiac enlargement, it may reduce ventricular dimensions (Fig. 28.1). These alterations will reduce myocardial oxygen consumption. Because of these conflicting actions, the use of digitalis must be individualized in patients with coronary artery disease, and it will probably only improve exercise performance in those patients with cardiomegaly and considerable reduction in ventricular function.

A few other drugs that may alter ventricular performance should be mentioned (Fig. 28.2). In patients with systemic hypertension, both guanethidine and reserpine will change exercise response. Both of these drugs will lower blood pressure and heart rate, with a resultant reduction in pressure-time per minute, and they will reduce cardiac output and contractility.[24, 25] These oxygen-sparing effects may be partly counteracted by an increase in ventricular dimensions. Antihypertensive diuretics will also lower systemic blood pressure and pressure-time per minute. In addition, they will reduce ventricular volume, cardiac output, and elevation of the left ventricular end diastolic and pulmonary artery pressures, and they will improve exercise performance in patients with noncoronary heart disease who have been in congestive heart failure.[26, 27] In the presence of

DRUG	ALTERED EXERCISE RESPONSE WITH DRUGS (Non-Cor. Art. Dis.)							
	SYST. BP	HR	PTI	LVV	dp/dt	CI	PAP↑	LVEDP↑
Guanethidine	↓	↓	↓	↑	↓	↓		
Reserpine	↓	↓	↓	↑	↓	↓		
Anti-hypertensive Diuretics	↓	→	↓	↓		↓	↓	↓
	May Improve Exercise Performance May Decrease Anginal Pain (In Combined ASHD & Ess. Hyper.) May Decrease "Ischemic" EKG Changes							

FIG. 28.2. Alterations of systemic blood pressure (Syst. BP), heart rate (HR), pressure-time index (PTI), left ventricular volume (LVV), rate of rise of left ventricular pressure (dp/dt), cardiac index (CI), pulmonary artery pressure (PAP), and left ventricular end diastolic pressure (LVEDP) during exercise with antihypertensive drugs in cardiac patients with noncoronary artery disease (Non-Cor. Art. Dis.). ↑, increase; ↓, decrease; →, no change.

combined coronary heart disease and systemic hypertension, these drugs should have an efficacious effect on exercise performance, anginal pain, and ischemic electrocardiographic changes.

The drugs that I have mentioned will alter the electrocardiographic response to exercise as well as ventricular performance. The electrocardiogram plays an important role in stress testing in terms of diagnosing coronary artery disease, confirming coronary insufficiency during exercise, and evaluating the results of physical conditioning programs. Drug alterations of the electrocardiographic response may significantly interfere with proper interpretation of the exercise electrocardiogram (Table 28.4). This presents practical problems, particularly when drugs are added to or withdrawn from a patient's medical regimen while he is in a physical training program. Both nitroglycerin and propranolol, by their oxygen-sparing effects, may decrease the ischemic S-T changes of the exercise electrocardiogram.[28, 29]

Table 28.4. *Drugs altering the ECG response to exercise*

Drug	Effect
Nitroglycerin	Decreased ischemic changes
Propranolol	Decreased ischemic changes
Digitalis	False-positive ischemic changes
Quinidine	False-negative ischemic changes
Hypokalemia	False-positive ischemic changes

During exercise-induced tachycardia, S-T abnormalities produced by digitalis may be indistinguishable from changes attributed to coronary insufficiency, producing false-positive exercise tests.[30] In contrast to digitalis, quinidine may prevent the appearance of S-T depression after exercise and thus may contribute to a false-negative response to exercise.[28] Hypokalemia may also cause false-positive exercise tests.[31]

Since the cardiac drugs will alter hemodynamics and the electrocardiogram during exercise, their interaction with physical training may present numerous problems (Table 28.5). The vasoactive drugs will alter maximal aerobic capacity, reduce maximal heart rate, and affect the response to submaximal exercise testing. These changes will make it more difficult to assess cardiovascular function and to determine target levels for training.[32, 33] Among the general principles of a conditioning program, there must be an overload of the muscles (skeletal and heart), a gradual progression of exercise, and a building of both strength and endurance.[34] The cardiac drugs may reduce the desired exercise stress of the cardiovascular system and interfere with these goals. Altered hemodynamics and electrocardiographic changes will also make it more difficult to evaluate the results of training. Finally, potentially dangerous drug side effects may affect the ability of any patient to participate successfully in a conditioning program. These side effects may include therapeutic actions that may disproportionately lower blood pressure, heart rate, and cardiac output response, leading to possible hypotension, syncope, congestive heart failure, coronary or cerebral insufficiency, cardiac arrhythmias, myocardial infarction or cerebral vascular accidents.[32, 34] In addition, toxic drug effects may lead to dangerous cardiac arrhythmias such as heart block, ventricular fibrillation or arrest, and myocardial depression with secondary heart failure.

The final question to be considered is, what is the place of the cardiac drugs in an exercise training program in patients with coronary artery

Table 28.5. *Problems with interaction of drugs with exercise training*

Difficulty in determining target levels for training
alterations in maximal aerobic capacity
reduction in maximal heart rate
Reduction in desired exercise stress of cardiovascular system
Interference with evaluation of training results
altered hemodynamics
altered ECG changes
Dangerous drug side effects
therapeutic: low blood pressure, heart rate or output response, possible syncope, heart failure, arrhythmias, possible coronary or cerebral insufficiency
toxic: cardiac arrhythmias-PVCs,* heart block, cardiac arrest, myocardial depression-congestive heart failure

* PVC, premature ventricular contraction.

disease? In the patient with minimal symptoms, the ideal physical conditioning regimen should exclude cardiac drug therapy. This would avoid any of the potential problems with hemodynamic or electrocardiographic interactions that I have discussed. It is unreasonable and impractical, however, to eliminate rigidly all patients from physical training who are taking one or more of these drugs. This policy would exclude a large group of symptomatic patients who might benefit from a carefully supervised training program. In patients with significant angina, the judicious use of nitroglycerin and/or propranolol might improve exercise performance to a level that would allow some degree of physical conditioning. In patients with premature ventricular contractions, exercise training may only be feasible with the concomitant use of antiarrhythmic drugs. In our own experience, patients taking digitalis, propranolol, and nitroglycerin may be stress-tested and may undergo physical training. What remains to be answered is whether the concomitant use of drugs and exercise training will be as beneficial as physical conditioning alone. Since our knowledge in this area is still limited, there is room for a great deal of research on the concomitant use of these two modalities of therapy. With awareness of the potential interactions, and with proper precautions and observation for side effects, it is reasonable to expect that many patients on cardiac drugs can participate in and benefit from physical conditioning programs.

This work was supported by Grant RD1994-M from the Social and Rehabilitation Service of the United States Department of Health, Education and Welfare.

REFERENCES

1. Muller, O., and Rorvik, K.: Hemodynamic consequences of coronary heart disease with observations during anginal pain and on the effect of nitroglycerin. Brit. Heart J. 20: 302, 1958.
2. Wegria, R., Nickerson, J. L., Case, R. B., and Holland, J. F.: Effect of nitroglycerin on the cardiovascular system of normal persons. Amer. J. Med. 10: 414, 1951.
3. Bernstein, L. F., Friesinger, G. C., Lichtlen, P. R., and Ross, R. S.: The effect of nitroglycerin on the systemic and coronary circulation in man and dogs. Circulation 33: 107, 1966.
4. Gorlin, R., Brachfeld, N., MacLeod, G., and Bopp, P.: The effect of nitroglycerin on the coronary circulation in patients with coronary artery disease or increased left ventricular work. Circulation 19: 705, 1959.
5. Mason, D. T., Spann, J. F., Jr., Zelis, R., and Amsterdam, E. A.: Physiologic approach to the treatment of angina pectoris. New Engl. J. Med. 281: 1225, 1969.
6. Sonnenblick, E. H., Ross, J., Jr., and Braunwald, E.: Oxygen consumption of the heart. Amer. J. Cardiol. 22: 328, 1968.
7. Sarnoff, S. J., Braunwald, E., Welch, G. H., Jr., Case, R. B., Stainsby, W. N., and Macruz, R.: Hemodynamic determinants of oxygen consumption of the heart with special reference to the tension-time index. Amer. J. Physiol. 192: 148, 1958.

8. Sonnenblick, E. H., Ross, J., Jr., Covell, J. W., Kaiser, G. A., and Braunwald, E.: Velocity of contraction as a determinant of myocardial oxygen consumption. Amer. J. Physiol. 209: 919, 1965.

9. Parker, J. O., DiGiorgi, S., and West, R. O.: Hemodynamic study of acute coronary insufficiency precipitated by exercise. Amer. J. Cardiol. 17: 470, 1966.

10. Wiener, L., Dwyer, E. M., Jr., and Cox, J. W.: Left ventricular hemodynamics in exercise-induced angina pectoris. Circulation 38: 240, 1968.

11. Robinson, B. F.: Relation of heart rate and systolic blood pressure to onset of pain in angina pectoris. Circulation 35: 1073, 1967.

12. Clausen, J. P., Larsen, O. A., and Trap-Jensen, J.: Physical training in the management of coronary artery disease. Circulation 40: 143, 1969.

13. Frick, M. H., and Katila, M.: Hemodynamic consequences of physical training after myocardial infarction. Circulation 37: 192, 1968.

14. Hellerstein, H. K., Burlando, A., Hirsch, E. Z., Plotkin, F. H., Feil, G. H., Winkler, O., Marik, S., and Margolis, N.: Active physical reconditioning in coronary patients. Circulation 37 (Suppl. 2): 110, 1965.

15. Varnauskas, E., Bergman, H., Houk, P., and Bjorntorp, P.: Hemodynamic effects of physical training in coronary patients. Lancet 2: 8, 1966.

16. Williams, J. F., Jr., Glick, G., and Braunwald, E.: Studies on cardiac dimensions in intact unanesthetized man. V. Effects of nitroglycerin. Circulation 32: 767, 1965.

17. Najmi, M., Griggs, D. M., Jr., Kasparian, H., and Novack, P.: Effects of nitroglycerin on hemodynamics during rest and exercise in patients with coronary insufficiency. Circulation 35: 46, 1967.

18. Wiener, L., Dwyer, E. M., Jr., and Cox, J. W.: Hemodynamic effects of nitroglycerin, propranolol, and their combination in coronary heart disease. Circulation. 39: 623, 1969.

19. Battock, D. J., Alvarez, H., and Chidsey, G. A.: Effects of propranolol and isosorbide dinitrate on exercise performance and adrenergic activity in patients with angina pectoris. Circulation. 39: 157, 1969.

20. Russek, H. I.: Propranolol and isosorbide dinitrate synergism in angina pectoris. Amer. J. Cardiol. 21: 44, 1968.

21. Parker, J. O., West, R. O., Ledwich, J. R., and DiGiorgi, S.: The effect of acute digitalization on the hemodynamic response to exercise in coronary artery disease. Circulation 40: 453, 1969.

22. Malmborg, R. O.: A clinical and hemodynamic analysis of factors limiting the cardiac performance in patients with coronary heart disease. Acta Med. Scand. 177 (Suppl. 426), 1965.

23. Covell, J. W., Braunwald, E., Ross, J., Jr., and Sonnenblick, E. H.: Studies on digitalis. XVI. Effects on myocardial oxygen consumption. J. Clin. Invest. 45: 1535, 1966.

24. Kahler, R. L., Gaffney, T. E., and Braunwald, E.: Effects of autonomic nervous system inhibition on the circulatory response to exercise. J. Clin. Invest. 41: 198, 1962.

25. Cohen, S. I., Young, M. W., Lau, S. H., Haft, J. I., and Damato, A. N.: Effects of reserpine on cardiac output and A-V conduction at rest and controlled heart rates in patients with essential hypertension. Circulation 37: 738, 1968.

26. Stampfer, M., Epstein, S. E., Beiser, G. D., and Braunwald, E.: Hemodynamic effects of diuresis at rest and during intense upright exercise in patients with impaired cardiac function. Circulation 37: 900, 1968.

27. Lal, S., Murtagh, J. G., Pollock, A. M., Fletcher, E., and Binnion, P. F.: Acute hemodynamic effects of furosemide in patients with normal and elevated left atrial pressure. Brit. Heart J. 31: 711, 1969.
28. Surawicz, B., and Lasseter, K. C.: Effects of drugs on the electrocardiogram. Progr. Cardiovasc. Dis. 13: 26, 1970.
29. Gianelly, R. E., Treister, B. L., and Harrison, D. C.: The effect of propranolol on exercise-induced ischemic S-T segment depression. Amer. J. Cardiol. 24: 161, 1969.
30. Kawai, C., and Hultgren, H. N.: The effect of digitalis upon the exercise electrocardiogram. Amer. Heart J. 68: 409, 1964.
31. Georgopoulos, A. J., Proudfit, W. L., and Page, I. H.: Effect of exercise on electrocardiograms of patients with low serum potassium. Circulation 23: 567, 1961.
32. McDonough, J. R., and Bruce, R. A.: Maximal exercise testing in assessing cardiovascular function. J. S. Carolina Med. Ass. 65 (Suppl. 1): 26, 1969.
33. Sheffield, L. T., Roitman, D., and Reeves, T. J.: Submaximal exercise testing. J. S. Carolina Med. Ass. 65 (Suppl. 1): 18, 1969.
34. Hellerstein, H. K.: Techniques of exercise prescription and evaluation. J. S. Carolina Med. Ass. 65 (Suppl. 1): 46, 1969.

29

Loafer's Heart

OTTO A. BRUSIS, M.D., M.P.H.

When the late Professor Wilhelm Raab in 1958 first used the term "loafer's heart,"[1] he referred to the heart of the physically inactive and sedentary individual. The term was intended to characterize major degrees of inertia-induced cardiac inefficiency and problems, short of the appearance of conventionally recognized heart disease.[2] For the purpose of this presentation, I believe it justifiable to consider the so-called "normal" heart in a population like ours by and large as representative of "loafer's heart." Further, we may assume that the effect of inertia and training upon cardiac morphology and function depends on the degree of physical activity as defined by the type of activity and its intensity, duration, and frequency. Thus the spectrum ranges from the heart of the permanently bedridden individual to that of the highly trained endurance athlete. In comparing the two extremes, the differences in structure and function become most obvious. Therefore I would like to discuss loafer's heart primarily by demonstrating the superiority of the heart of the physically well-trained individual in contrast to the less efficient state and, in fact, the inferiority of loafer's heart.

Morphologically, athlete's heart is characterized by a true hypertrophy of the myocardial muscle cells, resulting in an increase in the length of the heart, as well as in an increase in the size of all chambers. Consequently, the heart volume is increased. It has been found to range from 724 to 1437 cc. with a mean volume of 1008 cc., versus the heart of the untrained individual which ranges from 465 to 980 cc. with a mean of 737 cc.[3] Interestingly enough, however, the weight of the heart rarely ever exceeds the critical weight of 500 g. As long as this critical limit is maintained, the number of the muscle fibers does not increase.[4-6] As the heart increases in size, one observes a decrease of kymographically registered pulsations at the apex at rest, a phenomenon which disappears completely during and after physical exercise.[7]

The blood supply to the increased muscle mass is not impaired. Already

343

in 1935, Petren and coworkers were able to demonstrate an augmentation of myocardial capillaries after prolonged physical training.[8] This increase in vascularization has been observed even in hearts which did not undergo a measurable hypertrophy after extensive yet less strenuous physical training.[9] Recently Tomanek[10] reported an increase in the ratio of capillaries to muscle fibers in exercised versus inactive albino rats after 12 weeks of training. This increase was more pronounced in young animals than in older ones. His report confirmed earlier work by Tittle and others, who reported an increase of up to 44 per cent of this ratio in male rats.[11] In Eckstein's classic experiments,[12] exercised dogs showed an even more significant increase in coronary flow after 6 to 8 weeks of training than did their inactive counterparts who only had an experimentally caused stenosis of their circumflex coronary artery. The relative anoxia caused by exercise stress seems to be a stimulus for the augmented formation of coronary anastomosis.[13]

Probably the single best known parameter of the well-trained heart is its slow rate. This is invariably a sinus bradycardia. The bradycardia can vary with the degree of training, the kind of training, the kind of exercise and the age of the individual; nevertheless, it always can be demonstrated. Concomitant with this phenomenon is a lengthening of the ejection period and the tension period, together with a considerable lengthening of the diastole.[14] This in turn provides for an increased myocardial circulation with an improved oxygen supply to the myocardial cell.[15] It has been shown that capillary flow during systole comes to an almost complete standstill. The inflow into the coronary arteries, as well as the return from the coronary sinus, on the other hand, is increased during diastole,[16] thus providing more blood as diastole lengthens. In addition, the end systolic or residual volume is increased in the trained heart. It has been calculated that the ratio of end systolic volume to stroke volume in the athlete can reach $3:1$,[17] thus providing a reserve of arterialized blood which is available immediately upon demand.

Cardiac output as a function of O_2 uptake at rest and during exercise is diminished in the well-trained heart.[14, 18] Comparing overall work, the trained heart works about 50 per cent less than the untrained one at a standard work load.[19]

It should be understood that not all of these characteristics are always present in the well-trained heart. This is especially true of the increased size and volume of the heart which only can be found in extremely well-trained endurance type athletes.

All of the changes presented are reversible and can be lost fairly rapidly during periods of rest and inactivity, as several investigators have pointed out.[20, 21] On the other hand, they all can be acquired by the normal untrained individual by prolonged training, engaging in aerobic or endurance type exercises.[18, 20, 22-24] Once acquired, they can be maintained by considerably less effort than is necessary to get them in the first place.[19, 25]

Already strikingly superior at rest, the trained heart is capable of performing submaximal and maximal work at significantly higher levels than is the untrained one or, expressed differently, it can perform the same amount of work at considerably lower energy costs than can loafer's heart. In addition, it is able to return more rapidly to the resting state after exercise.[14, 15, 18, 20, 22-25]

What are the mechanisms by which physical training causes these changes in the performance of the heart? The chronotropic features are generally ascribed to an increased vagal tone. It is probable that central sympathoinhibitory mechanisms are also involved.[26, 27] The combination of these two separate antiadrenergic mechanisms seems the more likely as the negative chronotropic effects of training are accompanied by a negative inotropic phenomenon, namely, a marked prolongation of the tension period of the left ventricle.[28] To explain this as being due to purely vagal action would be difficult, since the ventricles are devoid of vagal fibers, in contrast to the atria. Accordingly, the tension period is much less altered by anticholinergic atropine than is the heart rate, and the acetylcholine content of the ventricles of trained animals is not augmented, whereas that of the atria is.[29] Thus, the neurovegetative state of the trained heart may be described as being dominated by vagal cholinergic and sympathoinhibitory antiadrenergic mechanisms. This predominance of antiadrenergic autonomic nervous factors is extremely important for the metabolic, structural, and functional superiority of the trained over the untrained heart. The adrenergic catecholamines waste oxygen,[30] impair energetic efficiency, and tend to produce myocardial hypoxia, whereas sympathetic inhibition and vagal acetylcholine cause the opposite, thus guaranteeing a better energetic economy of cardiac work.[31, 32] Recent work by DeSchryver and coworkers[33] shows that the catecholamine concentration in hearts of rats was decreased by 34 per cent after prolonged training. This training effect disappeared after 6 days. Saltzmann *et al.*[34] could demonstrate that the uptake of labeled epinephrine by the myocardium was 26 per cent lower in trained mice than in the untrained controls.

How are these advantages of the trained over the untrained heart related to the development of arteriosclerotic ischemic heart disease? Raab suggested a model (Fig. 29.1), which he called a "structural formula of pluri-causal pathogenesis of so-called coronary heart disease." [35] In this model he attempted to bring together what is known *de facto* and what can be deducted from related studies in regard to the pathogenesis of arteriosclerotic ischemic heart disease. Three compartments contribute to and/or

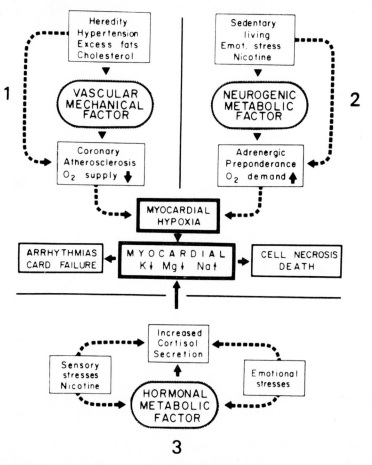

FIG. 29.1. Structural formula of pluricausal pathogenesis of so-called coronary heart disease. (From Raab, W.: Pluricausal pathogenesis and preventability of ischemic heart disease. Dis. Chest 53: 629, 1968.[35] Reproduced with permission.)

cause electrolyte imbalance in the myocardial cell. This leads directly to the well-known final manifestations of the disease: arrhythmia, cardiac failure, and cell necrosis and death.

The vascular mechanical factor (factor 1) is manifested by coronary atherosclerosis, which is influenced and/or aggravated by heredity, arterial hypertension, and excess fats and cholesterol in the diet. It leads to a diminution and occasionally to a complete occlusion of the coronary lumen and, consequently, to an insufficient oxygen supply to a circumscribed area of the myocardium.

The neurogenic metabolic factor is characterized by an adrenergic preponderance of the vegetative system. It can be caused and is influenced and aggravated by sedentary living, emotional stress and tension, and nicotine. It leads to an increased oxygen demand in the myocardium which when accompanied by factor 1, can prove fatal.

Finally, the hormonal metabolic factor whereby, through sensory and emotional stresses[36-38] and nicotine, cortisol secretion is increased can lead directly to a disturbance of the potassium, magnesium, and sodium equilibrium in the myocardium.

It should be understood that all of these factors may work together. Their interrelations are not quite understood yet. Nevertheless, they have been shown to exist and must be taken into consideration when we contemplate the prevention of arteriosclerotic ischemic heart disease. In Figure 29.2, three main targets for prevention are identified according to the categories which are considered most important in the pathogenesis of the disease.[39]

Target 1. The retardation of coronary atherosclerosis is a quite controversial issue concerning its susceptibility to the influence of exercise. No good studies are known which convincingly indicate a direct effect of physical training on the development of coronary arteriosclerosis. On the other hand, recent reports by Siegel and coworkers[23] have shown that prolonged physical training in formerly sedentary middle-aged men can significantly reduce serum cholesterol and triglycerides. No significant weight changes occurred in their subjects. Hanson and Nedde[40] demonstrated that both labile and essential hypertensive males can achieve a physically trained state and improve their cardiac parameters much the same as normal men can. More important yet for our discussion, abnormally high systolic, diastolic, and mean values of blood pressures can be significantly reduced and normalized. This can be observed during rest as well as during exercise. Whether the just cited influences of physical training on cholesterol and blood pressure have any preventive or therapeutic effect on atherosclerosis remains to be seen.

Target 2. The prevention of myocardial adrenergic preponderance by physical training can be postulated since we have seen that the trained heart becomes more and more dominated by vagal influences as training increases. By considerably enhancing sympathoinhibitory autonomic nervous mechanisms,[28] physical activity further contributes to the prevention or reduction of adrenergic preponderance in the myocardium. Bajusz[41, 42] demonstrated that acutely exercised rats showed a significantly higher resistance to cardiotoxic catecholamines and other agents than did controls. This effect lasted up to 24 hours after the cessation of exercise. Whether inferences for humans are possible in this regard needs further study.

The active, continuously training individual is less likely to smoke cigarettes than is his sedentary counterpart, simply because endurance type

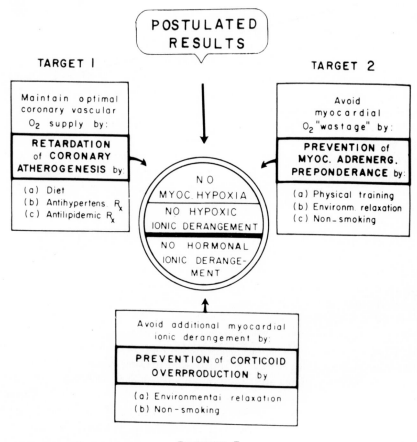

TARGET 3

FIG. 29.2. Schematic representation of the three interrelated main targets of prevention of arteriosclerotic ischemic heart disease. (From Raab, W.: *Preventive Myocardiology, Fundamentals and Targets.* Charles C Thomas, Publisher, Springfield, Ill., 1970. Reproduced with permission.)

training is not possible with one to two packs of cigarettes per day.[43] It is further generally accepted, based on empirical information rather than on scientific evidence, that emotional stress and tension can be reduced and even eliminated by vigorous physical activity.

Target 3. To what extent physical training will reduce overproduction of corticoids and thereby reduce their deleterious effect on myocardial electrolyte equilibrium is not yet investigated. Work by Frenkl and co-workers, however, seems to indicate that this might be possible.[44, 45]

Epidemiological data seem to confirm the advantages of the trained heart as compared with loafer's heart.[46] On the other hand, very little additional activity appears to be necessary to influence the incidence of and mortality from arteriosclerotic ischemic heart disease and to shift the balance toward the more favorable side.[47]

In conclusion, it seems reasonable and wise to avoid cardiac toxins such as nicotine, emotional stress and tension, and high cholesterol and fat intakes. At the same time, adopting and maintaining living patterns which include as an essential component regular cardioprotective physical exercise seems even more reasonable. By doing so we would provide the myocardial cell with a certain resistance against the few known, and probably even greater number of unknown, cardiac stressor agents. Further, by continuously ongoing training one would maintain an oxygen economy of the myocardium which would enable it to handle stress and emergency situations far better than the untrained or loafer's heart.

REFERENCES

1. Raab, W., "Loafer's heart." Arch. Intern. Med. 101: 194–198, 1958.
2. Kraus, H., and Raab, W.: *Hypokinetic Disease*. Charles C Thomas, Publisher, Springfield, Ill., 1961, p. 69.
3. Reindell, H.: Grösse, Form und Bewegungsbild des Sportherzen. Arch. Kreislaufforesh. 7: 117, 1940.
4. Linzbach, A. J.: Die Anzahl der Herzmuskelkerne in normalen, überlasteten, atrophischen und mit Corhormon behandelten Herzkammern. Z. Kreislaufforsch. 41: 641, 1952.
5. Kirch, E.: Herzkräftigung und echte Herzhypertrophie durch Sport. Z. Kreislaufforesh. 28: 893, 1936.
6. Kirch, E.: Anatomische Gundlagen des Sportherzen. Verh. Deutsch. Ges. Inn. Med. 47: 73, 1935.
7. Reindell, H.: Die Herzbeurteilung beim Sportsmann und die differentialdiagnostische Bewertung der Befunde im Elektrokardiogramm und Kymogramm. Deutsch. Med. Wschr. 65: 1369 and 1423, 1939.
8. Petrén, T.: Die totale Anzahl der Blutkapillaren im Herzen und in der Skelettmuskulatur bei Ruhe und nach langer Muskelübung. Verh. Anat. Ges. 43: 165, 1935.
9. Petrén, T., Sjöstrand, T., and Sylven, B.: Der Einfluss des Trainings auf die Häufigkeit der Kapillaren in Herz- und Skelettmuskulatur. Arbeitsphysiol. 9: 376, 1936.
10. Tomanek, R. J.: Effects of age and exercise on the extent of the myocardial capillary bed. Anat. Rec. 167: 55, 1970.
11. Tittel, K., Knacke, W., Brauer, B., and Otto, H.: Der Einfluss körperlicher Belastungen unterschiedlicher Dauer and Intensität auf die Kapillarisierung der Herz- und Skelettmuskulatur bei Albinoratten. In *Proceedings of the Sixteenth World Congress of Sports Medicine*, Hannover, Germany, 1966, p. 181.
12. Eckstein, R. W.: Effect of exercise and coronary narrowing on coronary collateral circulation. Circ. Res. 5: 230, 1957.
13. Zoll, P. M., Wessler, S., and Schlesinger, M. J.: Interarterial coronary anastomosis in the human heart with particular reference to anemia and relative cardiac anoxia. Circulation 15: 14, 1957.
14. Reindell, H., Weyland, R., Klepzig, H., Musshoff, K., and Schildge, E.: Das Sportherz. Ergebn. Inn. Med. Kinderheilk. 5: 306, 1954.

15. Hollmann, W.: *Der Arbeits- und Trainingseinfluss auf Kreislauf und Atmung.* Steinkopff, Darmstadt, 1959, p. 74.
16. Sabiston, D. C., and Gregg, D. E.: Effect of cardiac contraction on coronary blood flow. Circulation 15: 14, 1957.
17. Reindell, H., and Delius, L.: Klinische Beobachtungen über die Hemodynamik bei gesunden Menschen. Deutsch. Arch. Klin. Med. 193: 639, 1948.
18. Hanson, J. S., Tabakin, B. S., Levi, A. M., and Nedde, W.: Longterm physical training and cardiovascular dynamics in middle-aged men. Circulation 38: 783, 1968.
19. Mellerowicz, H.: Vergleichende Untersuchungen über das Okonomieprinzip in Arbeit und Leistung des trainierten Kreislaufs. Arch. Kreislaufforsch. 24: 70, 1956.
20. Saltin, B., Blomquist, G., Mitchell, J. H., Johnson, R. C., Wildenthal, K., and Chapman, G. B.: Response to exercise after bed rest and after training. Circulation 37 and 38 (Suppl. 7): 1968.
21. Taylor, H. L., Henschel, A., Brozek, J., and Keys, A.: Effects of bed rest on cardiovascular function and work performance. J. Appl. Physiol. 2: 233, 1949.
22. Leon, A. S., and Bloor, C. M.: Effects of exercise and its cessation on the heart and its blood supply. J. Appl. Physiol. 24: 485, 1968.
23. Siegel, W., Blomquist, G., and Mitchell, J. H.: Effects of a quantitated physical training program on middle aged sedentary men. Circulation 41: 19, 1970.
24. Ekblom, B.: Effects of physical training on oxygen transport system in man. Acta Physiol. Scand. (Suppl. 328), 1969.
25. Rosskamm, H., Brandts, W., and Reindell, H.: Zur Trainierbarkeit der Herz- und Kreislaufleistungsfähigkeit in Abhängigkeit von Alter und Geschlecht. Cardiologia 48: 441, 1966.
26. von Brücke, E. T.: Über die reziproke reflektorische Erregung der Herznerven bei Reizung des N. depressor. Z. Biol. 67: 507, 1917.
27. Folkow, B.: Hypothalamic inhibition of sympathetic tone. Paper presented at the Symposium on Central Nervous System Control of the Cardiovascular System, National Research Council, Washington, D. C., Nov. 1–3, 1959.
28. Raab, W., DePaula e Silva, P., Marchet, H., Kimura, E., and Starcheska, Y. K.: Cardiac adrenergic preponderance due to lack of physical exercise and its pathogenic implications. Amer. J. Cardiol. 5: 300, 1960.
29. Herrlich, H. C., Raab, W., and Gigee, W.: Influence of muscular training and of catecholamines on cardiac acetylcholine and cholinesterase. Arch. Int. Pharmacodyn. 129: 201, 1960.
30. Chandler, B. M., Sonnenblick, E. H., and Pool, P. E.: Mechanochemistry of cardiac muscle. 3. Effects of norepinephrine on the utilisation of high energy phosphates. Circ. Res. 22: 729, 1968.
31. Scott, J. C., and Balourdas, T. A.: An analysis of coronary flow and related factors following vagotomy, atropine, and sympathetomy. Circ. Res. 7: 102, 1959.
32. Raab, W.: The adrenergic-cholinergic control of cardiac metabolism and function. Advan. Cardiol. 1: 65, 1956.
33. DeSchryver, C., Mertens-Strythagen, J., Bescei, I., and Lammerant, J.: Effect of training on heart and skeletal muscle catecholamine concentration in rats. Amer. J. Physiol. 217: 1589, 1969.
34. Salzman, S. H., Hirsch, E. Z. Hellerstein, H. K., and Bruell, J. H.: Adaptation to muscular exercise: myocardial epinephrine-^{3}H uptake. J. Appl. Physiol. 29: 92, 1970.
35. Raab, W.: Pluricausal pathogenesis and preventability of ischemic heart disease. Dis. Chest 53: 629, 1968.

36. Raab, W., and Krzyvanek, J.: Cardiovascular sympathetic tone and stress response related to personality patterns and exercise habits. Amer. J. Cardiol. 16: 42, 1965.
37. Raab, W.: Correlated cardiovascular adrenergic and adrenocortical responses to sensory and mental annoyance in man. Psychosom. Med. 30: 809, 1968.
38. Raab, W., Chaplin, J. P., and Bajusz, E.: Myocardial necrosis produced in domesticated rats and in wild rats by sensory and emotional stresses. Proc. Soc. Exp. Biol. Med. 116: 665, 1964.
39. Raab, W.: *Preventive Myocardiology, Fundamentals and Targets.* Charles C Thomas, Publisher, Springfield, Ill., 1970.
40. Hanson, J. S., and Nedde, W. H.: Preliminary observations on physical training for hypertensive males. Circ. Res. 26 and 27 (Suppl. 1), July 1970.
41. Bajusz, E.: *Electrolytes and Cardiovascular Disease,* Vol. I. The Williams & Wilkins Company, Baltimore, 1965, p. 267.
42. Bajusz, E.: An ionic shift through which non specific stimuli can increase the resistance of the heart muscle. Cardiologia 45: 288, 1964.
43. Cooper, K. H.: Effects of cigarette smoking on endurance performance. J. A. M. A. 203: 189, 1968.
44. Frenkl, R., Csalay, L., Csákváry, G.: A study of the stress reaction elicited by muscular exertion in trained and untrained men and rats. Acta Physiol. Acad. Sci. Hung. 36: 365, 1969.
45. Frenkl, R., Csalay, L., Jákó, P., Budavari, I., and Zelles, T.: Effects and elimination of Prednisolone in physically trained and untrained subjects. Int. Z. Angew. Physiol. 28: 131, 1970.
46. Fox, S. M., III: Cardioprotection through physical activity. Paper presented at the Preventive Myocardiology meeting of the American College of Cardiology, Stowe, Vermont, June 1970, in press.
47. Haskell, W. L.: Physical activity and the prevention of coronary heart disease: what type exercise might be effective. J. S. Carolina Med. Ass. 65 (Suppl. 1): 41, 1969.

30

Patterns of Coronary Collateral Circulation in Angina Pectoris: Relation to Exercise Training

ALBERT A. KATTUS, M.D., AND
JULIUS GROLLMAN, M.D.

That the exercise tolerance of patients with angina pectoris may be greatly improved with regular exercise has been documented in our laboratory and in others.[1-3] To explain this phenomenon, it has been suggested that the ischemic human heart may respond in the same way that the dog heart responds to coronary ligation: with a rapid development of the collateral circulation, which is greatly enhanced in those dogs that are subjected to regular exercise.[4] The question then which we seek to answer in this chapter is: does the improved performance of patients with angina pectoris who participate in active training result from enhancement of the coronary collateral circulation? The evidence bearing on this question is derived from the study of 14 patients whom we have followed over extended periods of time and who have had coronary angiograms performed on two or more occasions separated by 1 year or more. Each of these patients had serial treadmill exercise tolerance tests. Six of the subjects had significant improvement in exercise capacity associated with a program of regular walking exercise. Four subjects failed to increase exercise capacity despite faithful adherence to a walking exercise program, and four had continued poor performances while remaining sedentary.

The findings suggest that the development of coronary collateral patterns is determined primarily by the degree of obstruction in the artery being fed by collaterals and by the availability of an unobstructed neighboring vessel which may serve as a source of supply to the obstructed segment. No enhancement of coronary collateral pattern was found that could be attributed solely to the exercise program.

METHODS

The patients were all men who had been referred to members of the Division of Cardiology at the UCLA Medical Center for evaluation of angina pectoris. They ranged in age from 33 to 58, the average being 46 years. The severity of angina was evaluated by a method of standard treadmill testing which has been developed in our laboratory. The treadmill test requires the patient to walk on a motor-driven treadmill with an upward tilt of 10 per cent. Walking is begun at 1 or $1\frac{1}{2}$ mph, and every 3 minutes the speed is accelerated by $\frac{1}{2}$ mile per hour. The test continues in 3-minute stages of walking at $1\frac{1}{2}$, 2, $2\frac{1}{2}$, 3, $3\frac{1}{2}$, 4, and sometimes $4\frac{1}{2}$ mph. A normal person has no difficulty completing the 4 or $4\frac{1}{2}$ mph stage. The patient with angina continues walking until he is stopped by symptoms that have reached a degree of intensity which he judges to be moderately severe, or 3+ on a scale of 4+. A single bipolar transthoracic electrocardiogram (ECG) lead is monitored throughout the test. Ischemic ST segment depression identifies the limiting symptom of chest pain as originating in the hypoxic myocardium. This test has been shown to be highly reproducible and quite sensitive in documenting changes in exercise tolerance in response to therapeutic measures.[5]

The coronary arteriograms were performed selectively by the techniques of Sones and Shirey[6] or Judkins,[7] sometimes employing a percutaneous entry into an arm or leg artery and sometimes employing arterial cut-down in the arm. Most studies were recorded on 35 mm. film which was subsequently reviewed and studied in detail. A few of the studies were recorded on roll film. Sketches were made to display the anatomy that had been defined by the angiographic studies. Figure 30.1, A displays photographs of views of selective cineangiograms from which the sketches were made. The right coronary artery is best visualized in the left anterior oblique projection, while the left coronary system is best viewed in the right oblique projection. Thus the sketches that are used for the basis of our report display the right coronary artery as though it were being seen in the left anterior oblique projection while the left coronary artery is presented as it is viewed in the right anterior oblique projection. The sketches derived from Figure 30.1, A relate to Patient 1, whose findings are displayed in Figure 30.1, B.

CASE REPORTS

Patients 1 through 6 are those who had improved exercise capacity as demonstrated by the treadmill test after a period of daily walking exercise.

Case 1. Patient I. L. was a 58-year-old man whose angina permitted him to complete only 2 minutes at the 2 mph stage of the treadmill test. One and one-half years later, after faithfully adhering to a training pro-

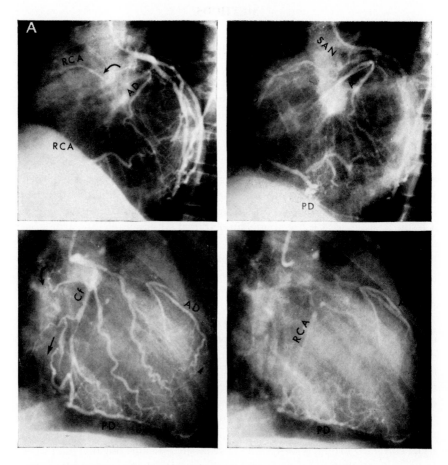

Fig. 30.1. Patient 1. A, single frames of cut film angiogram of left coronary artery injection in left oblique view above and right oblique view at bottom. To the left are early phases of injection and to the right, late phases. SAN, sinus node artery; RCA, right coronary artery; AD, anterior descending artery; PD, posterior descending artery; CF, circumflex artery; AVN, atrioventricular node artery. Arrows indicate pathways of collateral flow. B, diagrams of coronary arteriograms of 1966 and 1968. The right coronary artery is shown on the left and the left coronary artery on the right. Dotted segments are portions of arteries fed by collaterals. Arrows indicate directions of flow. At bottom are diagrams of treadmill tests. A full block is equal to 3 minutes of walking at the speed indicated at the top of the block. ST segment depression is indicated by check marks, and severity of angina is indicated by dots (1+ to 3+). Pulse rates at the end of exercise stages are indicated inside the blocks. EKG strips for various stages of exercise tests are displayed. See text for discussion.

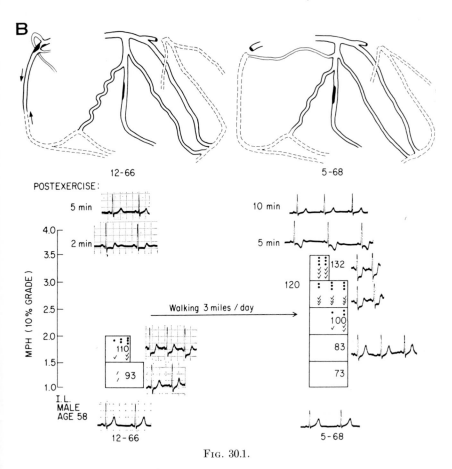

FIG. 30.1.

gram in which he walked 3 miles per day in 1 hour, his performance was much improved and he was then able to complete 2 minutes at the 3½ mph stage of the test. The coronary arteriogram in the original study showed a high grade stenosis of the right coronary artery with some primary filling from the right but also with collateral filling coming in from a visible branch of the circumflex system. The anterior descending coronary was completely occluded and was being fed by collateral from its diagonal branch and also from the marginal branch of the circumflex. After the improvement in capacity, the repeat study disclosed that the right coronary had then closed off completely and the right was being filled exclusively by collateral circulation. At this time, a small atrial branch could be seen coming from the circumflex system and entering the right coronary distal to the occlusion; the circumflex feed-in remained as before, as did the collateralization of the anterior descending. The development of the small atrial collateral channel feeding into the proximal right coronary would appear to be primarily related to the complete closure of the right coronary. The major pathways of collateralization through the circumflex and anterior descending systems did not appear to be altered. Thus, no changes in collateral pattern could be seen that would be attributable to the exercise training program.

Case 2 (Fig. 30.2). M. P., a 49-year-old man, was first studied in 1963, but the first treadmill test was recorded in 1964. This was not a standardized treadmill test but in it he was able to walk for 7 minutes at 3 mph. Two years later after following a walking program consisting of 3 to 4 miles of brisk walking at least 5 days a week, he had improved his performance so that he was able to complete the 4 mph stage of the treadmill test. The original coronary angiogram showed a complete occlusion of the anterior descending with collateral feeding in from the right side. Local stenotic lesions were present in the right coronary artery. Two and one-half years later, when the improved exercise capacity was documented, the coronary arteriogram was repeated and at this time an atrial branch of the proximal

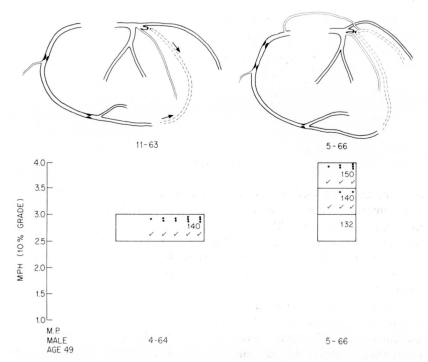

Fig. 30.2. Patient 2. Coronary angiograms of 1963 and 1966 are shown above, treadmill tests below. The first treadmill test was not done in the standard manner. The patient performed for 7 minutes at 3 mph. The second test was done in a standard manner and permitted completion of the 4 mph stage.

right coronary could be seen feeding into the proximal anterior descending coronary just beyond the area of obstruction. It was then noted that a new major stenotic area had appeared in the proximal right coronary artery, presumably reducing the effective pressure head feeding into the distal left anterior descending collateral system. The appearance of the auxiliary pathway of collateralization would seemingly have been necessitated by the progression of the disease in the collateral feed-in system, namely, the right coronary artery. There seems no justification for attributing this new collateral pathway specifically to the exercise program.

Case 3 (Fig. 30.3). Patient C. V., a 48-year-old man, had moderate impairment of his exercise capacity when he was first studied in 1967, being able to complete 1 minute at the 3 mph level of the treadmill test. About 1 year later, after pursuing a vigorous walking program covering 6 miles almost every day, he was able to complete the $3\frac{1}{2}$ mph stage of the treadmill test. The initial coronary arteriogram showed complete obstruction of the right coronary artery with only poor collateral filling of the distal portions of this vessel through a small branch of the circumflex artery. A severe

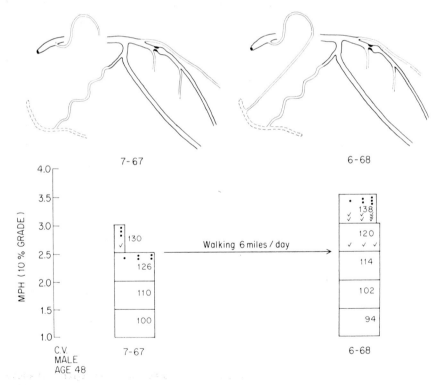

Fig. 30.3. Patient 3. Coronary angiograms of 1967 and 1968 are diagrammed above and standard treadmill tests are shown below.

stenosis in the anterior descending system was also present. One year later
when the improved performance was documented, there was a slight change
in the collateral pattern in that a proximal right atrial branch was then
seen to connect up through a very fine channel into the distal right coronary, presumably adding slightly to the perfusion of this vessel. But there
was no improvement in the extent of filling of the distal right coronary
artery, and one could hardly attribute the improved performance to enhancement of the collateralization of the right coronary system.

Case 4 (Fig. 30.4). H. S. was a 55-year-old man with very severe effort
as well as decubitus angina requiring as many as 40 to 50 nitroglycerin
tablets a day. When he was first seen in 1963, he was able to complete only
2½ minutes on the treadmill at 1½ mph. Because of his severe degree of
incapacity, he was offered surgery but turned it down in favor of an exercise program. He faithfully adhered to the training program, at first being
able to walk only about 100 feet at a time, later on gradually improving
his walking capacity until at the end of 1 year he was able to walk 1½ miles
each day in 45 minutes. The second treadmill test was not done in the
standard manner, but at that time he was able to complete 15 minutes of

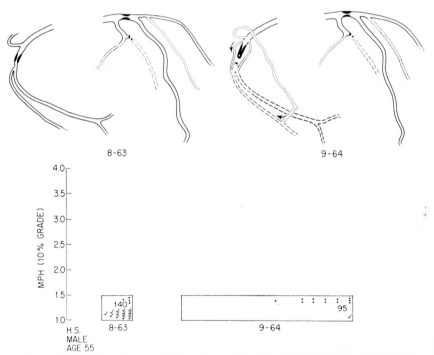

FIG. 30.4. Patient 4. Coronary angiograms of 1963 and 1964 are diagrammed above
and treadmill tests are shown below. The 1964 treadmill test was not standard: 1½
mph for 15 minutes.

walking at 1½ mph. The coronary anatomy during the initial study showed very high grade stenosis in the right coronary system and in the anterior descending coronary, with total occlusion of a marginal circumflex branch and faint collateralization of this vessel. One year later the right coronary stenosis had gone to complete occlusion and was being bridged by local collaterals, as well as by connections through a right ventricular branch. The anatomy of the left coronary system had not changed at all. Thus the enhancement of the collateralization of the distal right coronary would appear to be more reasonably determined by the progression of the stenotic lesion to complete closure, thus providing the hemodynamic pressure gradient leading to the development of collateralization. One could hardly attribute the change to the exercise itself.

Case 5 (Fig. 30.5). R. E., a 46-year-old carpenter who was disabled because of frequent and severe angina of effort, was followed over a 5-year period. A daily walking program, consisting of 4 miles a day covered in 1 hour, was pursued faithfully. This resulted in a dramatic improvement in his exercise tolerance, permitting him to complete 2 minutes of walking at 4½ mph before being stopped by fatigue, but with no sign of angina and no ischemic manifestations in the electrocardiogram. At the same time, the angina had completely disappeared from his daily life and he was able to resume his usual occupation without restriction. Coronary arteriograms recorded at the beginning and the end of this period disclosed two areas of local stenosis in the mid right coronary artery and one area of local stenosis at the origin of the anterior descending coronary artery. One year later when he was completely free of angina and had an excellent exercise tolerance, the coronary arteriogram disclosed that the original stenotic lesions remained as before and a new one had appeared in the distal portion of the right coronary artery. Thus, despite the fact that this patient had shown dramatic improvement in exercise capacity, there was no alteration in the obstructive disease and, indeed, there appeared to be progression. No sign of collateralization could be found. The patient's state of improved performance continued until February of 1969, at which time he suffered an acute anterior myocardial infarction from which he recovered. One year later the angiogram was repeated because the patient found that his exercise tolerance had been significantly diminished and he was no longer able to carry out his regular occupation without considerable distress from fatigue and occasional anginal episodes. His exercise tolerance had significantly deteriorated, but the treadmill test did not elicit anginal pain or ST segment depression. He was forced to stop at the 3 mph level because of fatigue. The arteriogram showed that the anterior descending coronary artery had become occluded but was filled slowly through a hairline opening, as shown by the injection of contrast media into the left coronary artery. The right coronary injection also resulted in retrograde filling of the anterior descend-

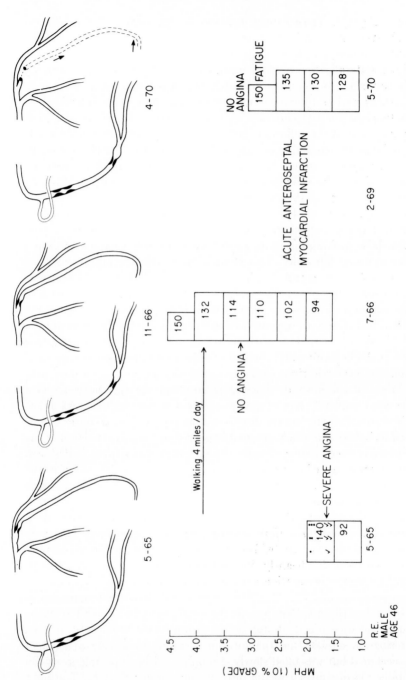

FIG. 30.5 Patient 5. Coronary angiogram diagrams appear above and treadmill tests below. This patient showed a great improvement in exercise capacity without the development of collaterals. Myocardial infarction was followed by the development of collateral circulation to the obstructed artery.

ing coronary from the distal branches of the posterior descending branch of the right. Thus this man's collateral pattern appeared to have been generated by the occlusion of the proximal anterior descending coronary. In this particular case, a certain insight into the physiology of the coronary collaterals may be deduced because it is clear that the local stenotic lesions in the right coronary were not sufficiently occlusive to prevent the flow of contrast material from the right to the anterior descending through the collaterals. This would suggest that a sufficient head of pressure could be transmitted through this partially occluded vessel to overcome the small head of pressure that was feeding into the distal portion of the anterior descending through the tiny hairline lumen, presumably occurring through recanalization of the thrombus that led to the infarction 1 year before. The finding is strongly indicative of the concept that the collateral filling of an occluded vessel is a result of an adequate pressure gradient between the low pressure occluded vessel and the higher pressure entering from the vessel that supplies the collateral. Thus, if there were high enough pressure in the donor vessel to provide collateralization, then the obstructive disease may not be as severe as is apparent from the angiogram, and the fact that this obstruction was not severe is what may have permitted the patient to improve his performance on the exercise program prior to the onset of his myocardial infarction.

Case 6 (Fig. 30.6). C. K. was a 38-year-old building contractor who had a 3-month history of anginal pain waking him from his sleep at night, despite the fact that his exercise tolerance was excellent, permitting him to go deer hunting at 7,000 feet altitude with no distress whatsoever. Holter tape recordings made while the patient was sleeping disclosed marked ischemic ST segment depression in the electrocardiogram, coinciding with the anginal distress that would waken him from sleep. On the other hand, treadmill performance was excellent, with anginal pain and ischemic ST segment depression appearing only at high levels of exercise. This syndrome corresponds to the inverse angina syndrome first described by Prinzmetal *et al.*[8] The coronary arteriogram disclosed a high degree of stenosis in the proximal portion of the anterior descending coronary artery and no other lesions anywhere in the coronary circulation. No collateral circulation was present. On a daily exercise program consisting of 2 miles a day of brisk walking which was completed in less than 30 minutes, the patient gradually lost all symptoms either of nighttime angina or angina with high levels of exercise. When he was studied 1 year later, he was able to complete 4½ mph on the treadmill without the appearance of substernal distress or of ischemic ST segment depression. Thus, the exercise program had resulted in a complete disappearance of the anginal syndrome. A repeat coronary arteriogram at that time disclosed that the local stenotic segment remained exactly as

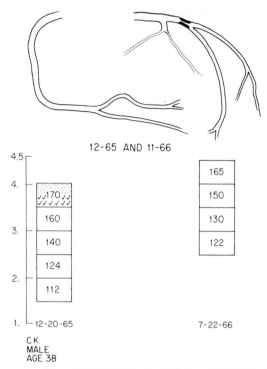

FIG. 30.6. Patient 6. The coronary angiogram diagram above shows that the single local stenosis of the anterior descending coronary artery had not changed, even though the patient was completely relieved of angina. No collateral circulation was present.

before, and no change whatsoever in the coronary anatomy could be discerned. In this man, then, an exercise program which resulted in complete alleviation of anginal disease did not lead to the development of collateral circulation, nor did it produce any discernible alteration of the coronary anatomy.

The next group of four patients is composed of individuals who faithfully adhered to an exercise program but showed no improvement in exercise capacity.

Case 7 (Fig. 30.7). D. M. was a 35-year-old male school teacher whose angina of effort permitted him to complete 2 minutes of walking at the 3 mph level before he was stopped by 3+ anginal pain. A walking program was instituted, consisting of 3 miles a day of brisk walking at a speed of approximately 4 mph. In the space of 1 year, his performance was improved to the point where he could complete 2 minutes at 4 mph befo:e being stopped by 3+ angina. During the next 4 years, however, he deteriorated steadily, and by 1970 his exercise tolerance had declined until he was able

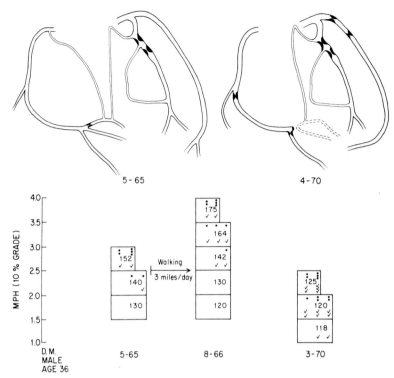

Fig. 30.7. Patient 7. Coronary angiograms show collateral development after total occlusion of the distal right coronary artery. Advancing disease was associated with reduced exercise capacity.

to complete only 2 minutes at the $2\frac{1}{2}$ mph stage of the treadmill test. A repeat coronary arteriogram at that time disclosed that the severe local stenotic lesions in the marginal circumflex branch remained unchanged but the distal right coronary artery was then occluded, new stenotic lesions had appeared in the anterior descending, and new stenotic lesions were present in the mid portion of the right coronary and in the proximal posterior descending branch of the right. The distal right coronary was receiving collateral input from an atrial branch originating in the circumflex artery; a right ventricular branch that had been visible in 1965 going from the proximal right coronary to the distal was no longer visible. During the intervening 4 years, the patient had adhered faithfully to his daily walking program but he found he was having more angina and frequently required nitroglycerin in order to complete his daily walk. The coronary collateral pattern feeding the distal right coronary artery beyond the site of occlusion was entering via visible pathways that were present before the occlusion had taken place; thus, the exercise did not have anything to do with the appearance of his collateral pattern, and the deterioration of his condition following an initial improvement was clearly explainable on the basis of advancing atheromatous disease in both the right and anterior descending coronary arteries.

Case 8 (Fig. 30.8). V. S. was a 55-year-old man with severe effort angina and a very low exercise capacity requiring him to stop treadmill walking in the 1½ mph stage. A 2-year program of weight reduction and regular walking exercise failed to result in any significant degree of clinical improvement or in increased exercise tolerance. Coronary arteriograms carried out 2 years apart disclosed complete occlusion of the right coronary artery with collateralization through its own atrial branch. There was no alteration of this pattern in 2 years. The total occlusion of the circumflex and its secondary marginal branch resulted in collateralization from its own primary marginal branch. This pattern also remained unchanged. However, severe stenotic disease had appeared in the intervening time in the anterior descending system. It appears likely that any improvement that might have been achieved from the walking program was nullified by the development of significant stenosis in the one remaining open coronary artery

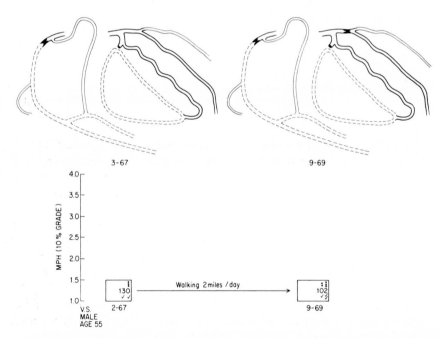

Fig. 30.8. Patient 8. Coronary angiograms of 1967 and 1969 above show that the collateral pattern was unchanged, but that stenosis of the anterior descending branch was advancing. The patient's very low exercise tolerance was indicated by treadmill tests, shown at bottom.

Exercise therefore failed to have any effect on the collateral patterns in this example.

Case 9 (Fig. 30.9). B. B. was a 48-year-old milkman who had to stop working because he could not carry his containers of milk up stairways because of anginal distress. His exercise capacity was poor, and he had to stop in the 2½ mph stage of the treadmill test. He subsequently had a Vineberg type of implantation operation, which failed to improve his function. He continued with a walking program of 1½ to 2 miles each day, which also failed to improve his symptoms or his exercise capacity. Three years after his original study, his exercise capacity was unchanged. Coronary arteriograms, which originally showed a high degree of stenosis in the right coronary artery, subsequently disclosed a second area of stenosis more proximally, but the collateral connection between the proximal branch and the distal right coronary artery was unchanged. On the left side, stenotic disease in the anterior descending artery remained unchanged. The circumflex was totally occluded to begin with but showed slight collateralization.

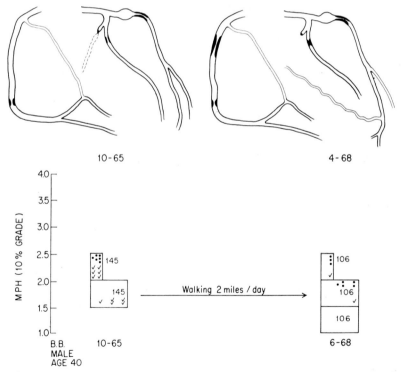

FIG. 30.9. Patient 9. Coronary angiograms of 1965 and 1968 show the advance of obstructive disease and the disappearance of the previously existing circumflex collateral. No change in treadmill exercise tolerance occurred.

This could no longer be visualized in the second study, and a new area of high grade stenosis in the marginal branch of the circumflex became apparent. In the second study, a far distal branch of the anterior descending coursing toward the right ventricle could be seen, but this did not seem to connect with any of the major coronary branches. Thus, in this patient the exercise program did not result in any enhancement of collateral formation. There was clear evidence of progression of the primary disease in the major coronary arteries.

Case 10 (Fig. 30.10). L. H. a 42-year-old male truck driver who was unable to work because of severe effort angina which permitted him to complete only 2 minutes of the 2 mph stage of the treadmill test. On an exercise program of 3 miles a day walking at a brisk pace, his exercise tolerance dramatically improved so that in the space of 9 months his performance carried him into the $3\frac{1}{2}$ mph stage of the test. Over the next 2 years, however, there was a gradual deterioration until in February 1970 his exercise tolerance had declined to the level at which he had begun in 1967, with termination of the exercise test in the 2 mph stage. A repeat angiogram in 1970 showed that the areas of local stenosis previously present

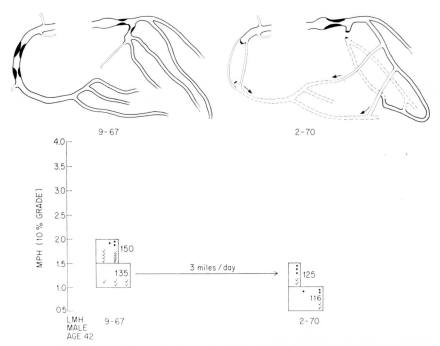

Fig. 30.10. Patient 10. Coronary angiograms of 1968 and 1970 show the development of collateral circulation following complete occlusion of the right coronary and circumflex which had previously been stenotic. Treadmill exercise capacity has deteriorated as collateral has developed.

in the right coronary artery had gone on to complete occlusion with the collateral now entering the right coronary from the left-sided injection. The local stenotic lesion in the left main coronary remained the same. Furthermore, the left circumflex was occluded at its origin and filled only partially by way of retrograde flow from the anterior descending through a marginal branch. In this man, then, the original improvement in exercise capacity was nullified by the progression of the atheromatous disease, resulting in complete occlusion of both the right and the circumflex coronary arteries then being filled by collaterals. It would appear from this observation that the development of the collateral filling was obligatory, following the total occlusion of the mainline branches. Since there was steady deterioration as these collaterals developed, we can document no suggestion of enhancement of collateral function by the exercise program.

In the foregoing group of four individuals in whom exercise training programs did not result in improved performance, it was found that collateral circulation appeared to generate in response to advancing degrees of coronary occlusion. No relation to exercise therapy could be discerned.

In the final group of four patients, we report observations on subjects who remained sedentary and made no attempt to enhance their capacity by exercise training programs.

Case 11 (Fig. 30.11). R. A. was a 43-year-old man who was observed over a period of 7 years. When he was first seen in 1963, his exercise tolerance required him to stop exercise in the $2\frac{1}{2}$ mph stage of the test. On a walking program over the next 2 years, his exercise tolerance greatly improved until he was able to complete the 4 mph stage of the test. This was achieved through regular walking exercise, 2 miles per day. Between 1965 and 1966, however, he had a steady worsening during a period when he had abandoned his exercise program. By November of 1966, his exercise tolerance had been reduced two stages and he was then required to stop in the 3 mph stage of the test. Angiograms taken in 1963 and 1966 both showed that the circumflex coronary system was totally occluded and being fed richly by collaterals from the right coronary. The deterioration in function seen in 1966 appeared to be due to the development of a high grade stenosis in the proximal right coronary, along with an additional area of stenosis in the more distal right coronary. As this was the main feeder channel for the collateral to the circumflex system, it appeared that this collateralization source was being throttled. In 1968 a Vineberg type of arterial implantation operation was carried out because of increasingly severe angina. In the following year, the patient's exercise tolerance was not significantly improved, being terminated in the $2\frac{1}{2}$ mph stage of the test. At this time, a repeat angiogram showed that the Vineberg implant was not functioning, the proximal stenosis in the right was more advanced, and new collateralization could be seen coming through an atrial branch from the right to the

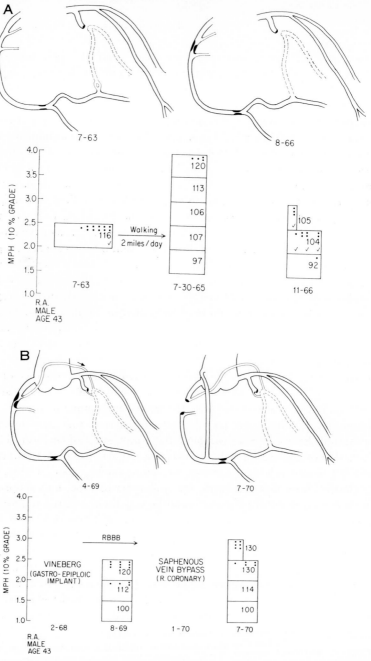

Fig. 30.11. Patient 11. A, coronary angiograms in 1963 and 1966 show complete obstruction of circumflex and collateral filling from the distal right coronary artery. As treadmill exercise capacity declined after cessation of the walking program, new stenosis appeared in the proximal right coronary artery. B, after gastro-epiploic implant surgery, function was not improved and proximal right stenosis was worse. New bridging collaterals are seen and new collateral has appeared in an atrial branch. Finally, a saphenous vein bypass graft was functional. The proximal right coronary artery had closed off, but maximal function of the graft was impeded by distal right stenosis.

circumflex and also local bridging collaterals from the proximal circumflex to the distal vessels beyond the area of occlusion. In January 1970, a saphenous vein bypass graft was carried out from the root of the aorta to the more distal right coronary artery. Only slight improvement in function was demonstrated over the next several months, and in July of 1970 a repeat angiogram showed that the bypass graft was indeed open and perfusing the distal right coronary artery, which had totally occluded at the area of the proximal stenosis. Optimal function of the right coronary system was prohibited by the presence of a local stenotic lesion in the distal right coronary just proximal to its bifurcation. Collateralization of the circumflex system remained the same as before via the proximal right coronary atrial branch and also via the distal right coronary.

In this series of four observations, then, it is seen that collateral function was throttled by the appearance of new stenotic disease in the donor artery. This was compensated for to some extent by the development of new collateral, but it is clear that this new collateral development cannot be attributed to exercise since no exercise program was followed; rather it was due to hemodynamic factors resulting from the closing off of the primary collateral supply by advancing atheromatous disease in the donor branch. The appearance of the vein graft indicates that it was functioning, but it was not functioning optimally because of a significant stenotic lesion between it and the vascular bed feeding the ischemic area.

Case 12 (Fig. 30.12). J. G., a 54-year-old male, had a poor exercise tolerance in 1963 when he was able to complete only the 2 mph stage of the treadmill test. When he was restudied in 1970, he could walk only on the level rather than the 10 per cent grade and was able to complete 4 minutes at 2 mph before stopping with 3+ angina. The original study in 1963 showed that the coronary lesions consisted of a high degree of stenosis in the mid right coronary artery and in the circumflex coronary system. In 1970 the right coronary and the circumflex had been completely occluded and were being fed by collaterals. In addition, a new area of high grade stenosis had appeared in the anterior descending coronary system. In this example, then, elaborate coronary collateral systems had been established in the absence of any exercise training program. These systems would appear to be related to the hemodynamic facts of total coronary occlusion demanding collateral flow.

Case 13 (Fig. 30.13). R. B. was first studied in 1960 when he was found to have angina at a time when he was referred for repair of an aortic coarctation. His exercise tolerance permitted him to complete the 2 mph stage of the treadmill test at that time. The coronary obstructive lesions did not appear to be far enough advanced to interfere with the proposed coarctation surgical repair, which was successfully carried out in 1961. His angina was markedly improved in the next several months, but thereafter it again

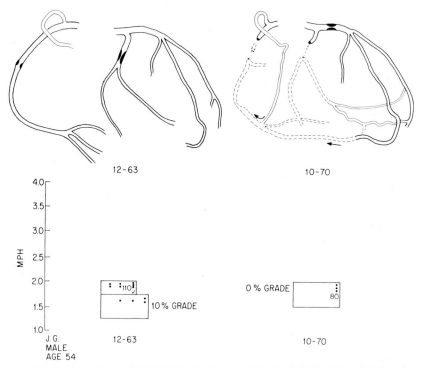

Fig. 30.12. Patient 12. Coronary angiograms of 1963 and 1970 show the development of an elaborate collateral system following total occlusion of right and circumflex systems. Treadmill exercise capacity deteriorated since the initial test was done at a 10 per cent upgrade, while the 1970 treadmill test could only be done with level walking.

began to deteriorate, and by the middle of 1963 his exercise tolerance was again at the 2 mph level. Repeat coronary arteriography disclosed that the stenotic lesion in the anterior descending system had gone to complete occlusion and was being fed by collaterals. A distal occlusion occurred in the right coronary, resulting in collateralization of the distal right coronary system, and a local area of stenosis in the mid right coronary remained unchanged. In this situation, then, the collateralization appears to have been related primarily to total occlusion of the coronary arteries. Since no exercise program was followed, this collateral development cannot be attributed to this cause.

Case 14 (Fig. 30.14). H. G. was a 44-year-old male whose exercise capacity was sharply reduced by severe angina pectoris, permitting him to complete only the 2 mph stage of the treadmill test. When he was restudied 4 years later, there was no change in his exercise capacity. Coronary arteriograms made in 1963 and 1967 showed no discernible change. In each

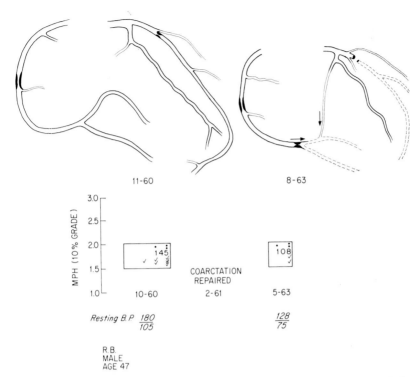

FIG. 30.13. Patient 13. Initial coronary angiogram and treadmill test carried out prior to repair of aortic coarctation. Blood pressure was high at first and low later on. Collateral circulation appeared after occlusion of the anterior descending coronary and distal right coronary artery. Treadmill exercise tolerance remained low.

there was total proximal right coronary occlusion with collateral filling beyond and anterior descending total occlusion with collateral filling beyond. The left coronary system was filling the distal right coronary via the circumflex branch, while the anterior descending system was being filled by right coronary branches which arose from this vessel proximal to its total occlusion. Thus there was reciprocal filling from right to left and left to right, which resulted in a stable situation that did not change over a period of 4 years. This well-developed collateral system could not be attributed to exercise training, since no such training was carried out.

DISCUSSION

In this study of 14 patients, we have attempted to relate the patterns of coronary collateral circulation to the improvement or nonimprovement of exercise capacity as determined by treadmill testing. This was done to test the hypothesis that exercise training improves the performance of the

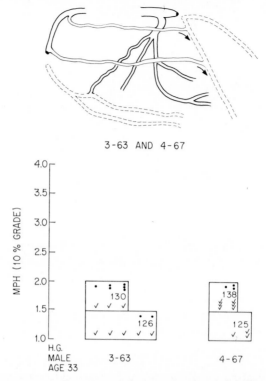

FIG. 30.14. Patient 14. Coronary angiograms in 1963 and 1967 appear exactly the same. Occlusions were complete and collateral patterns remained stable. Exercise tolerance on treadmill testing remained unaltered.

ischemic heart through the mechanism of enhancement of the coronary collateral circulation. Examination of the data as summarized in Table 30.1 requires rejection of the hypothesis. While patients 1 through 6 all showed improved exercise capacity in response to a training program, two of them did so without collateral circulation being present at all. Of the four who did demonstrate increased collateral, three had advancing occlusive disease to explain the increased collateral. In one, collateral developed only after a complete occlusion led to infarction.

In the group of four subjects (Patients 7 through 10) who failed to improve performance despite faithful adherence to an exercise program, advancing obstructive disease in the major coronary arteries was found to be the principal explanation for failure to improve. Collateral circulation was actually reduced in two of these subjects. Thus there was no evidence of collateral enhancement resulting from exercise in this group.

In the Patients 11 through 14, who did not exercise, an increased collateral pattern was observed in three, despite reduced or unchanged exercise capacity. In all three of these patients, the collateral enhancement was clearly due to the development of complete obstructions in major coronary arteries and not to exercise, since exercise was not performed.

The evidence strongly indicates that complete or almost complete obstruction of a coronary artery is the major stimulus to the development of collateral channels. It has been pointed out by James[10] that the development of collateral circulation may be limited by obstructive disease in the potential donor vessels, but we have found that some donor arteries continue to feed the collateral system despite what appear to be high degrees of stenosis as seen on the coronary angiograms (Cases 1, 5, 11, and 12). This finding indicates the difficulty of interpreting the degree of obstruction to flow offered by a stenotic lesion as seen on the cine-X-ray film. What appears to be a tight stenosis may in fact permit collateral filling of the other side (Cases 5 and 12). On the other hand, progressive stenosis on the donor side may compel the opening of alternate pathways of feeding the obstructed vessel (Cases 2 and 11).

The conclusion must be reached that the coronary collateral anatomy as visualized by the cineangiogram is not influenced significantly by exercise training programs, even though exercise capacity may be greatly improved. It is possible, however, that the blood flow through these collaterals may be increased by exercise training since flow is not measured by the angiographic technique.

The study does engender the strong impression that collateral coronary circulation, no matter how well developed, can never compensate completely for an obstructed major coronary artery. Most of the cases in this series in which the collateral system was well developed, feeding into an area beyond a total coronary occlusion, continued to have limitation of exercise capacity and marked ischemic changes in the exercise ECG. The two patients whose exercise performance became completely normal on following exercise training programs had major stenotic lesions but no occlusions and no collateral circulation.

The reason why the human patient with coronary artery disease does not behave like Eckstein's dogs with ligated coronary arteries is undoubtedly a species difference between canine arteries that are soft, pliable and free of disease, and human arteries encrusted with extensive atheroma.

CONCLUSION

Patients with angina pectoris who exercise regularly by walking 2 to 6 miles per day may improve their exercise capacity and reduce their anginal symptoms. This improvement cannot be attributed to an increase in the abundance of visible coronary collateral channels as detected by coronary arteriography. It is possible that blood flow may increase through collateral

Table 30.1

Patient	Sex	Age	Angina type	Duration of angina at first study	History of infarct	Change in degree of major artery obstruction	Change in collateral	Change in exercise capacity	Remarks
Exercise: improved									
1. I. L.	M	58	Effort + rest	12½ yr.	No	Advance	Increased	Improved 3 stages	Mild angina, 12 yr.; severe angina, 2 yr.
2. M. P.	M	49	Effort	3 yr.	No	Advance	Increased	Improved 2 stages	
3. C. V.	M	48	Effort	32 mo.	Yes	No change	Increased	Improved 1 stage	
4. H. S.	M	55	Effort + rest	7 yr.	Yes	Advance	Increased	Improved 3-15 min.	
5. R. E.	M	46	Effort	4 mo.	Yes	No change	No collateral	Improved 5 stages	Developed collateral only after infarct
6. C. K.	M	38	Inverse (rest)	3 mo.	No	No change	No collateral	Improved 1 stage	Angina completely relieved
Exercise: not improved									
7. D. M.	M	35	Effort	3 yr.	No	Advance	Reduced	Deteriorated 3 stages	
8. V. S.	M	55	Effort + rest	15 yr.	Yes	Advance	No change	No change	
9. B. B.	M	40	Effort	21 mo.	No	Advance	Reduced	No change	
10. L. H.	M	42	Effort + rest	6 yr.	Yes	Advance	Increased	Reduced	

No exercise: not improved								
11. R. A.	M	43	Effort	11 mo.	No	Advance	Increased	Reduced	Rest angina in recent 2 years
12. J. G.	M	54	Effort	15 mo.	No	Advance	Increased	Reduced	Rest angina in recent years
13. R. B.	M	47	Effort	6 mo.	No	Advance	Increased	No change	Coarctation repair, 1961
14. H. G.	M	33	Effort	1½–2 yr.	Yes	No change	No change	No change	

pathways without a visible change in the anatomic features as seen by X-ray. The most powerful stimulus to the development of collateral channels in the coronary circulation appears to be the occurrence of occlusion of major arteries.

Acknowledgements: The invaluable assistance of Mr. Paul Smokler and the UCLA Department of Academic Communications in preparing the illustrations and of Mrs. Frances Hetz in preparing the manuscript are gratefully acknowledged.

This study was supported by Grants HE-08470 and HE-11823 from the National Heart and Lung Institute of the United States Public Health Service and by USPHS Grant FR-00238 in support of the UCLA Clinical Research Center; also by the Reschke, Binnay Memorial Research Fund.

REFERENCES

1. Kattus, A. A.: Physical training and beta-adrenergic blocking drugs in modifying coronary insufficiency. In Marchetti, G., and Taccardi, B. (eds.): *Coronary Circulation and Energetics of the Myocardium.* S. Karger, Basel, 1967, p. 302.
2. Hellerstein, H. K.: Exercise therapy in coronary disease. Bull. N. Y. Acad. Med. 44: 1028, 1968.
3. Kaufman, J. M., and Anslow, R. D.: Treatment of refractory angina pectoris with nitroglycerin and graded exercise. J. A. M. A. 196: 137, 1966.
4. Eckstein, R. W.: Effect of exercise and coronary artery narrowing on coronary collateral circulation. Circ. Res. 5: 230, 1957.
5. Kattus, A. A., Alvaro, A. B., and MacAlpin, R. N.: Treadmill exercise tests for capacity and adaptation in angina pectoris. J. Occup. Med. 10: 627, 1968.
6. Sones, F. M., and Shirey, E. G.: Cine coronary arteriography. Mod. Concepts Cardiovasc. Dis. 31: 735, 1962.
7. Judkins, M. P.: Percutaneous transfemoral selective coronary arteriography. Radiol. Clin. N. Amer. 6: 467, 1968.
8. Prinzmetal, M., Kennamer, R., Merliss, R., Wada, T., and Bor, N.: Angina pectoris. I. A variant form of angina pectoris. Amer. J. Med. 27: 375, 1959.
9. Kattus, A. A., Hanafee, W. N., Longmire, W. P., MacAlpin, R. N., and Rivin, A. H.: Diagnosis, medical and surgical management of coronary insufficiency. Ann. Intern. Med. 69: 115, 1968.
10. James, T. N.: The delivery and distribution of coronary collateral circulation. Chest 58: 183, 1970.

31

The Physiology of Physical Fitness: A Relevant Curriculum for the Cardiac Patient

ROY J. SHEPHARD, M.D., Ph.D.

In these days of dissent, a university professor is lucky if he completes a lecture without a verbal or even a physical confrontation on the relevance of the material he is presenting. Dissent is now spreading to scientific meetings and, in order to forestall excessive audience participation, I will myself ask the stock question: is the physiology of physical fitness a relevant item of curriculum for the cardiac patient—or indeed for his physician?

The objectives of both the patient and the physician should be twofold: to halt the disease process and to restore as rapidly and as completely as possible the total adaptation of the patient to his environment. Exercise has little relevance to the first objective; indeed, it is contraindicated in the acute phases of cardiac disease. It has considerable relevance to the second objective, however, since fitness itself may be defined as "the physical, social, and psychological adjustment of the human organism to his environment."[1] No one would deny the tremendous importance to the cardiac patient of social and psychological problems but, lest our energies be dissipated over the entire field of human ecology, the present discussion is restricted largely to physical fitness.

PHYSICAL FITNESS

Physical fitness is itself a broad concept: "a vague malaise, accompanied by feverish activity, lasting about 3 weeks, and readily resolved by therapeutic doses of alcohol."* A committee of the World Health Organization spent almost a week of heated discussion, to conclude with the earth-shak-

---

* I believe this definition of physical fitness was first proposed by Dr. Warren R. Guild.

< 1 MIN	1 - 60 MIN	> 60 MIN
STRENGTH	AEROBIC POWER	FOOD
SKILL		FLUID
COORDINATION		HEAT LOSS
MOTIVATION		
O_2 DEBT		

FIG. 31.1. The relationship between the duration of physical activity and the necessary physical attributes.

ing discovery that fitness was "the ability to perform muscular work satisfactorily."[2]

For the younger man, it implies fitness for a place on the varsity team. With advancing years, the concept changes to control of a bulging waistline, prevention of cardiorespiratory disease, and even the maintenance of sufficient working capacity to meet the demands of office or factory, home and leisure. Women in general are less interested in development of skeletal or cardiac muscle but desire a good figure, good posture, and good body carriage. No one definition of fitness could cover all of these concepts. It is helpful to think in terms of the duration of activity (Fig. 31.1). If this is less than 1 minute, muscle strength, coordination, agility, motivation, and tolerance of oxygen debt are important. If the activity lasts for 1 minute to 1 hour, physical fitness is still influenced by these factors, but they become progressively subordinate to the ability of the body to transport oxygen from the atmosphere to the working tissues. If exercise is continued for longer than 1 hour, the extent and availability of food and fluid and the maintenance of the heat balance in turn become of increasing importance.

The sprint athlete is interested in fitness for brief effort. The marathon runner is interested in periods of more than 1 hour. But the ordinary cardiac patient who wants to earn his living, to enjoy his leisure, and to control his weight is interested mainly in moderate periods of activity. He seeks what I have called cardiorespiratory or endurance fitness.[1]

ENDURANCE FITNESS

The prime feature that determines endurance is the quantity of oxygen that can be transported from the atmosphere to the active tissues: this is the maximal oxygen intake, or aerobic power. One may envisage oxygen transport as proceeding through a series of bottlenecks (Fig. 31.2). These include, in turn, ventilation, wastage of ventilatory effort in the dead

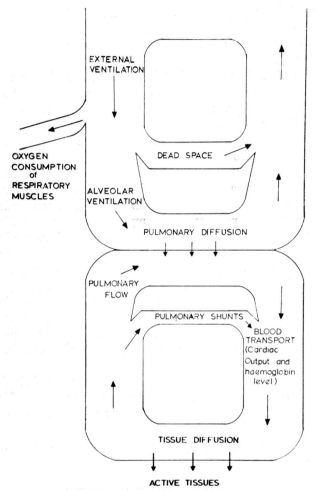

Fig. 31.2. Successive links in the oxygen transport chain from the atmosphere to the working tissues. (Reproduced from the *Ontario Medical Review* by permission of the publishers.)

space, consumption of oxygen by the chest muscles, the exchange of gas between lungs and blood, transport in the circulation, and the exchange of gas between the blood and active tissues.

One can represent the same sequence of events by a rather complex mathematical equation:

$$\frac{1}{\dot{U}} = \frac{1}{\dot{V}_A} + \left(\frac{B}{1-B}\right)\frac{1}{\lambda\dot{Q}} + \frac{1}{\lambda\dot{Q}} + \left(\frac{K}{1+K}\right)\frac{1}{\lambda\dot{Q}}$$

Here, $\dot{U}$ represents the overall transport, and the four terms on the right hand side of the equation are the respective contributions of alveolar ventilation, an interaction between pulmonary diffusion and blood transport, blood transport, and an interaction between tissue diffusion and blood transport.

In a normal, healthy person, the third term is by far the most important; oxygen transport depends largely on blood transport. Notice that the blood transport term has two parts: $\dot{Q}$, the maximal cardiac output, and λ, the solubility of oxygen in unit volume of blood. The latter depends in turn upon the hemoglobin level: a person with a low hemoglobin reading cannot expect to achieve a good oxygen transport.

In cardiac disease, several links in the oxygen transport chain may be impaired. Pulmonary congestion or edema may limit ventilatory effort and cause a poor intrapulmonary distribution of gas, thus reducing $\dot{V}_A$. Edema or changes in pulmonary capillary structure may modify diffusing capacity, thus restricting the second term. The maximal cardiac output may be reduced by valvular leakage, myocardial weakness, or the onset of symptoms and signs of myocardial oxygen lack. Tissue diffusion may also be restricted by degenerative changes in the vessels supplying the active muscles. At the same time, many patients show some polycythemia; this increases the value of λ, at the expense of a substantial increase in blood viscosity and thus cardiac work load. The net result of all these changes is a considerable decrease of maximal oxygen intake and thus of work tolerance.

The overall reduction in oxygen transport can often be elicited by simple clinical questioning.[3] But sometimes a remarkably healthy looking patient may swear that he is unable to walk as fast as his grandmother. He may seek compensation or have some other motive (perceived or partially perceived) for maximizing his symptoms. An objective test of the oxygen transport mechanism is then invaluable.

MAXIMAL OXYGEN INTAKE

If our intention were to test a young and athletic person, it would be a simple matter to take him to a laboratory, start him running on a treadmill, and increase either the speed or the slope of the running surface every minute until exhaustion was reached. Expired gas would be collected in large meteorological balloons, and the oxygen consumption would be calculated minute by minute. Let us watch such a test. As exhaustion is approached, the subject staggers along with a ghastly ashen gray pallor, uncertain whether he is speaking in English or Spanish, and eventually the point is reached where a further increase in the work performed no longer leads to an increase of oxygen consumption (Fig. 31.3). The directly measured maximal oxygen intake has been achieved.

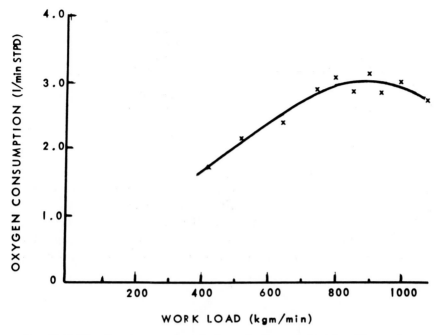

Fig. 31.3. The direct measurement of maximal oxygen intake. The work performed on a treadmill is increased in 5 per cent stages until a further increment of work load does not lead to any increase of oxygen consumption.

There are laboratories that use this approach with patients. Unfortunately, it works poorly on the type of patient who thinks he is more breathless than his grandmother; he just jumps off the treadmill. With more willing patients, there is a finite mortality, perhaps as high as one in 3000 tests on middle-aged men.

SUBMAXIMAL TESTS

It is more usual to assess cardiac patients from the response to submaximal effort. A bicycle ergometer or a step test may be used,[2, 4-6] and to advocate either procedure is a sure method of creating a confrontation (Fig. 31.4). The patient is exercised at three or four increasing work loads. In the absence of heart disease, 3 minutes at each load provides adequate time to attain a steady state but, if the circulation time is prolonged, 4 or more minutes may be required at any one intensity of exercise.

The pulse rate and electrocardiogram (ECG) waveform are monitored throughout exercise. An international committee has reviewed the possible placements of leads during exercise[7] and has recommended the CM_5 position as the best single placement of leads (Fig. 31.5). The oxygen consump-

Step	Bicycle
Familiar	Less familiar
Cheap	Costs $300 to $3000
No calibration	Calibration needed
Ancillary measurements difficult	Ancillary measurements easy
Looks simple	Looks impressive
Local fatigue unlikely	Local fatigue likely
Easy to lie down	Difficult to dismount

FIG. 31.4. A comparison of the step and the bicycle ergometer as means of performing submaximal exercise tests.

tion is best measured directly, but a family physician can predict it roughly from the work that is performed. On the bicycle ergometer, the effort is proportional to the loading of the belt and the number of pedal revolutions per minute. It is usually assumed that the patient attains a mechanical efficiency of 23 per cent. On the step test, the work performed is calculated from the product of step height, body weight, and the number of ascents

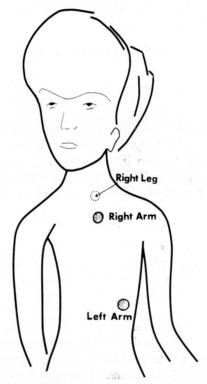

FIG. 31.5. Recommended placement of leads for exercise electrocardiography. (Reproduced from the author's book *Endurance Fitness*[1] by permission of the publishers.)

A. Work performed   = Weight (kg.) $\times$ step height (meters) $\times$ ascents per min.

                              = $75 \times 0.457 \times 20$

                              = 686 kg. m./min.

B. Work expenditure   = $\dfrac{686 \times 100}{16}$ = 4288 kg. m./min.

C. Oxygen expenditure   = $\dfrac{4288}{2135}$ = 2.01 l./min. STPD

D. Resting O_2 expenditure = 0.31 l./min. STPD

E. Total O_2 expenditure   = 2.32 l./min. STPD

FIG. 31.6. Estimation of oxygen consumption for patient weighing 75 kg. and ascending 18-inch (0.457 meter) step 20 times per minute. A, work performed; B, work expenditure (16 per cent efficiency); C, oxygen expenditure (2135 kg. m. = 1 liter of oxygen); D, resting oxygen expenditure (from tables); E, total oxygen expenditure = C + D.

per minute (Fig. 31.6). An efficiency of 16 per cent is assumed. Two factors may distort such calculations when they are applied to hospital patients. Lack of familiarity with the bicycle ergometer or the step test may lead to a certain clumsiness, reducing efficiency by 1 to 2 per cent[4]; on the other hand, an abnormally large proportion of the total effort may be sustained by anaerobic mechanisms, thus decreasing the apparent oxygen cost of a given effort.[8]

Data may be interpreted in several ways. With healthy patients, it is common to extrapolate the pulse-oxygen consumption line to the individual's presumed maximal heart rate, and from this to deduce the corresponding maximal oxygen intake (Fig. 31.7). Such an approach may work quite well for a symptomless patient who is recovering from a coronary attack. However, it is not applicable to the individual who has a tachycardia due to anxiety. Nor is it appropriate for the patient whose effort and thus maximal pulse rate are limited by arrhythmia, angina, or symptomless myocardial oxygen lack. The oxygen supply of the heart muscle is probably one determinant of maximal heart rate. Certainly, the maximal rate falls with the oxygen lack of high altitude,[9] and these changes are to some extent reversed by the administration of oxygen. Less is known about the maximal heart rate in patients with cardiac disease; the maximal attainable heart rate is often low for the individual, but it is less certain how far this limitation is physiological, how far it is symptomatic, and how far it is attributable simply to poor motivation.[10]

Irrespective of mechanisms, it is plainly wrong to extrapolate the pulse-oxygen intake line to a heart rate that can never be achieved. The alternative is to report responses at a measured or closely interpolated pulse rate. One well-known example of this is the PWC_{170}, the steady state rate of working at a pulse of 170 beats per minute. Here again, we have a difficulty. If a fixed pulse rate of 170 is chosen, the task is relatively easy for a

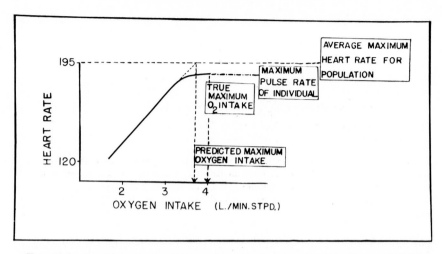

FIG. 31.7. Procedure for prediction of maximal oxygen intake. The straight-line relationship between heart rate and oxygen intake is extrapolated to the average maximal heart rate for the population in question, and a perpendicular is dropped to the oxygen intake scale. Any asymptote of oxygen intake or deviation of maximal pulse rate leads to inaccuracies in this prediction. L./MIN., liters per minute. (Reproduced from the author's book *Endurance Fitness*[1] by permission of the publishers.)

Age (years)	Target pulse rate (beats per minute)
20 - 30	160
30 - 40	150
40 - 50	140
50 - 60	130

FIG. 31.8. Age-related target pulse rates. The figures quoted correspond to an oxygen intake that is approximately 75 per cent of a normal individual's aerobic power.

young and healthy man but may well be impossible for an older cardiac patient. Physiologists are thus moving towards the idea of reporting responses—working capacity, oxygen intake, ST segmental depression and so on—at age-related target pulse rates (Fig. 31.8). These targets correspond to 75 per cent (or in some studies 85 per cent) of the aerobic power of a healthy individual.

WORK TOLERANCE

How do such figures relate to a patient's tolerance of daily work? Here, the guiding principle is a 50 per cent underload. It is unwise to run an

LIGHT WORK	$<$ 3.3 KCal/min
MODERATE WORK	3.3 - 5.4 KCal/min
HEAVY WORK	5.4 - 9.0 KCal/min
VERY HEAVY WORK	$<$ 9.0 KCal/min

FIG. 31.9. Rating of industrial activity in terms of energy expenditure.[11]

electric motor at more than 50 per cent of its rated power, and the same is true of man. Even if effort is not limited by symptoms of cardiac origin, attempts to sustain loads of more than 50 per cent of aerobic power over an 8-hour working day lead to fatigue, an increased incidence of injuries, and possibly (in the diseased heart) to decompensation.

Let us suppose that a patient has an oxygen consumption of 1.5 liters per min. when exercising at his target pulse rate. If this is 75 per cent of his aerobic power, he is unwise to develop an average daily oxygen consumption of more than 1 liter per min. The corresponding ceiling of daily energy expenditure is five times this reading, or 5 Kcal. per min. This would be sufficient to perform what the industrial physician would rate as light or moderate work (Fig. 31.9). It is about three times the resting energy expenditure. Fortunately, a greater energy demand is rare in the highly automated industrial plants of North America.

Interpretation of the 50 per cent loading is flexible and should take into account not only the average demands of an 8-hour shift but also any adverse factors in the working environment such as sudden peaks of more intense activity, isometric effort, awkwardness of posture, and a high environmental temperature.

CHANGES OF FITNESS WITH TRAINING

It is currently fashionable to propose training regimes for patients with a variety of cardiac and respiratory disorders. These regimes supposedly increase the aerobic power and thus the patient's effort tolerance. However, the physiological evidence for an improvement of physical condition is at best shaky. It is based on a change in the response to submaximal exercise; for instance, the pulse rate at a work load of 600 kg. per min. may have diminished from 140 to 120 beats per min., or the work performed at the target pulse rate may have increased from 750 to 900 kg. per min. To equate this unreservedly with an increase of aerobic power is to ignore the powerful effect of anxiety upon the pulse rate during submaximal exercise. The pulse rate of a normal, healthy patient may decline by 5 to 10 beats per min. as he becomes conditioned to the forbidding environment of treadmills, bicycles, and spirometers.[2, 12] How much larger the change in a patient who initially has fears regarding his cardiac status! This point is well brought out in recent controlled studies from this laboratory.[13] Post-myocardial infarction patients have been followed for a total of 24 months; some of our younger exercised patients are now pulling ahead but, over the first 12 months of rehabilitation, the improvement in exercise responses induced by regular physical training was no greater than that induced by an equivalent course of hypnotherapy.

This is not to deny that regular exercise can be of benefit to every cardiac patient; it can certainly help in controlling his weight, it may also modify the coagulability of the blood, stimulate the development of collateral blood vessels, reduce the stress imposed by exercise in an emergency, and help in a number of other ways. But conclusive documentation of most of these supposed benefits has yet to be obtained.

Sometimes, exercise to the level needed for an improvement of aerobic power cannot be attained. The patient may be afraid to exercise vigorously when away from a defibrillator and an attendant physician. Warning signs such as increasing angina and arrhythmias may indicate that the potential limit of an exercise program has been reached. Dr. Kavanagh and I have kept careful diary records of the activity of our coronary patients, and we have been surprised at how long it took for many of our exercise group to achieve the 30 points per week proposed by Cooper[14] for the establishment of even a minimal level of cardiorespiratory fitness.

LIFE STYLE

Perhaps the most important lesson from our study was the change in life style of the two groups. Some of the exercised patients became quite obsessional about achieving their daily points score. If this was not possible because of business commitments or for other reasons, they became even more tense and miserable than normal. On the other hand, the patients who dreamed of exercise under the guidance of the hypnotherapist became progressively more relaxed and a delight to both their office colleagues and their families.

The hypnotherapy patients also improved in physiological terms. Going back to our horrendous equation for oxygen transport, the limiting factor in many coronary patients is a poor maximal cardiac output. Symptoms prevent the attainment of the full potential maximal heart rate in the coronary patient. These symptoms are caused by a disproportion between cardiac work load and myocardial blood supply. Now, the work load of the heart depends much more upon the systemic blood pressure than on the volume of blood expelled per beat. Thus, if hypnotherapy controlled blood pressure more effectively than regular exercise, it could even be a better form of treatment. The same type of argument applies to muscle-building regimes. Normally, I am somewhat opposed to specific development of the skeletal muscles. Bulging biceps look very impressive on the cover of a magazine, but they add to the weight that must be carried by the heart. However, some development of the body musculature can help a coronary patient, particularly if his employment calls for intermittent activity of the isometric type, as in the carriage of heavy weights. The rise of blood pressure that occurs during isometric work is proportional to the force exerted, expressed as a percentage of maximal strength. If I have had a coronary attack, I shall avoid lifting pianos; but if this were my livelihood, studied inactivity might be more difficult. The remedy then would be to strengthen the muscles so that the same activity could be tolerated with a smaller rise of blood pressure.

RELEVANCE OF FITNESS

How relevant, then, is physical fitness to the life of the average cardiac patient? It may make him live a few years longer, but this has yet to be proven. It may improve the quality of his life. Many patients have been unnecessarily restricted in the past, and moderate activity will make for a happier and more useful life. But I am doubtful whether an obsessive search for fitness is either needed or desirable, particularly for the older patient. Certainly, we have no conclusive evidence that it is more rewarding to the patient or his family than a combination of more moderate activity and a relaxed attitude toward the total environment.

REFERENCES

1. Shephard, R. J.: *Endurance Fitness.* University of Toronto Press, Toronto, Ontario, Canada, 1969.
2. Shephard, R. J.: Rapporteur. Exercise tests in relation to cardiovascular function. World Health Organization Tech. Rep. 388, 1968.
3. Kellerman, J. J., Mann, A., and Kariv, I.: Functional evaluation of cardiac work capacity by spiro-ergometry in patients with rheumatic heart disease. Arch. Phys. Med. Rehab. 50: 189–193, 1969.
4. Shephard, R. J., Allen, C., Benade, A. J. S., Davies, C. T. M., diPrampero, P. E., Hedman, R., Merriman, J. E., Myhre, K., and Simmons, R.: Standardization of submaximal exercise test. Bull. W. H. O. 38: 765–776, 1969.
5. Weiner, J. S., and Lourie, J. A.: *Human Biology—A Guide to Field Methods.* Blackwell Scientific Publications, Oxford, England, 1969.
6. Larson, L.: Physical fitness measurement standards. Report of 1969 Conference, Tel Aviv, Israel, of International Committee on the standardization of physical fitness tests, 1970.
7. Blackburn, H., Taylor, H. L., Okamoto, N., Rautaharju, P., Mitchell, P. L., and Kerkhof, A. C.: Standardization of the exercise electrocardiogram. A systematic comparison of chest lead configurations employed for monitoring during exercise. In Karvonen, M. J., and Barry, A. J. (eds.): *Physical Activity and the Heart.* Charles C Thomas, Publisher, Springfield, Ill., 1967.
8. Ford, A. B., and Hellerstein, H. K.: Energy cost of the Master two-step test. J. A. M. A. 164: 1868–1874, 1957.

9. Pugh, L. G. C. E.: Physiological and medical aspects of the Himalayan Scientific and Mountaineering Expedition 1960–1961. Brit. Med. J. 2: 621–633, 1962.
10. Grimby, G., Bjure, T., and Helander, E.: Radio-transmitted ECG and measurements of energy expenditure during exercise therapy in patients with myocardial infarction. Mal. Cardiovasc. 10: 143–151, 1969.
11. Brown, J. R., and Crowden, G. P.: Energy expenditure ranges and muscular work grades. Brit. J. Industr. Med. 20: 277–283, 1963.
12. Shephard, R. J.: Learning, habituation, and training. Int. Z. Angew. Physiol. 28: 38–48, 1969.
13. Kavanagh, T., Doney, H., Pandit, V., and Shephard, R. J.: Comparison of exercise and hypnotherapy in the rehabilitation of patients following myocardial infarction. Paper presented at meeting of the Canadian Cardiovascular Society, Quebec City, Oct. 23–25, 1969.
14. Cooper, K. H.: *Aerobics*. Evans, New York, 1969.

32

*Periontogenic Diseases**

DWIGHT EMARY HARKEN, M.D.

This subject, **Periontogenic Diseases,** may have disturbed some of you and you may have looked fruitlessly in the dictionary for its meaning. It is of no use to try to find this word in the dictionary. It was created recently for just this sort of discussion and is defined below.

Intensive care units have allowed patients to survive elective surgical stress that was formerly uniformly fatal when due to trauma or other accidental disease or illness. However, it does behoove us to look again at intensive care units and see if we have used these as well as we should, or if there is, in this complicated environment, a set of disadvantages that we should correct. In other words, let us have a new look at the intensive care unit.

With our sophisticated monitoring and intensive care, day and night with strange sights, smells, the feeling of timelessness, artificial lights and constant never-ending activity on the part of conscientious nurses, doctors, and paramedical personnel, we have created a science fiction world. The sights, sounds, smells, and impression of timelessness upset normal human rhythms, diurnal (daily variation) or circadian (moon) rhythms. Man was meant to be awake at certain periods and asleep at certain periods. He becomes accustomed to these diurnal rhythms, and he cannot readily tolerate sudden variations. The experiences of the airlines with their passengers and particularly with the disturbed cycles of their stewardesses are excellent examples of this inability of man to adapt instantly to changes in his life patterns and cycles.

Early in my experience with severely stressed, terminal patients undergoing heart surgery, I found that they indeed went through some interesting cycles themselves. When they had survived surgery and awakened, there was euphoria. Then after 36 to 72 hours they became depressed, agitated, generally paranoidal, and exhausted even unto death. *"We see*

---

* Original concept presented at the Society of Thoracic and Cardiovascular Surgeons of Great Britain and Ireland, September 1969, Belfast.

what we look for and we look for what we know." The psychiatrists, looking at this situation of grossly disturbed, psychotic patients, decided that they could have conferences with the patients for 10 or 12 days and, if properly managed, these patients recovered in that period of 10 or 12 days. The psychiatrists ascribed this improvement to their conferences. As surgeons interested in the internal environment of men, we noticed that these patients had low sodium levels, and we called this the low sodium syndrome. The medical people ascribed our problems to variations in various medications, particularly digitalis. It was perhaps a combination of all of these.

Now our psychologist and psychiatrist friends tell us that much of this could have been avoided had there not been a communication gap between medical practice and the behavioral sciences. Here again we repeat for emphasis, "We see what we look for and we look for what we know." In this context I am reminded of the elderly Englishman whose house was bombed while he was taking a bath in his fourth floor flat. The walls caved in and he fell from the fourth to the third to the second to the first floor, into the basement. Four days later he was dug up naked, covered only with brick and mortar dust. He interpreted this drama in his own way, much as we have all done under similar circumstances, by saying, "All I did was just pull the plug out of the bathtub." Much of man's thinking and many conclusions are similar to that.

Back to our discussion, much of this intensive care trouble might have been avoided had there not been a communication gap between medical practice and the behavioral sciences.

Inasmuch as we are discussing a new disease and a form of disturbance of man, we have had our Harvard Greek students create a new word to describe it. The word is not iatrogenic, which means produced by a physician. The word is not nosocomial or diseases of the house or hospital. We are referring to diseases produced by the immediate environment, its equipment, its conditions, and the factors of life in and around the patient. The Greek scholars have created the new word, **Periontogenic,** meaning having genesis in the surroundings or produced by the environment.

Let us now study this form of new disease. Let it assume the pattern of scientific development. The scientific method involves first, the collection of facts, second, arranging these facts into patterns, and third, deriving lessons and rules from these patterns. Our first step, therefore, is to classify periontogenic diseases. These diseases are: I, psychological; II, mechanical; III, electrical; IV, infectious and chemical; V, human.

Now let us look individually at these categories with a view toward treatment.

In this classification of diseases, the first, **psychological,** of course, has to do with sensory deprivation. As I have stated, I had not heard of sensory deprivation, diurnal rhythms, or circadian variations until recent years.

When we first recognized this patient pattern of euphoria, then agitation, exhaustion, depression, paranoia, and even death, we variously but logically ascribed the sequence to those things we understood. We must think, in addition, of the monotony of the sounds ("white noise") in an intensive care unit, the warning "beeps" and alarm sounds, the patient's fear of death, the loss of privacy, the offensive functions that he observes, his personal and other patients' exposure—this is enough to give him hallucinations of terrifying activity. All of this happens when the patient's defenses are at their lowest ebb.

Much can be done in the treatment of this condition by anticipation and warnings before the patient undergoes this experience if the surgery is elective. These warnings are given not only to the patient but to his family.

The sense of timelessness must be corrected by restoring diurnal cycles. There should be, if possible, windows in the intensive care units, clocks, calendars, lights, and radio, as well as regular visits by friends, physicians, the clergy, and others. Here understanding with simple corrective measures is both prophylactic and therapeutic.

The second category in periontogenic classification is the **mechanical** or **physical** group. Here, for example, the proper use of the respirator can correct or prevent the compacted lung or loss of compliance. The misuse of such equipment can be fatal. The patient is almost always physically restrained and encumbered by intravenous feeding and monitoring lines, by peroral and rectal sensing devices and external electrodes, and even by intravenous or transthoracic internal electrodes. Chest tubes and urinary catheters may make this encumbrance not only terrifying but painful and always extraordinarily restrictive. One is reminded of the kind of restriction that Gulliver must have felt when he awakened from his deep sleep and found himself tied down by the Lilliputians, or of Laocoön of Greek mythology, beset by snakes.

Electrical periontogenic diseases can run the spectrum from leakage currents that can produce arrhythmias to currents that can shock, burn, or even cause death by electrocution. Prevention lies in such spheres as proper use, common grounding, appropriate isolation transformers, and electrode terminal coverage. Absolutely vital is inspection, maintenance, and familiarity with correct usage of the complex electrical and electronic equipment. Here we must remember that electric beds and electric lights, as well as our monitoring and therapeutic equipment, are all potentially lethal electric shock hazards.

Infectious and chemical periontogenic diseases are prevented by the proper and careful use of reverse precautions, meticulous asepsis in the equipment that is inserted or injected intravenously, and the proper sterilization of equipment such as respirator and beds after use. Prevention also involves isolation of the medical and paramedical personnel caring for some patients.

Human factors comprise the fifth periontogenic class. Here we find that all individuals who have to do with the care of the patient, be it the cleaning woman, the electrical engineer, the oxygen therapist, all nurses, all physicians, students, clergymen, and family visitors, consider their services, and with some reason, absolutely essential. Furthermore, they have no idea that their visits represent a link in the chain of continuous disturbance of the patient, who is perhaps being allowed no opportunity to rest or sleep. It is incredible that these patients can be kept awake as if by Chinese flagellation torture for 48 to 72 hours. Here it is obligatory to have a quiet, calm, forceful special nurse in constant attendance who allows the patient to rest. This nurse must have the confidence and conviction that allows enforcement of the restriction of disturbance. Personally, I often find it useful, and sometimes even necessary, to put up a sign saying: "DO NOT DISTURB F. C. S.! THIS MEANS YOU!" Inevitably some visitor will ask what the F. C. S. means and you simply tell them that the sign says "DON'T DISTURB FOR CHRIST'S SAKE!" This is generally dramatic enough to bring visitors to re-evaluate their intrusions.

Other human factors involve proper interpretation of such things as monitoring signals so that the patient is not erroneously "resuscitated" because the electrode has become detached from his arm to produce a flat electrocardiographic pattern. Conversely, electrical interference must not be misinterpreted as ventricular fibrillation. The patient must not be asphyxiated because the oxygen line, the endotracheal tube, or the respirator becomes obstructed.

These categories are reviewed, *i.e.*, psychological, mechanical, electrical, infectious, and human. Perhaps there is an underlying thread or common denominator in what is called T. L. C. (tender loving care) for infants in hospitals or for an adult who, in his terrified, debilitated and weakened state, reverts to an infantile state and needs that same "tender loving care."

Thus is uncovered a whole new brand of diseases produced by our life-saving techniques, which are yet dangerous of and in themselves.

In all of this, we can expect more complications as more complicated material is evolved in monitoring, in recording, and eventually in the computerized care of our patients.

33

The Role of Emotions in the Rehabilitation of the Cardiac Patient

JOHN F. BRIGGS, M.D.

There is no adequate definition of the term emotions. Emotions play a major role in our lives. Through each day, emotions are major factors enabling us to meet the stresses and strains which confront us. When faced with an unsurmountable situation, one may become depressed, frustrated, hostile, or involved in rage reactions. Once the problem is solved, one's emotional pattern returns to normal. Emotions play a greater role when one is an invalid or ill, and the failure by the physician to recognize the role of emotions may delay or even prevent successful rehabilitation.

This is particularly true in the cardiac patient. Today, with the modern advances medically and surgically in the treatment of the cardiac patient, we are in a position to rehabilitate a greater number of these people so that they may return to a normal or near normal social, economic, and community life. The physician must be aware of his impact on the patient emotionally and he must recognize that the patient's emotions, when well-controlled and directed, will assist his rehabilitation.

This is usually easy in individuals who suffer from cardiac disease. Rehabilitation is developed around the etiology of the disease and to the highest degree of functional achievement. To this end, the functional capacity of the heart is most helpful.

CLASSIFICATIONS

1. Heart disease without any functional incapacity.
2. Heart disease which produces distress only when the patient exerts himself heavily.
3. Heart disease which produces distress on moderate exertion.
4. Heart disease which at rest or minimal exertion produces severe distress.

In most cardiac patients, the important emotional stresses are found in the areas of fear, anxiety, tension, frustration, hostility, depression, rage, hate, and love.

The treatment of the emotional role in rehabilitating the patient may be summarized using the letters of the word EMOTIONS.

"E" represents Education

The patient, his family, his relatives, his employer and all coworkers are involved with the patient's care. They must be taught that the patient, in order to recover from his illness and return to work, must have their help. Special emphasis in rehabilitation must be placed on the role of the family and the employer. Constant reassurance that he is to get better and return to work alleviates frustration, fear, hostility, and depression. The love of his family and the sincerity of their presence will help him to return to normal or near normal life. Education will dissipate the feeling of "why me, why should I have heart trouble?" It will help dispel the rage that he has against his affliction.

"M" represents Multiple Disciplines

Many disciplines are available to assist the patient and his family to overcome the emotional distress that is present. It must be reiterated that the patient is going to recover, that he will be able to return to some gainful occupation, and that he will return to a rewarding social, economic, and community life. To help achieve this end, there are available the trained physiatrist, physiotherapist, occupational therapist, dietitian, nutritional expert, employer, personnel director, union leader, attending physician, and all of the medical groups that can assist in his care. He has available to him the trained disciplines and knowledge of hospital personnel who can assist him concerning his insurance and his financial problems.

He also has at his disposal the trained skills of the social service department. Above all, the patient must know that the company physician, the industrial nurse, and his employer are interested in him, his progress, and his ability to return to work. A conference with his religious adviser can be of great help to him when he is under strain emotionally. During this period, the family must be made part of the treatment so that they will understand the patient and his problems. The use of these facilities alleviates fear, anxiety, tension, and worry, all of which handicap the patient.

"O" stands for Optimism in training the patient

The physician must recognize he too may have emotional insecurity and that he must disguise this insecurity when he cares for the acutely ill or chronically ill cardiac patient. He must be aware that his role as a physician requires him not only to cure but also to assist the patient in overcoming the latter's emotional problems. He must recognize the existing emotional problems, and he must act in a confident manner with self-assurance at all times. If there is doubt in the attending physician's mind as to whether the patient can be rehabilitated, the patient may recognize these doubts, which will worsen his condition. The family and relatives must be assured and reassured that optimism on their part is a predominant factor in the care of the patient. They should never display any signs of doubt or pessimism.

"T" represents Therapy

It is essential the patient know what is being done for him and why it is being done. He and his family must be informed of the medications used and the reason for their use. It is important they know that rest is imperative but that it is only a temporary measure and that, as soon as medically feasible, the patient will be encouraged to be up and around to determine the functional capacity of his heart. The patient, as well as the family, must learn that at first there are many "don'ts" which will be replaced by "do's" when he returns to more normal physical activity commensurate with the return of his cardiac function.

"I" has two Important Roles

First, there is an iatrogenic role. Occasionally, a physician does not have the emotional stability needed to care for the cardiac patient. He may radiate insecurity and uncertainty which are recognized by the patient, the relatives, and others concerned in the treatment. On self-analysis, if the attending physician finds it difficult to care for the cardiac patient, he should refer the patient to a doctor who does not have this instability or insecurity. The other factor concerns the individual. He must never be considered as the man in the third bed on the left in the general ward who has hypertensive cardiovascular disease in failure. He must not be considered as the individual who is 5 feet 10 inches tall, 186 pounds, blue eyes, etc. He must be thought of as a person with his own personality, remembering always that there is dignity in each of us, well or sick. He is Mr. Smith, who apparently presents a calm approach to his problems but is actually fearful, anxious, worried, and insecure. He has a right to be worried about his family, his financial problems, his job, etc. His world now seems to be falling in on him. Tact and understanding may reveal that the man is a smiling but depressive and disturbed person. No amount of medication or surgical procedure will assist him at this time. Only kindness, tact, and sympathy will allay his fears and anxieties, as well as those of his family. The physician must always radiate self-confidence and self-assurance.

"O" represents Opportunity

There are many opportunities today for the rehabilitated cardiac patient. The patient and his family again must be taught to understand that the great majority of cardiac patients do return to work and do enjoy a normal type of life.

Through job training, work rehabilitation, and education programs, most cardiac patients will find some type of gainful employment. Experience reveals that cardiac patients return to the same work or nearly the same type of work that they performed before their heart attack. Opportunity is there, and the physician and all of those helping in the patient's care will assist the individual and direct him to those opportunities.

"N" stands for the New Future he approaches

Because of the nature of his illness, certain restrictions are necessary. These restrictions in his new life should not be made arbitrarily by the attending physician but should depend upon the individual's functional classification. As individuals leave the hospital, they are often fearful, worried, anxious, and depressed. The sense of security found in the hospital is temporarily lost. By reviewing again the individual's problems with him, with his family, and with all those associated with him, the physician can lessen these anxieties, fears, and tensions and enable the patient to make the adjustment from hospital to home. The patient must be reminded that his rehabilitation will continue at home with the services of the various agencies that assisted him in the hospital, and that these services will continue until he is able to return to work. It is essential that his employer or personnel director be familiar with his hospital course and the plan for rehabilitation. At the proper time, the industrial physician and management can aid him in his return to work on a graduated program commensurate to his functional recovery.

"S" stands for Sex

Many patients who have sustained a heart attack fear that they will be impotent. When the patient recovers and is on periodic exercise before going home, it is well to explain both to the individual and to the spouse that sexual intercourse will be permissible. The love play should be the responsibility of the healthier individual. If the husband is the cardiac patient, the wife should be in the superior position and perform the physical work needed. If the wife is the patient, the upright position is still preferable. In those individuals having angina, nitroglycerin taken prior to the act will often prevent pain during coitus.

SUMMARY

Emotions play an important role in our normal everyday life, but they have an even greater role in the individual with heart disease. The physician must always be alert to the emotional pattern of his patient and do everything possible to teach the patient how to control his emotional outbursts. The physician must recognize that often the cardiac individual conceals his emotional upsets, particularly their reactive depression.

In recapitulation, the members of the family must be an integral part of training the individual to improve his emotional state. The physician always approaches the patient with assurance, confidence, and optimism concerning his future. The major emotional disturbances can be minimized by kindness, sympathy, and love. In the emotional rehabilitation of the individual with heart disease, it is important to enlist the aid of his employer and religious adviser. They can assist in controlling his existing emotional problems and can hasten his return to a normal or near normal life.

34

Surgical Advances in Congenital Heart Disease

FORREST H. ADAMS, M.D.

INTRODUCTION

Approximately 1 per cent of all neonates have congenital heart disease. Fifty per cent of those born with congenital heart disease do not reach their first birthday, and about 90 per cent of the deaths occur within the first 6 months of age. Cardiac failure and hypoxia are the two chief causes of death. Since accurate diagnostic techniques and palliative or corrective surgery are currently available to treat most of these malformations, many of the deaths can and should be prevented. To do so requires the early recognition that the newborn infant with cyanosis, respiratory distress, or failure to thrive may be suffering from congenital heart disease. When initial studies suggest the possibility of a cardiac lesion, prompt referral and transport to a cardiac center should be arranged immediately. Neonates with symptomatic heart disease, especially those with cyanosis, tend to deteriorate suddenly and require care in facilities where complete diagnostic studies and both medical and surgical treatment can be carried out 24 hours a day. Thus, in the decade of the 1970s, the major effort in the diagnosis and treatment of patients with congenital heart disease needs to be directed toward the infant and small child. The etiology, pathogenesis, and prevention remain to be studied in a systematic way.

NATURAL HISTORY OF CONGENITAL HEART LESIONS

In order to institute proper medical or surgical treatment in patients with congenital heart defects, it is important to know the natural history of the lesion being considered. That is, what will happen if no treatment is given? Unfortunately, *good* information regarding the natural history of the various congenital heart lesions is lacking. On the other hand, some information is available.

Table 34.1 shows the percentage of heart defects causing deaths in the

Table 34.1. *Percentage of heart defects causing death in the newborn**

	Toronto, 106 cases, 1953-1957	Boston, 100 cases, 1931-1954	Baltimore, 170 cases, 1927-1959	Buffalo, 165 cases, 1949-1964
TGV	10	27	16	15
VSD	7	19	18	2
CA	13	11	15	10
HLH	27	1	12	22
PS or PA	8	1	7	7
PDA	2	0	9	2
Tetralogy	5	4	4	7
TA	3	4	3	4
AV canal	5	0	3	4

* TGV, transposition of the great vessels; VSD, ventricular septal defect; CA, coarctation of the aorta; HLH, hypoplastic left heart syndrome; PS, pulmonary stenosis; PA, pulmonary atresia; PDA, patent ductus arteriosus; TA, tricuspid atresia; AV, atrioventricular.

newborn period at four major medical centers in the United States and Canada during the past several decades. The frequencies at the four centers were similar, with the major causes of death being transposition of the great vessels (TGV), ventricular septal defect (VSD), coarctation of the aorta (CA), and hypoplastic left heart syndrome (HLH). Such studies on patients referred to a medical center are of limited value, however, in answering the question concerning the natural history of specific lesions. In order to do so, the total population of infants born with congenital heart defects must be followed prospectively for a considerable period of time.

Two recent prospective studies on infants with congenital heart disease are of interest. The first is information accumulated from the perinatal study conducted by the National Institutes of Health in which 56,109 newborn infants were followed for a number of years or until death.[1] Table 34.2 shows the frequency of heart defects as well as their outcome in these 56,109 infants. The striking fact from this table is the high frequency (30 per cent) of VSD compared with all of the other lesions. Furthermore, approximately 30 per cent of the VSDs closed in those surviving the infancy period.

Another prospective study has been conducted at Einstein Medical Center by Hoffman *et al.*, and in this instance only those neonates suspected of having VSD were sequentially followed.[2] All neonates born at their medical center (39) and those referred from outside hospitals (36) were included. Table 34.3 shows the distribution of the neonates in the two groups according to the severity of their symptoms. It is interesting to note the differences between the two groups; *i.e.*, those referred in

Table 34.2. *Frequency of heart defects in 56,109 births*

Lesion*	Total	Stillbirths	Live births neonatal deaths	infant deaths	child- hood deaths	survivors
VSD	133	9	9	5	1	109†
PS, isolated	37	1	5			31
VSD + PS	11				2	9
ASD, secundum	34	3	7			24
ECD, partial	6	1	3			2
ECD, complete	14	4	1	2	1	6
PDA, isolated	35		1	10	1	23‡
CA, preductal isolated	12	2	10			
CA + ASD or VSD	7		5	1		1
Tetralogy of Fallot	16		2	2	1	11
Aortic stenosis	16					16
Aortic and mitral valve atresia	15	2	13			
Peripheral PS ± valve stenosis	11				1	10
EFE	10		1	3	4	2
Truncus	9	2	6			1
CA, postductal	11			1		10
TGV, isolated	8		2	3	1	2
TGV, complex	3		1	2		
Vascular ring	7		1	4	1	1
Single ventricle	4	1		2		1
Abnormality of coronary artery	7	2	2	2	1	
Double outlet RV	5	1		1	2	1
Pulmonary atresia	7	2	1	4		
Tricuspid atresia	5		2	2		1
Mitral insufficiency	3				1	2
EMF	3	2		1		
Miscellaneous	28	5	6	5	3	9
Total	457	37	78	50	20	272

* VSD, ventricular septal defect; PS, pulmonary stenosis; ASD, atrial septal defect; PDA, patent ductus arteriosus; CA, coarctation of the aorta; TGV, transposition of the great vessels; RV, right ventricle; ECD, endocardial cushion defect; EFE, endocardial fibroelastosis; EMF, endocardiomyofibrosis.

† Of whom 37 closed spontaneously.

‡ Of whom two closed spontaneously after 14 days.

from outside hospitals were generally sicker than those born in the Einstein Medical Center. This is as one might expect, since doctors are not as likely to refer for care neonates who are asymptomatic. The patients were thoroughly studied, including heart catheterization on several occasions. Many were followed as long as 7 years. Table 34.4 shows the outcome of the group according to their original symptom classification. Sixteen closed, 29 became smaller, 12 were well, and 57 of the 74 were classified as doing well. Table 34.5 shows the basis of the previous classification related to the resistance to the flow of blood across the ventricular defect. In this table, the larger the defect, the lower is the resistance value.

In summary, VSD is a very common congenital heart lesion in neonates, being four times as common as any other lesion. Over 40 per cent have symptoms in the infancy period, but eventually most close or get considerably smaller. Very few of the original group seen in the infancy period eventually required surgery according to present thinking.

Table 34.3. *Range of symptoms in infants with VSD**

Source	Severe	Moderate	None	Total
Einstein Medical Center	2	14	23	39
Referred	10	17	9	36
Total	12	31	32	75

* From Hoffman *et al.*[2]

Table 34.4. *Outcome of infants with VSD according to symptoms (7 years)**

	Total	Closed	Smaller	Well	Total doing well
Severe	12	0	2	0	2
Moderate	30	3	19	3	25
None	32	13	8	9	30
Total	74	16	29	12	57

* From Hoffman, *et al.*[2]

Table 34.5. *Relation of outcome to resistance across defect in infants with VSD**

R_{VSD}/m^2	Total	Closed	Smaller	Well	Total doing well
0–5	27	0	12	0	12
6–10	12	1	10	1	12
11–20	15	5	5	4	14
21–30	7	3	1	2	6
Over 30	13	7	1	5	13
Total	74	16	29	12	57

* From Hoffman *et al.*[2]

INDICATIONS FOR SURGERY

Most cardiologists agree that surgery should be considered if one or more of the following situations exist.

1. Persistent heart failure.
2. Excessive polycythemia.
3. Hypoxic spells.
4. Moderate to severe cardiomegaly.
5. Moderate to severe upper extremity hypertension.
6. Excessive pulmonary blood flow.
7. Decreased exercise tolerance.

The exact level of deviation of each of the above parameters requiring surgical intervention is still not determined and is a matter of individual preference of the cardiologist based on his previous experience.

PALLIATIVE SURGICAL PROCEDURES FOR THE INFANT

As already indicated, many infants with heart disease get into trouble and will die in spite of adequate medical treatment. Although definitive surgery can be successfully performed in infants with patent ductus arteriosus (PDA), CA, and pulmonary stenosis (PS), palliative surgery is indicated for the remaining lesions if it is judged that the patient cannot tolerate waiting until an older age.

The Rashkind balloon atrioseptostomy has proven to be a good procedure for increasing arterial oxygenation and relieving heart failure in neonates with TGV. However, if the cyanosis later increases and the arterial oxygen saturation drops much below 65 per cent, surgical creation of an atrial defect by the Blalock-Hanlon technique or definitive repair is required.

Patients with severe decrease in pulmonary blood flow and associated right to left shunting require some type of systemic to pulmonary artery shunt. In the small infant under 1 year of age with symptomatic tetralogy of Fallot (TF), pulmonary atresia (PA), tricuspid atresia (TA), etc., the Cooley (or Waterston) procedure has been most beneficial. In certain situations, such as PA and TA in the infant over 6 months of age, a Glenn vena cava-pulmonary artery shunt will also be of value.

Although most infants with VSD can be managed medically, some with excessive pulmonary blood flow and associated severe pulmonary hypertension with failure require pulmonary artery banding within the first 6 months of life. This procedure is also of value in certain forms of cyanotic heart disease with excessive pulmonary blood flow, such as truncus arteriosus and TGV with VSD.

OPTIMAL AGES FOR DEFINITIVE SURGERY

Little unanimity exists regarding the best time to do definitive surgery on patients with specific uncomplicated lesions. This is because no controlled studies have yet been performed to answer this question. Factors to be considered in the decision for operation include the following.

1. The natural history of the defect.
2. The time of development of pulmonary vascular obstruction.
3. The likelihood of cerebral vascular accident, brain abscess, and bacterial endocarditis.
4. Psychological factors.
5. Technical expertise.

Table 34.6 lists what are currently considered by us to be the optimal age ranges for definitive surgery of the common congenital heart lesions. This takes into account all of the factors listed above.

RECENT ADVANCES IN MANAGEMENT OF PATIENTS

It is important to indicate and to emphasize some of the recent advances in the treatment of patients with congenital heart defects. These include the following.

1. Early recognition and treatment of the neonate or infant in profound trouble: statistics indicate that this is where the major effort toward salvaging patients with congenital heart disease should be directed.
2. Monitoring of arterial blood gases and pH: metabolic acidosis is a frequent cause of morbidity and mortality both pre- and postoperatively, especially in the hypoxemic infant. An increased awareness of these derangements and prompt correction have saved many such infants.
3. Maintenance of body temperature: neonates and infants are incomplete homeotherms. Unintentional cooling of the distressed infant can lead to increased risk of morbidity and mortality.
4. Fluid and electrolyte balance: over-hydration and the development of electrolyte abnormalities can have serious consequences postoperatively.
5. Use of hyperbaric conditions: although few centers are yet able to perform

Table 34.6. *Optimal age for definitive surgery in heart disease*

Defect	Years
Patent ductus arteriosus	1–2
Coarctation of aorta	4–5
Ventricular septal defect	4–5
Atrial septal defect	4–5
Tetralogy of Fallot	6–10
Transposition of great vessels	3–10

Table 34.7. *Results of surgery in infants under hyperbaric conditions**

Defect	Total	Alive
Transposition of the great vessels	74	65
Tetralogy of Fallot	61	53
Ventricular septal defect	28	28
Tricuspid atresia	20	14
Pulmonary atresia	8	3
Aortic stenosis	12	10
Coarctation of aorta with complications	8	6
Atrioventricular canal	6	5
Truncus Type 1	6	3

* From Fyler *et al.*, Postgrad. Med., 1969.[3]

surgery under hyperbaric conditions, the group at Boston Children's Hospital has demonstrated not only the feasibility but also the good results that can be obtained on the small infant. Table 34.7 shows their most recent results.

6. Use of profound hypothermia: mild hypothermia is frequently used during prolonged cardiopulmonary bypass. Recently, certain groups have obtained good results with profound hypothermia.

7. Use of membrane oxygenator: several membrane oxygenators have recently been developed and are currently being tested in animals and man. The Lande and the Kolobow oxygenators are quite similar in principle and offer the potential advantage of prolonged extracorporeal support and small priming volume.

8. Aortic homografts: some patients with severe TF, PA, and Type I truncus arteriosus require extensive plastic reconstruction between the right ventricle and the pulmonary artery. Use of the aortic homograft has made such reconstruction possible, with very good early results.

9. Management of low cardiac output: it is not uncommon for certain types of patients to develop low cardiac output following cardiopulmonary bypass for definitive surgery. Its prompt recognition and early treatment have saved many lives.

10. Treatment of respiratory insufficiency: some patients have great difficulty in ventilating adequately postoperatively. This can be accomplished with proper usage of a nasotracheal tube or, in some instances, with a tracheotomy.

11. Treatment of hypoglycemia: some infants are liable to develop hypoglycemia. If promptly treated, myocardial function improves.

LONG-TERM COMPLICATIONS FOLLOWING SURGERY

Most patients who have had surgical repair of their congenital heart defects are greatly benefited. This can be measured by an increase in arterial oxygenation, a disappearance of heart failure, a decrease in heart size, a decrease in lung congestion, and an increase in exercise tolerance. Not all patients are completely restored to normal function, however.

A significant number of long-term complications still occur following surgery. They include the following.

1. Varying degrees of heart block or arrhythmia.
2. Residual shunts.
3. Persistence or progression of pulmonary vascular disease.
4. Residual gradients.
5. Valvular insufficiency.
6. Calcification and degeneration of homografts.
7. Development of ventricular aneurysm.

It is thus apparent that long-term follow-up of patients who have had surgical correction of their lesion is indicated in many instances. Repeat heart catheterization, even in the asymptomatic patient, is indicated in the presence of residual murmurs and cardiomegaly.

REFERENCES

1. Mitchell, S. C., Korones, S. B., and Berendes, H. W.: Congenital heart disease in 56,109 births. Circulation 43: 323, 1971.
2. Hoffman, J. I. E., *et al.:* Unpublished data.
3. Fyler, D. C., Nadas, A. S., and Bernhard, W. F.: Operable heart disease in the newborn period. Postgrad. Med. 46: 80, 1969.

35

Autologous Tissue Repair in Mitral and Aortic Valvular Disease

CHARLES P. BAILEY, M.D., TERUO HIROSE, M.D., AND FRANK S. FOLK, M.D.

Accumulating evidence that prosthetic devices replacing cardiac valves[1-6] provide, at best, only palliation for a limited period of time has led to efforts to replace cardiac valves with either fresh or preserved (devitalized) homologous (cadaver)[7-11] or heterologous (animal)[12-16] valves. Because these trials have been made only during the rather recent past, the long-term possibilities of such an approach cannot yet be fully evaluated. However, the later experiences of Lam *et al.*,[7] Binet,[12] and Ross[10] suggest serious limitations to the usefulness of the method.

Alternatively, efforts have been directed toward surgical reconstruction of the deformed natural valve. If the closed cardiac procedures are included, these attempts really were commenced in 1923 by Cutler and Levine.[17] Others followed.[18-25] With the advent of modern type open heart surgery in 1954, more adequate mobilization of both incompetent and stenotic valves under direct vision became feasible, and since then such procedures have become standard practice in many clinics.[26-31]

Unfortunately, both the closed and the open types of mobilization of stenotic valves amount essentially to merely surgical division of fairly classic fibrous strictures. The overwhelming propensity of such divided strictures to reform with the passage of time is reflected in an extremely high incidence of eventual recurrence of the valvular stenosis, an experience now admitted by practically all observers. Thus, these techniques must also be included among the palliatives.

The success of Johanson[32] in 1953 and of Devine and Horton[33] and others[34, 35] in "curing" urethral strictures by the interposition of skin grafts into the longitudinal axis of the incised stricture (Fig. 35.1) suggested to the authors that fibrous strictures in other areas similarly might be clinically curable by the interposition between their divided extremities of tissues which do not readily undergo scar transformation.

TISSUES

Interposition within the continuity of a mitral leaflet of an arcuate segment of autologous pericardium was tried by many[36-39] in an effort to lengthen this "cusp." The observed tendency of pericardium to become detached from the cut valve margins (Fig. 35.2), and the variability of its behavior with respect to subsequent shrinkage, thickening, and induration have finally led to the discontinuation of these efforts.

Absolom *et al.*[40] suggested the central tendon of the diaphragm as a tissue for valvular reconstruction. The difficulties associated with interruption of the continuity of the diaphragm (potential for herniation, the possibility of subdiaphragmatic bleeding or abscess formation) and the tendency of this tissue to become shrunken and retracted with the passage of time have deterred further trial.

The use of full thickness left atrial wall obtainable from the posterior lip of the atriotomy was tried in 1964.[41, 42] The friability and lack of inherent tensile strength of this tissue, its tendency to subsequent thickening and shrinkage, and its limited quantitative availability (although readily obtainable in small amounts from the posterior lip of the atriotomy) have combined to diminish its utilization.

In 1962, one of us (C. P. B.) utilized autogenous aortic wall to create individual aortic valve cusps.[43] The limited availability of this tissue in substantial quantity, as well as its lack of inherent strength, renders its use for valve reconstruction limited and generally impracticable (see Fig. 35.13).

Senning[44] was the first to utilize autogenous fascia lata to reconstruct or replace the aortic valve (1962). He experienced little or no thromboembolism.

Subsequently, fascia lata has been used more widely in reconstruction, especially of the aortic valve,[45-50] although there has been some effort also to employ this material in the mitral area.[51-55] Generally, these attempts have involved the utilization of frames or skeletons of plastic or metallic construction, on which the fascia is fitted for ease in valve formation and implantation.

Human fascia has been utilized in clinical surgery since the turn of the century, apparently being introduced by McArthur[56, 57] in 1901. Murphy[58] subsequently used fascia in arthroplasties. Kirschner[59, 60] was the first to use sheets of fascia lata as grafts. Gallie and le Mesurier[61-63] showed that fascia lata grafts buried within the human body retain their histological structure and their tensile strength for a period of at least 6 to 10 years. Foshee[64, 65] described regeneration of fascia lata. This observation was confirmed by Peer.[66] By 1917, Lewis,[67] had demonstrated the readiness with which grafted fascia becomes permeated by the body fluids. It so readily

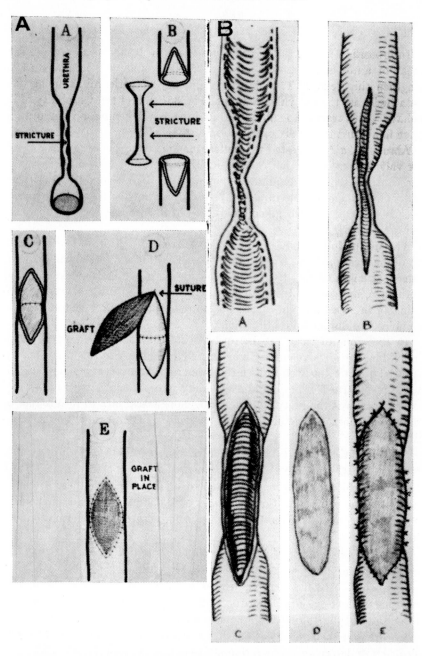

Fig. 35.1. Reproduction of the techniques of Devine *et al.* for "cure" of urethral stricture by interposition between (B) the margins of the longitudinally divided stricture of a graft of autogenous skin or (A) by widening of the site of anastomosis

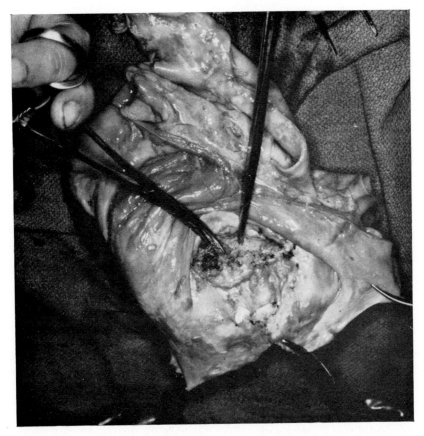

FIG. 35.2. Marginal detachment of a graft of pericardial tissue employed to lengthen the mural cusp of the mitral valve (7 months postoperative).

picks up sufficient blood supply from adjacent tissues that it undergoes little or no degenerative changes following transplantation.

Senning[44] has noted no deleterious histological changes in the fascia lata used for reconstruction of aortic valves even after the passage of 5 to 7 years. Evidently, fascia so used is able to absorb sufficient nutrition from the flowing blood.

All of this is in marked contrast with the observations of Gilbert and associates[68] and Zimmerman[69, 70] in the experimental construction of cardiac

with a skin graft after sleeve resection. (Reproduced with permission from Devine, P. C., Horton, C. E., Devine, C. J., Sr., Devine, C. J., Jr., Crawford, H. H., and Adamson, J. E.: Use of full thickness skin grafts in repair of urethral strictures. J. Urol. 90: 67–71, 1963; and from Devine, P. C., Sakati, I. A., Poutasse, E. F., and Devine, C. J., Jr.: One-stage urethroplasty: repair of urethral stricture with a free full thickness patch of skin. J. Urol. 90: 191–193, 1968.)

valves in dogs (but not in baboons). Their canine fascia lata grafts were subject to late degeneration, to fibrous replacement, and even to cartilaginous metaplasia or bone formation. These observations would appear to be but one more example of the difficulties associated with attempts to correlate biological observations in one species with the development of clinical methodology in another.

Shrinkage of free grafts of fascia lata after implantation would seem to be of fundamental importance in clinical utilization. Wierzejewski[71] has stated that human fascial grafts shrink after implantation by one-fifth to one-sixth of their cross-sectional area. However, the present authors have estimated from clinical cases that the shrinkage of fascia lata used in constructing cardiac valves approaches 30 per cent of each linear measurement of the grafted segment. This would amount to a reduction of approximately 50 per cent in the final cross-sectional area. It would appear that all of this shrinkage occurs within the first 18 to 24 months after implantation, the grafts thereafter remaining stable both grossly and microscopically.

Fascia lata, despite early reservations on the part of the authors with respect to its lack of any endothelial or even mesothelial covering, does not appear to be thrombogenic when implanted within the cardiac chambers. Perhaps this is related to the observations of Gilsdorf *et al.*[72] and Sawyer[73] with respect to the generation of a negative electrical charge upon the living tissue surfaces over which blood moves (flows). Whatever the real explanation may be, since 1967, when fascia lata has been used for valve construction, we have not felt it necessary to use anticoagulants either in the early or late postoperative period. We have observed no single instance of thromboembolism. This experience appears to be duplicative of that of others using tissue grafts within the cardiac chambers.

Having finally obtained a reasonably satisfactory reparative material which might be used for the reconstruction of damaged cardiac valves, it was logical to attempt to develop appropriate principles for such reconstruction and to support them by suitable surgical techniques. As a matter of fact, such design development had already been in progress following the earliest efforts at valve reconstruction with pericardium, atrial wall, etc.

While the various procedures employed might well be grouped under the general designation of "dressmaker" techniques, it is a fact that some of the early ones, although eminently qualifying for such designation, actually proved disappointing in practice.

The clinically encountered types of valve malformation are widely variable, depending upon causation (congenital, rheumatic, syphilitic, infarctional, or iatrogenic) and the interplay of certain pertinent associated or consequent elements, such as hypertension, combinations of valve involvement, deficiencies in bodily collagen formation (Marfan's syndrome), and

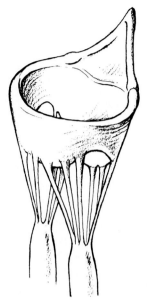

Fɪɢ. 35.3. Fundamental structure of the mitral valve mechanism (after Zimmerman[77]). Note its similarity to a woman's girdle.

coexisting myocardial involvement. Hence, considerable individualization is essential in planning the proper corrective procedure for the individual case. We describe below those techniques which have proved valuable in our hands.

THE MITRAL VALVE

Although Wolff[74] and Henle[75, 76] have described the essential anatomic features of the mitral valve in fairly accurate detail, apparently Zimmerman[77] and Zimmerman and Bailey[78, 79] were the first to recognize the essentially sleeve valve (skirtlike) nature of this structure. Perhaps it would not be amiss to say that the valve structure more closely simulates that of a woman's girdle (Fig. 35.3). With such a basic design, it is easy to visualize the effect of superimposition of the individual and group pathological features which contribute to the development of valvular stenosis, insufficiency, or some combination thereof. If one considers the development of rheumatic mitral stenosis, one will readily appreciate that there often will be seen a significant element of shortening of the skirtlike structure from "hemline" to "waist" as well as a purse-string type of narrowing of the "hemline." The funnel-like mitral valve which so often has been described[23, 80, 81] will then be seen to be but an intermediate stage between the individual extremes of these processes. A variable amount of thickening of the valve margin, induration, or even calcification may become superimposed.

The shortening of the valve sleeve from free margin to base may not be symmetrical. It may be limited to one cusp (mural or septal valve component) or it may involve unipolar portions of both. A variable degree of chordal incorporation within the thickened or even lengthened valve substance may be seen, even to the point of direct papillary attachment, as described so well by Brock.[80]

For permanently effective tissue reconstruction of the stenotic mitral valve, at least three primary surgical objectives must be satisfied and a fourth must be considered. (1) The two valve components must be widely separated at the time of surgery (Fig. 35.4). This must include splitting of any cross-fused portions of the chordopapillary supporting system, essentially by the method previously described under the term neostrophingic mobilization.[82] (2) If the valve sleeve or skirt has become shortened sufficiently to impose a complicating element of valvular incompetence in the present or to threaten the development of insufficiency in the foreseeable future, it must be lengthened appropriately. (3) In order to prevent eventual reformation of what is essentially a fibrous stricture following surgical division, it is essential that some living tissue which will not become converted into a scar should be interposed between the extremities of the widely divided structure. Fascia lata, particularly in the form of a suspending sheet,

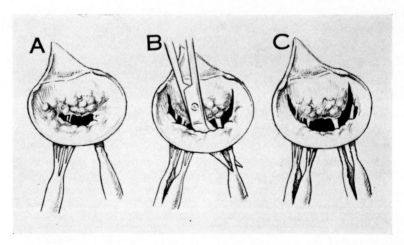

Fig. 35.4. Neostrophingic mobilization of the stenotic mitral valve. A, typically strictured valve. B, dividing the valve poles in the direction of the right and left fibrous trigones, respectively. C, if the subvalvular structures are cross-fused, this subvalvular secondary stenosis must be relieved by extensively splitting the supporting structures into two separate groups.

appears to perform this function admirably. (4) In some cases in which the valve has become excessively thickened (usually because of heaped up and infiltrating calcific salts) it may also be necessary to excise much or all of the extremely pathological tissue, hopefully preserving at least enough of the valve margin to permit reattachment of the chordae tendineae to the tissue of replacement (again fascia lata) (Fig. 35.5, A to C). If it is not feasible to so preserve the valve margin, a fan-shaped fascial suspensory attachment may be required to maintain valve competence, much as in the repair of that type of valvular incompetence which is due to chordal or papillary rupture (described later; see Fig. 35.9).

In applying these separate or combined surgical principles to the clinical problem of mitral stenosis, we have proceeded as follows.

1. First the stenotic valve is divided as completely as possible, utilizing the technique of neostrophingic mobilization.[82, 83] The individual valve components are separated anatomically by carrying the cleavage of the valve poles or commissures fully to the target points—practically to the lower margins of the respective fibrous trigones (Fig. 35.4). Simultaneously, any cross-fusion of the supporting chordae tendineae is surgically relieved by splitting. Should there be direct adherence of the papillary muscles or of any complex chordopapillary fusion masses to the free margin of the valve, they must be split anatomically, perhaps as far as their ventricular origin, thereby creating two hemipapillary supports.

2. If the valve is so shortened from "hemline" to "waist" as to produce present or impending incompetence, circumferential elongation[52] of the valve "miniskirt" with a strip of fascia lata is indicated (Fig. 35.5, D) and will in itself prevent or overcome the insufficiency. Should the shortening be asymmetrical—limited to one valve cusp or to the same polar extremity of both cusps—a semicircular or crescentic inlay of fascia lata placed so as to lengthen this shortened portion of the valve circumference[52, 84] will serve the same purpose (Fig. 35.6, A to C).

In cases of "pure" mitral stenosis in which there is a rather small left ventricular chamber, even though the valve may have undergone significant apico-basal shrinkage, extreme caution must be exercised with respect to complete circumferential lengthening. Implantation of too wide a circumferential strip of fascia will result in a marked reduction in the left ventricular stroke output, probably because of an excessively large systolic deflection of the now elongated valve structure into the left atrial chamber which detracts from the expulsive volume much as does an internal ventricular aneurysm.

Probably a strip of fascia 1.5 cm. in width is the maximum safely tolerable in such cases. It is preferable to insert a crescentic inlay at each valve pole (Fig. 35.6, D).

While our position may change in the future, in the average case of pure

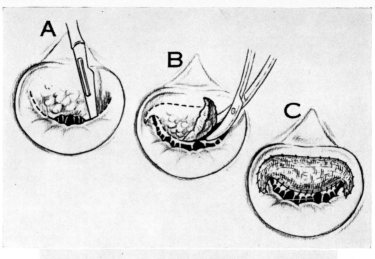

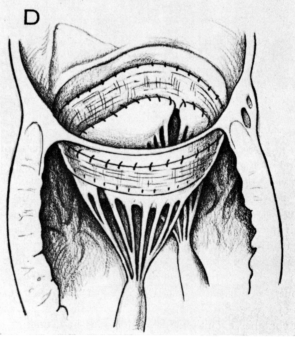

Fig. 35.5. Resection of calcific or otherwise extremely pathological tissue and replacement with fascia lata. A, extensively calcified valve. B, excision of the pathological tissue, hopefully preserving enough of the free margin for reconstruction. C, reconstructed valve. As long as sufficient marginal tissue (or fragments thereof) remains attached to the chordae, they can be reattached in such a manner as to maintain valve support (see Fig. 35.9). D, if the valve skirt is generally shrunken from margin to base, it may be lengthened by interposition of a circumferential strip of fascia lata. However, the completely separated mural and septal valve components must be separately suspended from the fascia margin.

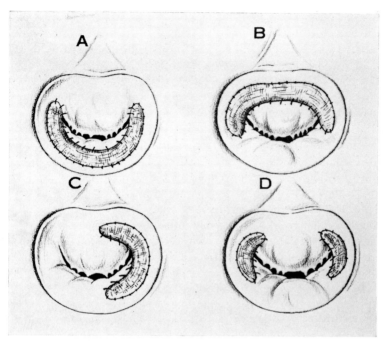

Fig. 35.6. Methods of interposing crescentic grafts of fascia lata to lengthen asymmetrically shrunken mitral valves. Note that in each instance the operative separation of the valve elements is rendered permanent by bridging the margins of the divided stricture with autogenous grafted tissue (fascia lata) in accordance with the Johanson-Devine principle. A, lengthening of the shrunken mural leaflet; B, lengthening of the shrunken septal leaflet; C, lengthening of the shrunken tissues limited to one pole of the stenotic valve; D, permanent separation of the two valve components at both poles in cases of pure stenosis (with a small left ventricle) in order to prevent eventual reformation of the stricture.

mitral stenosis in which the valve skirt has undergone marked shortening, it is not our policy to interpose a lengthening circumferential strip.

3. Once the valve components have been fully separated by a proper neostrophingic mobilization, provision must be made to prevent later reformation of the valve stricture (restenosis). As stated before, this can be accomplished reliably by the interposition of new healthy tissue between the extremities of the divided valve.[54, 85] Such an effect is conveniently accomplished when a circumferential or crescentic inlay extends past a valve pole. The cut extremities of the two fully divided valve components (mural and septal) are then suspended separately at sites 4 mm. apart from the medial edge of the fascial graft (see Figs. 35.5 and 35.6). A hiatus of this distance in the effective support of the fascial margin will not produce incompetence, and the achieved anatomic separation of the valve margins will be a permanent one.

When no serious degree of symmetrical or asymmetrical shortening of the valve is present, small crescentic inlays of fascia lata, measuring no more than 3 cm. in length and 1.5 cm. in mid-width (reduced by the actual suturing to effective measurements less than two-thirds of these) may be interposed at either divided valve pole, or both (Fig. 35.6, D). Again the separate suspension of the extremities of the two valve components from the medial fascial margin will preclude reformation of the valve stricture.

4. In cases of extensive encrustation of bone or of both valve components with calcific material, the excess sometimes may simply be cut away or debrided from the remaining intact valve substance. Then the previously described techniques for management of the stenotic process may be applied. Of course, there can be no guarantee with this method of management that the calcific lesions will not reform.

When the calcium salts extensively infiltrate and thicken the valve substance, it usually will be necessary to excise the involved area. At times this will create a significant deficit in the continuity of the valve ribbon. A portion of the valve margin may require excision, thereby creating a greater or lesser degree of chordal detachment. Since it rarely is practicable to attempt direct suture repair of such detached chordae tendineae (unless they are significantly thickened), it is urged that every effort be made to preserve the actual valve margin if at all possible, even to the point of preserving separated individual fragments of marginal tissue. These fragments, along with their attached chordae, can then be resutured, perhaps with hiatal intervals 4 mm. in width, to the medial edge of a locally implanted graft of fascial tissue used to replace the excised portion of the valve (Fig. 35.5, A to C). In most cases, a wider than usual strip or crescentic inlay of fascia lata will readily compensate for the loss of the excised tissue. When the resulting chordal detachment is extensive and direct suture repair is not feasible, resort must be made to the method of marginal suspension described below in the treatment of primary mitral insufficiency resulting from chordal detachment. Since fascia lata is inherently inelastic, no internal ventricular aneurysmal effect will be caused by replacement of the excised valve substance per se.

Mitral Insufficiency

The possible causes of incompetence of the mitral valve are legion. They include congenital clefts and deficiencies in valve continuity, various iatrogenic lacerations and excisions of valve substance, shortening (symmetrical or asymmetrical) of the valve skirt, usually in association with coexistent stenotic lesions, widening or dilatation of the atrioventricular junction ("pure insufficiency"), and finally, loss of marginal support of the valve, whether as a result of lengthening or of actual rupture or detachment of the chordae tendineae or one of the papillary muscles.

Congenital valve clefts often may simply be sutured. Because of the risk of subsequent cutting through of the sutures in the ever-moving and probably immature valve, it is best to buttress the lines of repair with strips of autogenous fascia lata. Gross deficiencies in the continuity of the cusps may be overcome by the interposition of fascial grafts (patching). Such a procedure may not be in itself sufficient, however, unless marginal support is simultaneously provided. Similarly created lacerations and punctures may be repaired by direct suturing with or without graft reinforcement.

Shortening of Valve Skirt

Unless this is of congenital origin, nearly all of these patients will be recognized to suffer from an element of concomitant mitral stenosis, although the latter process may not yet have attained sufficient severity to have become clinically or hemodynamically evident. Whereas the former type of "miniskirt" may be treated by simple elongation of the valve with a circumferential graft of fascia lata,[52] the latter type of lesion will also require a permanent anatomic separation of the divided valve components by separate suspension of their polar extremities from the medial margin of the circumferential lengthening graft[54, 85] at sites 4 mm. apart (Figs. 35.5 and 35.6). In patients with a significant element of mitral insufficiency, with or without concomitant stenosis, there is very little risk associated with the interposition of even a rather wide circumferential fascial strip (up to 3 cm. in width), since any subsequent dynamic loss of ventricular blood from the bolus of ejection because of an element of created "internal ventricular aneurysm" will be less than the actual previous ejection loss due to the regurgitation.

Pure Mitral Insufficiency

In this condition, the essential adverse factor is such a generalized widening of the atrioventricular junction that an otherwise entirely normal mitral valve is unable to defend it. It may be due to generalized dilatation of the left ventricle resulting from a toxic cause such as rheumatic fever, to intrinsic myocardial weakness (preventing normal "sphincteric" reduction in the atrioventricular passageway during systole) as in the various myocardiopathies, or to compensatory dilatation and hypertrophy of the ventricle such as is seen in cases with associated major aortic insufficiency. Since the essential problem is a relative dearth in the amount of available normal valve tissue with respect to the size of the atrioventricular passage to be defended, simple enlargement of the valve with a circumferential graft of fascia lata should be—and is—an ideal solution. Providing that there is no other cause for the insufficiency, simple elongation of the valve skirt with a sufficiently wide (up to 4 cm. in width) strip of fascia lata (Fig. 35.7)

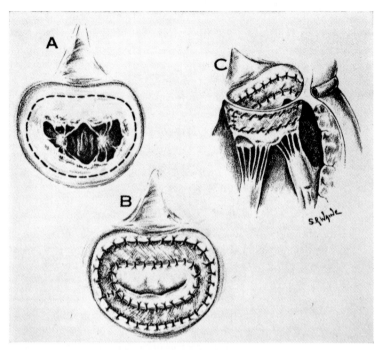

FIG. 35.7. Lengthening of the mitral skirt in insufficiency caused by simple enlargement of the atrioventricular junction, no stenosis being present. In such cases, it is not necessary to separate the mural and septal components anatomically. A, circumferential valvulotomy; B, repaired valve, top view; C, repaired valve, side view.

always abolishes the incompetence. But a narrower strip may not, for obvious reasons. Surgical separation of the otherwise normal components at the poles is not necessary in this group of patients.

Chordopapillary Dysfunction

Not infrequently at operation for repair of mitral insufficiency, the cause of the incompetence will be seen to be symmetrical or asymmetrical elongation of the chordae tendineae. In the former instance (Fig. 35.8, A to C), the valve edges do not make secure systolic contact because the elongation of the chordae causes the valve structure to be displaced during systole farther than normally into the left atrial chamber, the coapting margins of the respective valve components then being not the true valve margin but the lattice-like subvalvular mesh of chordae attached to the valve margin. While there may well be other equally effective ways to deal with this situation, we have found simple elongation of the valve skirt with a circumferential strip of fascia lata to be immediately and highly effective

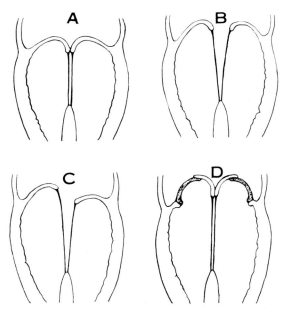

FIG. 35.8. Correction of mitral insufficiency resulting from symmetrical or asymmetrical pathological elongation of the chordae tendineae. A, normal cusp suspension; B, symmetrically elongated chordae tendineae; C, asymmetrically elongated chordae tendineae; D, correction by elongation of the valve skirt with a circumferential strip of fascia lata. Note that the enlarged valve intrudes into the atrial chamber during systole like an internal ventricular aneurysm. However, since more of the bolus of ejection would be lost if the valve were incompetent, a net hemodynamic advantage or gain is provided.

(Fig. 35.8, D). Of course, it is conjectural whether the weakened chordae subsequently will continue to elongate, perhaps eventually restoring the incompetence.

This procedure is equally effective in cases of asymmetrical elongation of the chordae in which the essential element in the causation of the leak is the difference in the levels of the valve margins at the moment of closure (Fig. 35.8, C). Although we have always utilized the method of circumferential elongation in each case encountered so far, it may be that some type of asymmetric lengthening of the valve would be equally effective.

Actual rupture of the papillary muscle, as seen in cases of inadvertent (iatrogenic) division during surgery and in the early period after acute myocardial infarction, produces immediate overwhelming and usually fatal mitral insufficiency. Such patients sometimes have been saved by emergency surgery with the insertion of a prosthetic valve. To date, we are aware of no successful effort to reconstruct such a valve with a proper fascial support. We feel confident that this can be done, however, and we await such an opportunity.

What is often called papillary muscle dysfunction (appearance of murmur and other evidences of mitral insufficiency following an episode of myocardial infarction) would appear to be a misnomer. Miller[86] has reported his inability to produce detectable mitral insufficiency by experimental infarction of the papillary muscles in dogs. While the papillary muscle becomes thin and tendon-like (but not elongated) following infarction when there has been no actual rupture, the valve margin remains satisfactorily supported, and no regurgitation occurs. Apparently, synchronous contraction of the papillary muscles during ventricular systole is not essential to mitral valve competence.

In several clinical instances in which we have been called upon to operate for papillary muscle dysfunction, we have in each case found a marked localized thinning and dilatation of the ventricular wall, involving a portion of the mural part of the mitral valve circumference. This is really a limited aneurysmal dilatation of the ventricular wall which fortuitously involves the atrioventricular junction, causing an outbulging and distortion of the base of the otherwise normal mitral valve. Conceivably, resection of these areas of ventricular scarring would have solved the problem of valvular dysfunction in each of these patients. However, since simple elongation of the mural component of the mitral valve by the interposition of a crescentic inlay of fascia lata (Fig. 35.6, A) successfully eliminated the incompetence in the first such patient operated, we have continued to follow this course, which has continued to be clinically satisfactory. However, if there were an associated enlargement, a noticeable outward bulging of the left ventricular surface, or a history of previous thromboembolic episodes, undoubtedly excision of the ventricular scar and immediate ventriculoplasty would be preferable.

Rupture or Detachment of Chordae Tendineae

Probably there are many causes for chordal rupture or detachment. Steering wheel accidents[87-89] may be causative. Although lesser grades of chordal detachment (limited to one or two or only a few chordae) may pass unnoticed, more massive detachments presumably might be immediately fatal. In most cases, the immediate appearance of a previously nonexistent systolic murmur following thoracic trauma will bear sufficient notice to the examiner of the occurrence of this type of injury. This murmur is often extremely loud, may be either of a harsh or a musical ("sea gull") quality, and sometimes is maximal over the aortic area. Cineventriculography readily will identify the specific valvular dysfunction.

At operation the full extent of chordal detachment readily will be seen,

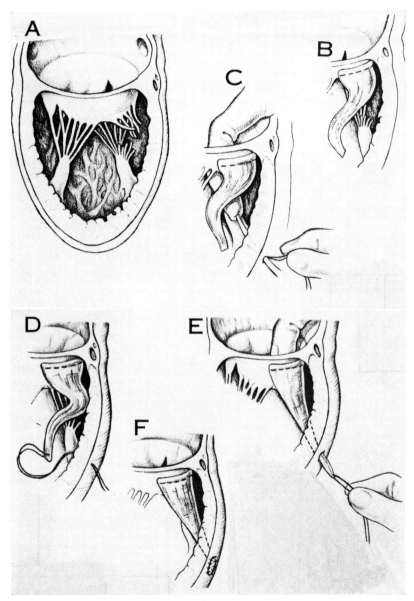

FIG. 35.9. Steps in resupporting a mitral valve partially flail because of rupture of supporting chordae tendineae. Note that, in the stage of surgery represented in E, the intracardiac finger can appreciate the degree of tension on the new support required to bring about valvular competence, the heart having resumed its function.

with the corresponding extent of "flail" movement of the unsupported valve margin. Since direct suture reattachment nearly always will be impracticable, most authorities have recommended prosthetic replacement of the valve.[90, 91] We have been gratified, however, with the results obtained by resupporting the previously flail valve margin by suspension with a fan-shaped graft of fascia lata,[89] the tapering end of which is drawn completely through the left ventricular wall by transmyocardial passage of a suture-bearing probe digitally directed in proximity to the base of the appropriate papillary muscle (Fig. 35.9). The proper amount of tension to be applied to support the valve margin is determined by digital examination of the functioning valve after closure of the atriotomy. The protruding end of the fascial strip is then sutured externally to the ventricular epicardium at such tension as will maintain optimal competency.

Results of Mitral Reconstruction

It can well be imagined that we have not been successful in every attempt at valve reconstruction, and that failure was more common during our earlier attempts. Naturally this would be expected in the course of a process which included actually coming to an understanding of the basic nature of the structure of the repaired valve, as well as efforts to devise suitable reconstructive techniques for the differing types of valvular deformity and dysfunction encountered clinically.

Indeed, this work has also embraced experimentation with different graft tissues, changes in the perfusion equipment and technique employed, choice of patients submitted to reparative surgery, and finally in the adoption of certain surgical short-cuts which reduce the operative and perfusion time required.

Accordingly, the series of 212 patients is divided chronologically into three groups with proper annotation as to the graft material used and as to the type of repair employed (Charts 35.1 and 35.2). Clinical and hemodynamic evidences of improvement are depicted in Charts 35.3 and 35.4.

THE AORTIC VALVE

If the structure of the mitral valve can be said to be similar to that of a woman's girdle, the aortic valve may with equal propriety be said to resemble a woman's brassiere—but with three cups. Indeed, much the same kind of physical forces apply to these respective fluid-holding structures, the diastolic blood surge or gravity acting upon the supported female breast (in the upright position) distending the cups.

Aortic Stenosis

The mechanisms by which the effects of the rheumatic process deform the aortic valve are similar to those seen in the pathogenesis of mitral

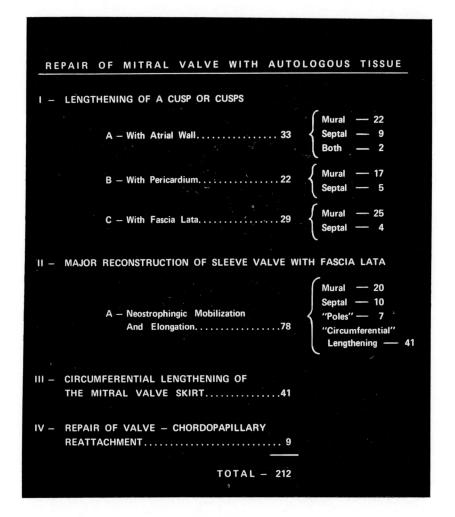

REPAIR OF MITRAL VALVE WITH AUTOLOGOUS TISSUE

I – LENGTHENING OF A CUSP OR CUSPS

A – With Atrial Wall............... 33
- Mural — 22
- Septal — 9
- Both — 2

B – With Pericardium............... 22
- Mural — 17
- Septal — 5

C – With Fascia Lata............... 29
- Mural — 25
- Septal — 4

II – MAJOR RECONSTRUCTION OF SLEEVE VALVE WITH FASCIA LATA

A – Neostrophingic Mobilization And Elongation...............78
- Mural — 20
- Septal — 10
- "Poles" — 7
- "Circumferential" Lengthening — 41

III – CIRCUMFERENTIAL LENGTHENING OF THE MITRAL VALVE SKIRT...............41

IV – REPAIR OF VALVE – CHORDOPAPILLARY REATTACHMENT...................... 9

TOTAL – 212

Chart 35.1

stenosis. Miliary vegetations appear upon the aortic (sinusoidal) surfaces of the aortic cusps (which in this valve, unlike the mitral, are indeed discrete structures), and particularly upon the zones of marginal coaptation, the respective lunulae and the corpora aurantii. Soon a variable amount of fibrinous exudate comes to coat the affected (roughened) surfaces. The adjacent portions of the cusps in the region of the natural valve commissures readily become adherent because of the agglutinating effect of this exudate, since the normally functioning aortic valve does not open fully except under conditions of maximal cardiac output (Fig. 35.10).

Chart 35.2

Period	Cases	Mortality		Survivors	Clinical evaluation: murmurs		
		early	late		none	1/16–3/6	4/6–↑
Aug. 22, 1963 to Dec. 31, 1967	46	13 (28%)	3 (6%)	30	18	8	4
Jan. 1, 1968 to Dec. 31, 1968	58	7 (12%)	2 (3.4%)	49	33	10	6
Jan. 1, 1969 to March 31, 1970	108	10 (9.4%)	4 (4%)	82	57	19	6
Total	212	30 (14.2%)	12 (5.7%)	161	108	37	16

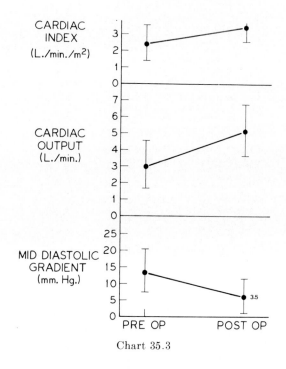

Chart 35.3

Subsequent organization of this agglutinating exudate by the invasion of fibroblasts results in thickening of the valve margins and in permanent cross-fusion of the adjacent basal portions of adjacent cusps (progressive, centripetally directed obliteration of the commissures). A subsequent inward rolling of the free valve margins and infiltration by calcific salts, especially in the regions of the cross-fused commissures, are extremely

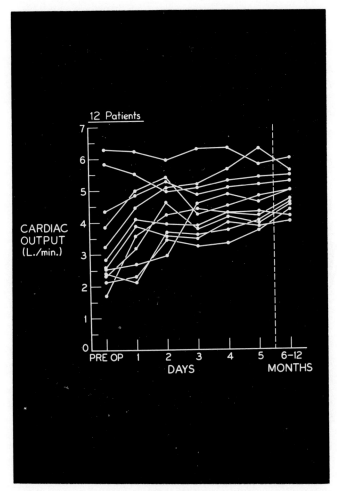

Chart 35.4

common (over 90 per cent). Often there is a heaping up of readily detachable (debridable) layers or masses of calcific material within the concavities of the cusps.

The net result of the foregoing processes is a marked reduction in the size of the effective aortic orifice, although if the processes are symmetrical a central equilateral "triangle of incompetence" simultaneously will be created (Fig. 35.11, A). This ensures a coexisting element of valvular insufficiency. On the other hand, if the process is asymmetrical with only one or two of the commissures becoming obliterated, bicuspid conversion of the valve orifice will take place. Here the residual passageway will be a slitlike opening, corresponding respectively to residual portions of one or

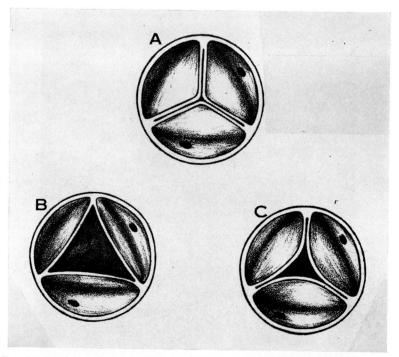

F<small>IG</small>. 35.10. Leonardo da Vinci showed 500 years ago that the normal aortic valve can open only to the size of an equilateral triangle. However, at less than maximal bodily activity, it only opens centrally, to a varying degree. Hence, the peripheral portions of the lines of cusp coaptation readily can become adherent without seriously reducing valve effectiveness.

two radii of the original circular aortic aperture. The degree of impedance to flow then will depend upon the rigidity of the margins of the slit (Fig. 35.11, B). Such stenotic valves may be completely competent.

Since these processes involve the entire structure of the aortic valve, it undergoes a total pathological conversion into a classic fibrous stricture (with or without extensive calcific infiltration). No operative procedure less than total excision and replacement of the entire valve structure would seem to be capable of bringing about a clinical cure. While many authorities have sensed this, most have construed it to mean prosthetic replacement of the valve. The finally evolved principles and techniques for reconstruction of a fascial valve to treat aortic stenosis do not differ materially from those utilized for aortic insufficiency. We discuss below the specific surgical measures for these respective conditions together.

Aortic Insufficiency

While the residual triangle of incompetence mentioned in conjunction with symmetrical aortic stenosis does represent one of the commonest

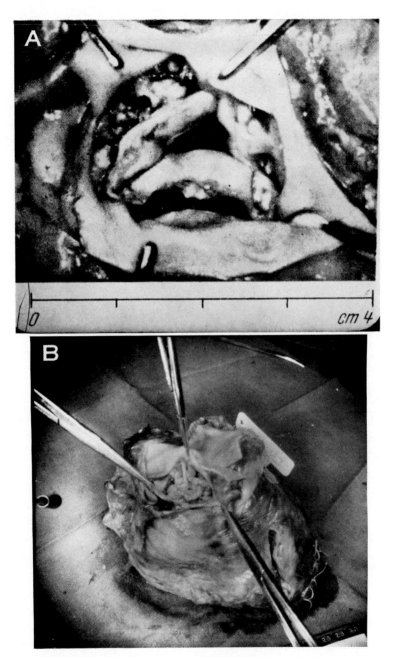

Fig. 35.11. A, symmetrical aortic stenosis. Note the central triangular "aperture of incompetence." Note rolling of valve margins and calcifications. (Reproduced with permission from Bailey, C. P.: *Surgery of the Heart*, Lea & Febiger, Philadelphia, 1955, Fig. 525 B, p. 758.) B, asymmetrical aortic stenosis. Because of obliteration of two of the lines of aortic cusp coaptation but not the third, the residual opening represents but a single radius of the original aortic root cross-section. Such a stenotic valve may be completely competent.

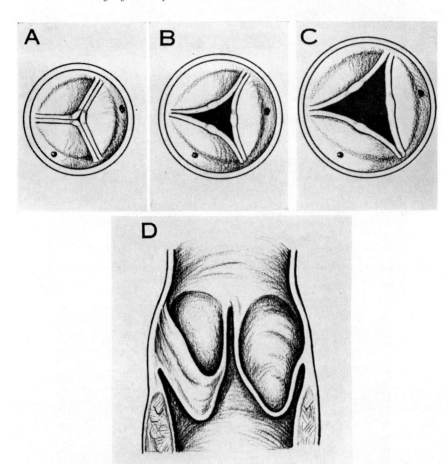

FIG. 35.12. Stages in the pathological widening of the aortic root which eventually render it impossible for even a normal valve to defend the enlarged passageway.

(although not the most severe) forms of aortic insufficiency, it is far from being the only type encountered. The most classic hemodynamic signs of aortic insufficiency (wide pulse pressure, bounding pulses) are seen in such conditions as luetic aortitis and in Marfan's syndrome, in which, as a result of weakening of bodily collagenous structures, the aortic root becomes dilated without compensatory enlargement of the valve cusps to defend the enlarged passageway (Fig. 35.12, A to C). Nearly equally severe insufficiency may result from ulcerative destruction of the valve cusps by bacterial endocarditis or by prolapse of individual cusps (Fig. 35.12, D). The latter condition may be caused either by apico-basal shortening of the cusps or by pathological elongation of their free margins. Similarity to the prolapse of the aged female breast is obvious.

A motley variety of other etiological factors contributes to produce a number of diverse types of insufficiency: rupture of a cusp such as may occur during extreme physical straining, iatrogenic insufficiencies associated with gunshot or stab wounds or with too vigorous efforts to dilate the stenotic valve surgically, various congenital malformations of the aortic valve, especially those involving bicuspid or supernumerary cuspid formation or abnormally low attachment of one of the aortic cusps (frequently seen in association with large ventricular septal defects), and dissecting aneurysm or other type of aneurysm involving the ascending aorta.

The first recorded successful effort to replace the entire aortic valve (thus excluding previous efforts to repair or replace less than all of the cusps) with autogenous tissue was made by one of us in 1962.[43] Three individual, larger than normal aortic cusps were created from a sleeve of resected ascending aorta (subsequently replaced with a prosthetic sleeve of crimped Teflon). While the created valve was nearly perfectly competent in this case, it was realized that the inherent friability of the aortic wall would not lend itself to consistent repetition of such a procedure (Fig. 35.13).

In 1967 Senning reported his early experiences with the reconstruction and replacement of aortic valves using autogenous fascia lata.[44] He used two basic techniques: strip lengthening of the margins of prolapsic cusps (Fig. 35.14) and creation of individual cusps of fascia lata (Fig. 35.13). In both techniques, the resulting valve cusps were larger than normal, requiring suspension from the aortic wall at sites placed well above the natural commissures. We soon followed Senning's lead.

While immediate complete valvular competence was the rule with strip lengthening of the aortic cusps, nearly every one of the valves that we reconstructed from individual cusps of fascia lata was at least minimally incompetent from the first. This was particularly marked when subtotal replacement of the valve had been carried out with preservation of one or two of the natural cusps that had appeared to be well formed and well supported. This difficulty in achieving initial competence was ascribed to minor elements of surgical inaccuracy in achieving perfect symmetry of the created cusps. The normally functioning aortic valve is truly a mechanism of precision, with a certain caveat to be mentioned below.

Moreover, after the passage of 3 or more months, the initially perfect competence nearly routinely achieved in those cases in which strip lengthening of the valve had been carried out began to deteriorate, with increasing evidence of returning insufficiency being noted. While the increment of regained incompetence often became established at a level less severe than

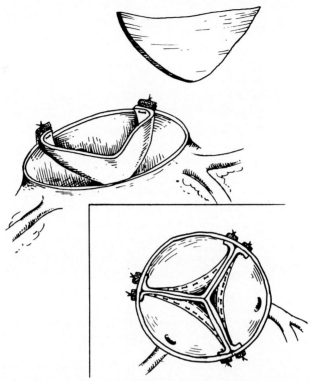

F<small>IG</small>. 35.13. Reconstruction of the excised aortic valve with individual cusps created from autogenous tissue and sutured in place. (Reproduced with permission from Bailey *et al.*[43])

that which existed prior to surgery, at other times all surgical benefit was lost.

Reoperation consistently revealed detachment of the elongating fascial strip from the two supracommissural areas which bound the left coronary cusp. This detachment had occurred despite the application of externally buttressed through-and-through attaching sutures. Evidently, sufficient fibrous union to withstand the incessant, repetitive diastolic surges (100,000 times a day) had not developed between the upper margin of the fascial strip and the approximating intimal surface of the aorta. Notably different was the situation with respect to the anterior commissure, the one lying between the noncoronary and the right coronary cusps. At the time of surgery, the free ends of the fascial strip had been left protruding through the long anterior aortotomy utilized to expose the valve to view. Upon closure of the aortotomy, these fascial ends had simply been incorporated within the reparative aortic suture line. Here there was no detachment,

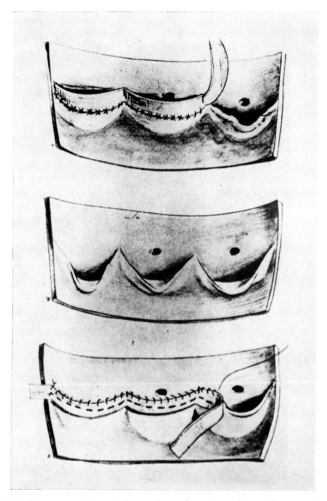

Fig. 35.14. Reconstruction of the prolapsed aortic valve with a continuous strip of fascia lata. (Reproduced with permission from Senning, A.: Reconstruction of the aortic valve with the patient's own tissues. In *Therapeutic Advances in the Practice of Cardiology* (Proceedings of the Second St. Barnabas Hospital Cardiovascular Symposium, New York, December 1967). Grune & Stratton, Inc., New York, 1970, Fig. 2, p. 188.)

dense collagenous welding together of the different tissues having taken place (Fig. 35.15).

In dealing with the instant surgical problem encountered at the time of secondary surgery, two longitudinally directed aortotomies 6 mm. long were created in the supracommissural areas bounding the left coronary

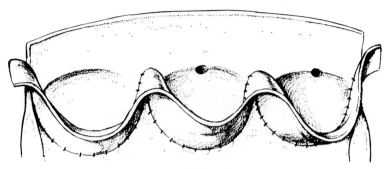

Fig. 35.15. Illustration depicting prolapse seen at reoperation or autopsy of aortic valve elongated with fascia lata because of detachment of the grafted ribbon of tissue from the supracommissural sites of attachment, despite through-and-through suturing. This did not occur at the commissure between the right and the noncoronary cusp where the ends of the fascial strip were incorporated within the suture line of the repaired aortotomy.

cusp. Two appropriate sites on the upper margin of the prolapsed fascial strip were caused to become extruded through the aortic wall, and sufficient external suture traction was applied to them to bring about symmetrical resuspension of the prolapsed valve (Fig. 35.17E). Reparative suturing of the newly created aortotomies rendered this situation permanent. Valvular competence was restored immediately and has persisted to date.

Subsequent favorable experience when this principle of transaortic suspension of the supracommissural portions of the fascial ribbon was employed at the time of initial surgery soon convinced us of its soundness.

In many cases, however, particularly those with associated aortic stenosis in which the entire valve substance is pathological, strip lengthening is inappropriate since the diseased cusps must be excised in their entirety. Since we have never been very successful in achieving aortic valvular competence when three individual aortic cusps have been created of grafts of fascia lata, it was thought that a modification of the strip grafting procedure might be preferable.

One of our associates, the late Warren Zeph Lane, created a biscuit cutter type of device capable of punching out a conjoint trilobate (gang valve) fascial graft (Fig. 35.16) in various sizes which it was thought might, after excision of the distorted natural cusps, simply be sutured appropriately to the scalloped line of natural aortic cusp origin, the upper fascial margin subsequently being suspended at the three appropriate sites by way of incorporation within the reparative suture lines of three supracommissural aortotomies.

Two unanticipated practical difficulties intruded. To our surprise, the aortic valve was not always found to be precisely symmetrical. The depths

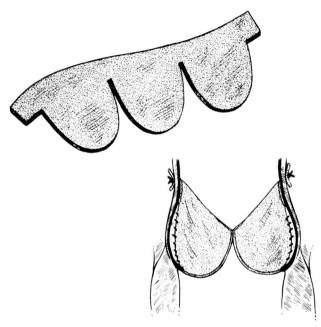

Fig. 35.16. Trilobate gang valve of fascia lata proposed by the late Warren Zeph Lane for replacement of an excised aortic valve.

of the individual cusps often differ, as do their widths. Hence the configuration of the scalloped line of valve origin varies from case to case, to a degree that completely vitiates the usefulness of the described punched out "gang valve" in fully half of all cases.

Moreover, variations and irregularities in the operator's hand sewing of the individual bulges of the graft to the scalloped line may easily result in too much or too little of the first fascial scallop being used up, with corresponding displacement of the other two fascial scallops. In our hands, therefore, this technique proved impracticable.

Finally it was realized that a simple fascial strip might be employed if the lower margin were made at the tme of definitive surgery to conform to the undulations of the scalloped line of valve origin by appropriate hand trimming with a pair of scissors (custom tailoring) as the suturing proceeded (Fig. 35.17, A to C). This principle proved to be entirely practicable and is currently in use. Once the entire custom-tailored lower margin of the fascial strip has been securely attached, suitable portions of the upper margin of the fascial strip are caused to become extruded through the three supracommissural aortotomies (the anterior longitudinal aortotomy being also supracommissural). While suture traction is being applied to the three extruded portions of the fascial ribbon (the beginning and end of the strip

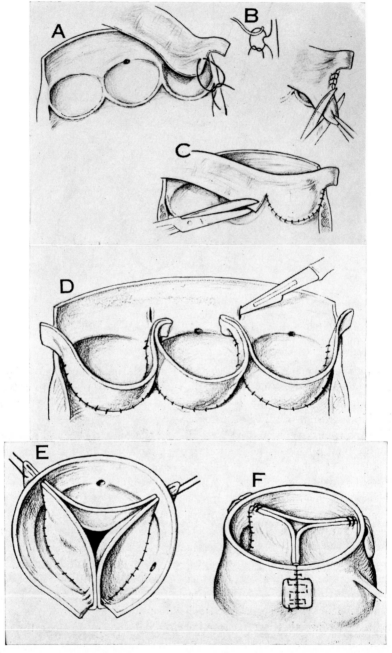

FIG. 35.17. Steps in the suturing on of a "king-sized" three-cusp aortic valve by custom contouring of the lower margin of a fascial strip to conform with the possibly

emerging from the anterior aortotomy being one of these portions), the valve is inspected for upper (marginal) symmetry (Fig. 35.17, E). Should this be found to be lacking initially, appropriate adjustment by varying the amount of traction applied to the sutures, or by removing one or more of them and replacing them at slightly different sites upon the fascial margin, will soon suffice to bring about "perfect" marginal symmetry (which seems to be about the way Nature herself accomplishes this in the often imperfectly structured natural valve). This symmetry then is rendered permanent by suture repair of the aortotomies, incorporating within them the protruding portions of the fascia (Fig. 35.17, F). In deference to the anticipated subsequent (perhaps 50 per cent in area) shrinkage of the fascial valve, an effort is made to provide a substantial excess of fascial "valve" tissue. The additional height of the over-sized cusps in itself contributes considerably to this effort while precluding subsequent prolapse.

In an attempt to mimic Nature's device to ensure instant competence of the natural aortic valve, the upper margins of the adjacent intra-aortic portions of the fascial loops as they emerge from the three supracommissural aortotomies are joined together with sutures placed at sites 3 to 4 mm. from the aortic wall (Fig. 35.17, F).

Such fascial replacements of the aortic valve nearly always are highly competent from the first, if the fascial strip has been made wide enough. In an adult, the strip needed will vary from 3 to 7 cm. in width, depending essentially upon the diameter of the aortic root. Late incompetence does not thereafter seem to supervene, in the absence of infection.

Since the performance of these painstaking reconstructive procedures may take appreciably longer than does simple prosthetic replacement of the valve, it is essential that proper coronary perfusion be provided throughout the course of the definitive surgery. A great deal of probably unnecessary morbidity and mortality was experienced during the developmental period of this effort because of failure properly to provide such support. Yet it can be most simply provided. A catheter inserted anywhere into the arterial circuit (femoral artery, usually) is connected by a line containing a Y connection to two Spencer or other coronary catheters of appropriate size. The tips of the catheters are then sutured snugly within the respective coronary ostia at the beginning of the definitive procedure and are removed at its end. No excess of coronary perfusion is possible with this arrangement, yet myocardial support always seems to be adequate.

---

asymmetric scalloped line of natural aortic valve origin. The upper margins of the fascial ribbon are drawn through small aortotomies created above the commissures bounding the left coronary cusp. Symmetry is provided by adjusting the suture traction upon the three extruded portion of the fascial strip (supracommissural portions and the extremities). Initial competence is ensured by cross-suturing the adjacent intra-aortic portions of the fascial loops close to the repaired aortotomies.

Table 35.1. *Replacement of aortic valve with fascia lata (October 26, 1967 to September 20, 1970)*

	Cases	Postoperative results*	Operative deaths
Three-cusp replacement	27	Five no AI Four 1+ AI Five 2+ AI	9
Two-cusp replacement	5	Three 1+ AI One 2+ AI	1
One-cusp replacement	3	Two 1+ AI One 2+ AI	0
Total	35	25	10

* AI, aortic insufficiency. Last eight consecutive cases showed no residual aortic insufficiency.

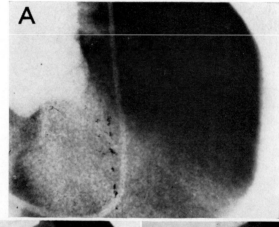

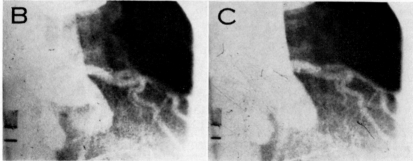

FIG. 35.18. Frames from a 35 mm. cineangiographic aortogram from Patient K. P., a 37-year-old white male with wide open aortic insufficiency resulting from marginal prolapse of the cusps. A, preoperative aortogram, diastolic phase. Note 3+ insufficiency. B, postoperative aortogram, systolic phase (strip lengthening of the aortic cusps). C, postoperative aortogram, diastolic phase. Note total competence of the aortic valve.

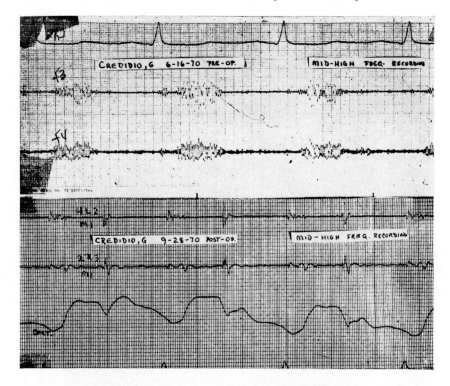

Fig. 35.19. Preoperative (above) and postoperative (below) phonocardiogram obtained from G. C., a 49-year-old white male with severe calcific aortic stenosis and insufficiency, treated by valve excision and implantation of a custom-contoured fascial valve.

Elective ventricular fibrillation by an appropriate device* is employed routinely.

Our early results with these procedures are given in Table 35.1. Representative pre- and postoperative frames obtained at aortography in K. P., a 37-year-old male white patient with pure aortic insufficiency, are shown in Fig. 35.18. Pre- and postoperative clinical findings (Chart 35.5), phonocardiographic tracings (Fig. 35.19), and catheterization findings (Fig. 35.20) in G. C., a 49-year-old white male with preponderant calcific aortic stenosis, are shown.

SUMMARY

In view of the accumulating evidence that long-term effective palliation is not routinely achievable with prosthetic valve replacement, a worldwide

---

* Medtronic fibrillator device, Medtronic, Inc., 3055 Old Highway 8, Minneapolis, Minnesota 55418.

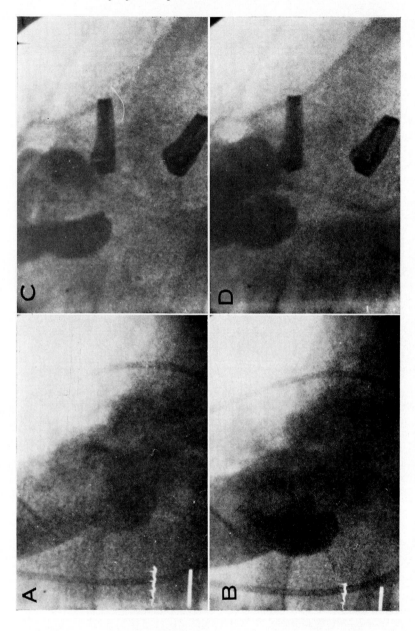

Fig. 35.20. Preoperative and postoperative aortographic frames from Patient G. C. A, preoperative, systolic phase; B, preoperative, diastolic phase; C, postoperative, systolic phase; D, postoperative, diastolic phase. Note abolition of aortic incompetence.

Chart 35.5

Patient: G.C. Age: 49 years	Preoperative 6/16/70	Postoperative 9/25/70
Right atrium	4/2 mm. Hg	4/2 mm. Hg
Right ventricle	20/3 mm. Hg	20/4 mm. Hg
Pulmonary artery	20/12 mm. Hg	20/8 mm. Hg
Pulmonary vein capillary	6/4 mm. Hg	6/4 mm. Hg
Left ventricle	170/4 mm. Hg	116/8 mm. Hg
Aorta	110/70 mm. Hg	110/80 mm. Hg
Cardiac index	2.67 l./min./m²	2.84 l./min./m²
Aortic insufficiency	2½+	None
Aorta systolic gradient	60 mm. Hg	3 mm. Hg

investigation of possible alternative methods of treatment for disease of the cardiac valves is now underway. Among the methods studied is the implantation of homograft (cadaver) and heterograft (animal) valves, both experimentally and clinically.

The increasingly favorable results obtained by reconstruction of mitral and aortic valves using autologous fascia lata, the concomitant avoidance of the problems of thromboembolization and of biological rejection, and the aggregated long-term experience with this tissue in other fields as well as in cardiac surgery have brought us to the conclusion that this probably represents the basic method of management to which all cardiac surgeons ultimately must turn.

REFERENCES

1. Hufnagel, C. A., Villegas, P. D., and Nahas, H.: Experience with new types of aortic valvular prostheses. Ann. Surg. 147: 636, 1958.

2. Harken, D. E., Taylor, W. J., Lefemine, A. A., Lunzer, S., Low, H. B. C., Cohen, M. L., and Jacobey, J. A.: Aortic valve replacement with a caged ball valve. Amer. J. Cardiol. 9: 292, 1962.

3. Starr, A., and Edwards, M. L.: Mitral replacement—clinical experience with ball-valve prosthesis. Ann. Surg. 154: 726, 1961.

4. Bjork, V. O., Cullhed, I., and Lodin, H.: Aortic valve prosthesis (Teflon); two-year follow-up. J. Thorac. Cardiovasc. Surg. 45: 635, 1963.

5. Magovern, G. J., and Cromie, H. A.: Sutureless mitral and aortic valve. Paper presented at the Forty-third Annual Meeting of the American Association for Thoracic Surgery, Houston, Texas, April 8, 1963. J. Thorac. Cardiovasc. Surg. 46: 726, 1963.

6. Bryant, L. R., Trinkle, J. K., Spencer, F. C., Danielson, G. K., Shabetai, R., and Reeves, J. T.: Cardiac valve replacement. J. A. M. A. 216: May 1971.

7. Lam, C. R., Aram, H. H., and Munnell, E. R.: An experimental study of aortic valve homografts. Surg. Gynec. Obstet. 94: 129, 1952.

8. Murray, A.: Homologous aortic segment transplants as surgical treatment for aortic and mitral insufficiency. Angiology 7: 466, 1956.

9. Beall, A. C., Jr., Morris, C., Jr., Cooley, D. A., and DeBakey, M. E.: Homotransplantation of the aortic valve. J. Thorac. Cardiovasc. Surg. 42: 497, 1961.

10. Ross, D. N.: Homograft replacement of the aortic valve. Lancet 2: 487, 1962.
11. Barratt-Boyes, B. G.: Homograft aortic valve replacement in aortic incompetence and stenosis. Thorax 19: 131, 1964.
12. Binet, J. P.: Heterologous aortic valve transplantation. Lancet 2: 1270, 1965.
13. Carpentier, A., Chanard, J., and Briotet, J. M.. Replacement of mitral valve with heterotopic heterografts. Presse Med. 75: 1603, 1967.
14. Ionescu, M. I., Wooler, G. H., and Smith, D. R.: Mitral valve replacement with aortic heterografts in humans. Thorax 22: 305, 1967.
15. O'Brien, M. F.: Heterograft aortic valves for human use. J. Thorac. Cardiovasc. Surg. 53: 392, 1967.
16. Ionescu, M. I., Mashhour, Y. A., and Wooler, G. H.: Reconstructed heterograft aortic valves for human use. Thorax 23: 221, 1968.
17. Cutler, E. C., and Levine, S. A.: Cardiotomy and valvulotomy for mitral stenosis. Boston Med. Sci. J. 188: 1023, 1923.
18. Souttar, H. S.: Surgical treatment of mitral stenosis. Brit. Med. J. 2: 603, 1925.
19. Pribram, B. O.: Die operative Behandlund der mitral Stenose. Arch. Klin. Chir. 142: 458, 1926.
20. Smithy, H. G.: An approach to the surgical treatment of valvular disease of the heart. Paper presented at the Sixteenth Annual Assembly of the Southeastern Surgical Conference, Hollywood, Fla., April 5–8, 1948.
21. Bailey, C. P.: Surgical treatment of mitral stenosis (mitral commissurotomy). Dis. Chest 15: 377, 1949.
22. Harken, D. E., Ellis, L. B., Ware, P. F., and Norman, L. R.: Surgical treatment of mitral stenosis. Valvuloplasty. New Engl. J. Med. 239: 801, 1948.
23. Baker, C., Brock, R. C., and Campbell, M.: Valvulotomy for mitral stenosis. Report of six successful cases. Brit. Med. J. 2: 1283, 1950.
24. Smithy, H. G., and Parker, E. F.: Experimental Aortic valvulotomy. Surg. Gynec. Obstet. 84: 625, 1947.
25. Bailey, C. P., Glover, R. P., O'Neill, T. J. E., and Redondo Ramirez, H. P.: Experiences with the experimental surgical relief of aortic stenosis. J. Thorac. Surg. 20: 516, 1950.
26. Creech, O., Jr.: Treatment of aortic insufficiency by obliteration of the posterior sinus of Valsalva utilizing extracorporeal circulation and temporary cardiac arrest. Bull. Tulane Univ. Med. Fac. 17: 73, 1958.
27. Bailey, C. P., and Zimmerman, J.: The surgical correction of aortic regurgitation—bicuspid conversion. Amer. J. Cardiol. 31: 6–21, 1959.
28. Effler, D. B., Groves, L. K., Martinez, W. V., and Kolff, W. J.: Open-heart surgery for acquired mitral insufficiency. J. Thorac. Surg. 36: 665, 1958.
29. Ellis, F. H., Jr., Brandenburg, R. O., Callahan, J. A., and Marshall, H. W.: Open-heart surgery for acquired mitral insufficiency. Arch. Surg. 79: 227, 1959.
30. Mulder, D. G., and Winfield, M. E.: Valvuloplasty for acquired aortic stenosis. Ann. Surg. 151: 203, 1960.
31. Bailey, C. P.: Surgery of the heart. In Gould-Sylvester, E.: *Pathology of the Heart.* Charles C Thomas, Publisher, Springfield, Ill., 1960, p. 1033.
32. Johanson, B.: Die Rekonstruktion der männlichen Urethra bei Strikturen. Z. Urol. 46: 361–375, 1961.
33. Devine, C. J., Jr., and Horton, C. E.: A one-stage hypospadias repair. J. Urol. 85: 166–72, 1961.
34. Kishev, S.: A new method of urethroplasty for urethral stricture. Brit. J. Urol. 34: 54, 1962.

35. Kaufman, J. J., Pearman, R. O., and Goodwin, W. E.: Complications of the Johanson operation in the repair of urethral strictures. J. Urol 87: 883–890, 1962.

36. Templeton, J. Y., III, and Gibbon, J. H., Jr.: Experimental reconstruction of cardiac valves by venous and pericardial grafts. Ann. Surg. 129: 161, 1949.

37. Frater, R. W. M.: Anatomical rules for the plastic repair of diseased mitral valve. Thorax 19: 458, 1964.

38. Sauvage, L. R., Wood, S. J., Bill, A. H., Jr., Logan, G. A., and Deane, P. G.: Pericardial autografts in clinical cardiac surgery. Surgery 53: 213, 1953.

39. Edwards, W. S., and Holdefer, J.: Partial and complete reconstruction of the mitral valve with pericardium. Paper presented at the Second National Conference on Heart Valves, Los Angeles, June 1968.

40. Absalom, K. B., Hunter, S. W., and Quattlebaum, F. W.: A new technique for cardiac valve construction from autologous diaphragm. Surgery 46: 1078, 1959.

41. Mulder, D. G., Miethke, J., and Charbonneau, T.: Atrial graft for right ventricular outflow tract roof. Arch. Surg. 88: 193, 1964.

42. Bailey, C. P., Hirose, T., and Zimmerman, J.: Reconstructing cardiac valves with patient's own tissues. New York J. Med., July 1, 1968, p. 1835.

43. Bailey, C. P., Carstens, H. P., Zimmerman, J., and Hirose, T.: Aortic valve replacement with autogenous aortic wall. Amer. J. Cardiol. 15: 367, 1965.

44. Senning, A.: Fascia lata replacement of aortic valves. J. Thorac. Cardiovasc. Surg. 54: 465, 1967.

45. Ionescu, M. I., and Ross, D. N.: Heart valve replacement with autologous fascia lata. Lancet 2: 335, 1969.

46. Edwards, W. S., Karp, R. B., Robillard, D., and Kerr, A. R.: Mitral and aortic valve replacement with fascia lata on a frame. J. Thorac. Cardiovasc. Surg. 58: 854, 1969.

47. Lincoln, J. C., Riley, P. A., Revignas, A., Greens, M., Ross, D. N., and Ross, J. K.: Viability of autologous fascia lata in heart valve replacement. Thorax 26: 277, 1971.

48. Kenneth, G.: Design and construction of fascia lata aortic valve prosthesis Thorax 25: 436, 1971.

49. Ionescu, M. I., Ross, D. N., Deac, R. C., Grimshaw, V. A., Taylor, S. H., Whitaker, W., and Wooler, G. H.: Autologous fascia lata for heart valve replacement. Thorax 25: 46, 1970.

50. Yates, A. K.: A fascial frustum valve for aortic valve replacements. Thorax 26: 184, 1971.

51. Flege, J. B., Jr., Rossi, N. P., Auer, J. E., and Ehrenhaft, J. L.: Technique of mitral valve replacement with autologous fascia lata. J. Thorac. Cardiovasc. Surg. 54: 222, 1967.

52. Bailey, C. P., Zimmerman, J., and Hirose, T.: Reconstruction of the mitral valve with autologous tissues. In *Therapeutic Advances in the Practice of Cardiology* (Proceedings of the Second St. Barnabas Hospital Cardiovascular Symposium, New York, December 1967). Grune & Stratton, Inc., New York, 1970.

53. Lincoln, C., Balcon, R., Emanuel, R., McDonald, L., Muir, J., Ross, D., Somerville, J., and Taylor, Jr.: Mitral valve replacement with fascia lata (abstract). Cardiovasc. Res. Suppl. 4: p. 200, 1970.

54. Bailey, C. P., Zimmerman, J., Hirose, T.; and Folk, F. S.: Reconstruction of the mitral valve with autologous tissue. Ann. Thorac. Surg. 9: 103, 1970.

55. Brownlee, R. T., and Yates, A. K.: A fascia lata mitral valve based on the "frustum" principle. Thorax 26: 284, 1971.
56. McArthur, L. L.: Autoplastic sutures in hernia and other diastases: preliminary report. J. A. M. A. 37: 1162, 1901.
57. McArthur, L. L.: Fascia lata. J. A. M. A. 43: 1039, 1904.
58. Murphy, J. B.: Ankylosis: arthroplasty, clinical and experimental. Trans. Amer. Surg. Ass. 22: 315, 1904.
59. Kirschner, M.: Über freie Sehen und Fascientransplantation. Beitr. Klin. Chir. 65: 472, 1909.
60. Kirschner, M.: Die pracktischen Ergegnizze der freien Fascien-Transplantation. Arch. Klin. Chir. 92: 888, 1910.
61. Gallie, W. E., and le Mesurier, A. B.: The use of living sutures in operative surgery. Can. Med. Ass. J. 11: 504, 1921.
62. Gallie, W. E., and le Mesurier, A. B.: Free transplantation of fascia and tendon. J. Bone Joint Surg. 4: 600, 1922.
63. Gallie, W. E., and le Mesurier, A. B.: The transplantation of the fibrous tissue in repair of anatomical defects. Brit. J. Surg. 12: 46, 1926.
64. Foshee, J. C.: Fascia lata regeneration. Surgery 14: 554, 1943.
65. Foshee, J. C.: Fascia lata regeneration; animal experimentation. Surgery 21: 800, 1947.
66. Peer, L. A.: *Transplantation of Tissues*, Vol. I. The Williams & Wilkins Company, Baltimore, 1955.
67. Lewis, D.: Fascia and fat transplantation. Surg. Gynec. Obstet. 24: 127, 1917.
68. Gilbert, J. W., Jr., Mansour, K., Sanders, S., and Gravanis, N. B.: Experimental reconstruction of the tricuspid valve with autologous fascia lata. Arch. Surg. 97: 149, 1968.
69. Zimmerman, J.: Personal communication to C. P. Bailey, 1967; unpublished observations on experiments in dogs.
70. Zimmerman, J.: Personal communication to C. P. Bailey, 1970; unpublished observations on experiments in baboons.
71. Wierzejewski, I.: Die freie Faszienüberflanzung. Munchen. Med. Wschr. 63: 875, 1916.
72. Gilsdorf, R., Bina, P. C., and Absalom, K. B.: Investigation on thrombosis using a new experimental model. J. A. M. A. 186: 932, 1963.
73. Sawyer, P. N.: Bioelectrical phenomena and intravascular thrombosis—the first 12 years. Surgery 56: 1020, 1964.
74. Wolff, C. F.: *Acta Acad. Scient. Pretopol*, Part I, 1781, p. 211.
75. Henle, J.: *Handbuch der Gefussleben des Menschen*. Braunschweig, 1876.
76. Henle, J.: *Handbuch der Systematischen Anatomie des Menschen*. Gefaesslebre Vol. III, Part I. Braunschweig, 1855–1871.
77. Zimmerman, J.: A new look at cardiac anatomy. J. Albert Einstein Med. Center 7: 77, 1959.
78. Zimmerman, J., and Bailey, C. P.: The surgical significance of the fibrous skeleton of the heart. J. Thorac. Cardiovasc. Surg. 44: 701, 1962.
79. Zimmerman, J., and Bailey, C. P.: The surgical anatomy of the cardiac valves. Hunterian Lecture. Ann. Roy. Coll. Surg. Engl. 39: 348–366, 1966.
80. Brock, R. C.: Surgical and pathological anatomy of the mitral valve. Brit. Heart J. 14: 489, 1952.
81. Harken, D. E., Ellis, L. B., Dexter, L., Farrand, R. E., and Dickson, J. F., III: The responsibility of the physician in the selection of patients for mitral surgery. Circulation 5: 349, 1952.

82. Bailey, C. P., and Hirose, T.: Maximal reconstruction of stenotic mitral valve by neostrophingic mobilization (rehinging of the septal leaflet). J. Thorac. Surg. 35: 559, 1958.

83. Bailey, C. P., Zimmerman, J., and Likoff, W.: The complete relief of mitra stenosis—ten years of progress toward this goal. Dis. Chest 37: 543–661, 1960.

84. Bailey, C. P., Zimmerman, J. Hirose, T. and DeVera, E.: Mitral valvular reconstruction with human tissues. Paper presented at the First St. Barnabas Symposium on Rheumatic and Coronary Heart Disease. J. B. Lippincott Company, Philadelphia, 1967.

85. Bailey, C. P., Zimmerman, J., Hirose, T., and Folk, F. S.: Use of autologous tissues in mitral valve reconstruction. Geriatrics 25: 119, 1970.

86. Miller, G. E., Jr., Cohn, K. E., Kerth, W. J., Seltzer, A., and Gerbode, F.: Experimental papillary muscle infarction. J. Thorac. Cardiovasc. Surg. 56: 611, 1968.

87. Soulié, P., Acar, J., Bernadou, A., and Caramanian, M.: Les ruptures de cordages de l'appareil mitral et leur étiologie; à propos de 27 cas. Arch. Mal. Coeur 58: 457, 1965.

88. Barger, H.: The effects of trauma, directly and Indirectly, on the Heart. Quart. J. Med. N. S. 13: 137, 1944.

89. Bailey, C. P., Vera, C. A., and Hirose, T.: Mitral regurgitation from rupture of chordae tendineae due to "steering wheel" compression. Geriatrics 24: 90, 1969.

90. Austen, W. G., Sanders, C. A., Averhill, J. H., and Freidlich, A. L.: Ruptured papillary muscles; report of a case with successful mitral valve replacement. Circulation 32: 597, 1965.

91. Sanders, C. A., Austen, W. G., Harthorne, J. W., Dinsmore, R. E., and Scannel, G.: Diagnosis and surgical treatment of mitral regurgitation secondary to ruptured chordae tendineae. New Engl. J. Med. 276: 943, 1967.

36

Direct Myocardial Revascularization by the Saphenous Vein Graft Technique: Three Years' Clinical Experience

RENÉ G. FAVALORO, M.D.

Since our first clinical application of the saphenous vein graft technique in May 1967 to November 30, 1970, 1,853 grafts have been performed in 1,445 patients. At present, the operative technique is well standardized. The great majority of the operations are performed under total cardio-pulmonary bypass with hemodilution technique and normothermia. In a sharply localized obstruction in a dominant right coronary artery, the operation can be performed without cardiopulmonary bypass. Induced fibrillation is used in most of the patients, and cross-clamping of the aorta for 15 to 20 minutes (enough time to perform one anastomosis) is utilized when anastomoses are performed to small distal coronary arteries. For anastomoses to the right coronary artery and anterior descending coronary artery, a vent is placed in the left atrium through the right superior pulmonary vein. Anastomoses to the circumflex coronary artery require a left ventricular vent in order to decompress fully the left ventricle and to expose any area of the circumflex coronary distribution with a routine midline anterior thoracotomy.

We can perform bypasses to the distal distribution of the right coronary artery, including the posterior descending and atrioventricular branches of the right coronary artery. Double bypasses can also be performed to the distal distribution of the right coronary artery. Also, we can perform bypasses to the main anterior descending branch of the left coronary artery, diagonal branches of the anterior descending branch of the left coronary artery, main circumflex coronary artery, lateral branches of the circumflex coronary artery, and diaphragmatic distribution of the circumflex coronary artery. Double bypasses can be performed to the right and anterior descending coronary arteries, right and circumflex coronary arteries, or anterior descending and circumflex coronary arteries. Triple and quadruple bypasses can also be performed when indicated. Our present operative technique allows us to perform saphenous vein graft bypasses at any site in the coronary circulation.

Approximately 80 per cent of the distal anastomoses are performed with interrupted 6-0 silk sutures. When the lumen of the artery is large enough, 6-0 Ethiflex running sutures are used. Anastomoses on the anterolateral wall of the aorta are performed with running 6-0 Ethiflex sutures. The indications for the operation are segmental localized obstruction above 70 per cent or totally occluded arteries with good distal runoff (beyond the site of the obstruction, the artery should show obstruction of less than 50 per cent). By coronary cineangiography, the ideal patient demonstrates severe diffuse coronary arteriosclerosis but still preserves a normal muscle. In a routine left cineventriculogram, which is performed in all of our patients, the ideal patient will show good contraction of the left ventricle with normal end diastolic pressure and normal cardiac output. Nevertheless, we are seeing increasingly more patients with abnormal ventricles, because they have previously suffered several myocardial infarctions. The end diastolic pressure is significantly elevated, and the cardiac output is greatly diminished.

Since our first attempt at revascularization in patients with abnormal ventricles early in 1966, I am firmly convinced that operations can be performed in those patients with an acceptably low operative mortality (2 deaths in the last 42 patients). Areas of significant scar tissue or true ventricular aneurysm can be resected to improve the overall contraction but, more important, multiple bypasses should be done in order to protect them for the future. For example, consider the case of a 48-year-old patient who showed overall impaired contraction of the left ventricle with an end diastolic pressure of 38. There was huge dilatation of the entire left ventricle. The patient was operated upon, and a triple saphenous vein graft bypass was accomplished (distal portion of the right coronary artery, lateral branch of the circumflex, and main anterior descending). The entire anterolateral wall was resected, and the postoperative coronary cineangiography showed good contraction of the diaphragmatic and lateral portions of the ventricle and scar tissue on the distal portion of the anterolateral wall where the reconstruction was done. The end diastolic pressure was 8. The patient is presently totally asymptomatic and working several months postoperatively. As I mentioned previously, operations in patients with abnormal ventricles can be performed with a low operative risk. We do not have a long followup, and only time will determine the benefit for this particular group of patients.

Another indication for the saphenous vein graft technique is in patients with acute coronary insufficiency. Coronary insufficiency can be divided as follows: (1) impending myocardial infarction, and (2) acute myocardial infarction with or without cardiogenic shock. In patients with impending myocardial infarction, I have no doubt that emergency coronary cineangiography should be performed and bypasses should be done in order to prevent damage to the left ventricle. Following this policy, 19 patients have been operated upon at the Cleveland Clinic with two hospital deaths. All of the survivors are free of angina and fully recovered. Patients with impending myocardial infarction are ideal candidates for the direct approach with the saphenous vein graft technique.

Acute myocardial infarction still accounts for a mortality of approximately 20 to 30 per cent, even though the patients are now being admitted to highly organized constant care units. If the patient is in cardiogenic shock, the mortality rises to between 85 and 100 per cent. Personally, I think that there will be a definite place for emergency operations in this group of patients. Partial cardiopulmonary bypass can be instituted, and we will then be able to maintain the patient with an acceptable systemic circulation. Emergency coronary cineangiography can be performed and, if saphenous vein graft bypass can be done after carefully reviewing the cineangiography, the operation should be performed in order to diminish the present mortality rate. Ten patients with acute myocardial infarction have been operated upon at the Cleveland Clinic, with one death. One patient was studied while suffering an impending myocardial infarction. The coronary cineangiography showed 90 per cent occlusion of the left main coronary artery, but beyond that point there was excellent circulation without significant obstruction in the anterior descending and circumflex coronary distribution. This patient was operated on that same morning, and a double saphenous vein graft bypass operation with one to the anterior descending and one to the circumflex was done. The postoperative studies showed excellent perfusion of the distal distribution of the left coronary artery with a normal left ventricle. The patient was discharged 2 weeks postoperatively and remained totally asymptomatic 4 months after the operation.

Another example concerns a patient with a severe obstruction at the beginning of the anterior descending branch of the left coronary artery. He had had an acute myocardial infarction. His blood pressure went to 90, he was sweating, and the electrocardiogram showed a typical pattern of an anteroseptal myocardial infarction. He was operated upon within 3 hours of the infarction, and a saphenous vein graft bypass was performed, resulting in good function of the graft with excellent perfusion of the distal distribution of the anterior descending artery. The left ventriculogram showed only minimal damage to the anterolateral wall of the left ventricle. More clinical experience is necessary to determine the exact place for the saphenous vein graft technique in the acute phase of coronary insufficiency.

I am convinced that this offers a tremendous future in this particular area, and I am quite optimistic about its application.

Up to November 30, 1970, we did 618 grafts to the right coronary artery with a hospital mortality rate of 3.8 per cent, 489 grafts on the left coronary artery with a hospital mortality rate of 2.5 per cent, and 338 multiple grafts (double, triple, and quadruple) with a hospital mortality rate of 3.5 per cent. In approximately 30 to 40 per cent of the patients, single or double internal mammary artery implants were performed simultaneously with the direct approach. I do not have enough space to discuss this aspect, but I do believe that there is still a definite place for indirect myocardial revascularization by internal mammary artery implantation. Thirty-five patients had aortic, mitral, or both valves replaced simultaneously, and approximately 10 per cent underwent reconstruction of the left ventricle.

The present low mortality rate must be attributed to the following factors. (1) High quality coronary cineangiography, which is the most important and which allows us to decide prior to the operation the precise location of the obstruction and where the distal anastomosis should be placed. (2) Standardization of the operative technique, which allows us to perform the operation in minimal time. (3) Anesthesia with methoxyflurane. (4) Careful evaluation of the blood volume by left atrial pressure. Venous pressure is not a reliable method for determining the exact blood volume. We are relying more on left atrial pressure and, for this reason, we place a catheter in the left atrium through the right superior pulmonary vein, which is left in place for 4 to 5 days. This is important in patients with abnormal ventricles. They do not tolerate high volume, and they are liable to develop pulmonary edema and concomitant left ventricular failure. (5) The prevention of hypokalemia, the most common cause of ventricular arrhythmias, including ventricular fibrillation. (6) Generous administration of coronary vasodilators, mainly nitroglycerin, during and after the operation.

Our long-term follow-up studies have shown that 85 per cent of the grafts remained open. So far, more than 400 grafts have been restudied. The majority of them were studied 6 months postoperatively, and the longest follow-up was 39 months after operation. A total of 87 per cent of the grafts to the anterior descending are open, 83 per cent on the right are patent, and 81 per cent on the circumflex coronary artery are patent. I have no doubt that these figures will improve, because some of the early pitfalls in our operative technique have been corrected. We have not seen as yet a single dilatation of a graft, and late thromboses are very rare 3 months postoperatively. I think it is worthwhile to mention that, of the first 300 patients operated upon, there are only 16 late deaths (5.3 per cent), and only 9 patients (3.3 per cent) had a myocardial infarction. This new approach has opened a new era in myocardial revascularization, and I believe that the natural course of the disease in a significant number of patients can be changed. The accumulative data have encouraged us to enlarge our indications because the great majority of patients are asymptomatic and able to work full time.

37

The Long-term Results of Human to Human Heart Transplantation

M. S. BARNARD, M.CH., AND
CHRISTIAAN N. BARNARD, M.D., PH.D.

This chapter presents our experience of the long-term results following heart transplantation in three of our five patients; two patients in this series were excluded from analysis because of their severe and fatal complications and limited survival (18 and 64 days).

PATIENTS

Of the three patients, two were male and one was female. Their ages were 59, 52, and 37 years. All three patients suffered Class IV disability, as the result of either ischemic heart disease (Case 2), cardiomyopathy (Case 3), or rheumatic heart disease (Case 5) (Table 37.1).

DONOR-RECIPIENT MATCHING

Donor pairs were matched for ABO compatibility and lymphocyte cross-match and by leucocyte typing. Because of the limited data and very small series, no correlation of apparent histocompatibility and clinical outcome can be made, but it is interesting to note that the worst match (Case 5) resulted in our longest survivor (now more than 20 months).

METHODS

Surgical techniques for clinical cardiac transplantation, the prevention, recognition, and treatment of rejection, and the prevention of infection have been previously described.[1-4]

FOLLOW-UP STUDIES

Once discharged, our patients attended the outpatient clinic twice weekly for 6 months and after that once a week. At each visit, a follow-up history

Table 37.1. *Recipients, age, cardiac disease, and other complications*

RECIPIENTS				
NO	SEX	AGE	CARDIAC DISEASE	OTHER COMPLICATIONS
1	M	53	ISCHAEMIC HEART DISEASE	DIABETES MELLITIS
2	M	59	ISCHAEMIC HEART DISEASE	ATHEROSCLEROSIS
3	M	52	CARDIOMYOPATHY	
4	M	63	RHEUMATIC HEART DISEASE AORTIC VALVE REPLACEMENT	MENTAL DEPRESSION SQUAMOUS EPETHELIOMA OF SCALP
5	F	37	RHEUMATIC HEART DISEASE AORTIC & MITRAL VALVE REPLACEMENT	

was obtained and a careful physical examination was made. In addition, a standard 12-lead electrocardiogram was taken. A summed peak to peak voltage of the QRS complexes in leads I, II, and III was recorded. Chest roentgenograms were obtained at regular intervals. Blood specimens were taken for hematological studies, as well as for evaluation of liver and renal functions.

Two patients were studied by routine right and left heart catheterization in the supine position under light anesthesia, 12 months (Case 5) and 18 months (Case 3) after transplantation. Left ventricular volumes were calculated from the left ventricular cine-angiograms in the right oblique projection. Changes in heart rate were studied in both cases following abrupt changes in blood pressure produced by amyl nitrite and phenyl-ephrine.

In one patient (Case 5) the hemodynamic changes induced by exercise were studied with the patient supine pedaling a bicycle ergometer at a work load of 200 kg. per min. for 3 minutes. In this patient, selective coronary angiography and a right endomyocardial biopsy were performed.

In two of the three patients, the heart and other organs were studied at autopsy (Cases 2 and 3).

CLINICAL STATUS

All of our long-term survivors returned to their homes and could live relatively normal lives. One could play active sports and returned to work. This result is shared by other centers. Stinson *et al.* report that four of the six patients who survived beyond 6 months have returned to work.[5]

COMPLICATIONS

Infectious diseases have occurred postoperatively in all three patients. We had to treat herpes simplex of the lips, mouth, and throat, bladder infections, septicemia, and, in one case, meningitis. Fortunately, none of our cases developed hyperglycemia or pancreatitis.

Two of our three cases developed signs of hepatic toxicity, as evidenced by jaundice, raised bilirubin, alkaline phosphatase, and lactic dehydrogenase levels. Both of these cases responded favorably when azothioprine was discontinued or reduced. Leukopenia occurred in two patients. Again, a discontinuation and reduction in the azothioprine dosage resulted in a normal white blood cell count after a very short period.

In one patient, severe serum sickness with arthritis and nephritis occurred while she was receiving antilymphocyte globulin (ALG). In spite of immediately discontinuing the ALG, these symptoms did not completely clear, and her creatinine clearance was still 50 to 60 ml. per min. In addition, her joints were abnormally enlarged and she had severe weakness of the lower limbs.

Two of the three patients developed intestinal bleeding. In addition, all patients developed neuropathy, symptomatic osteoporosis, and also muscular weakness in spite of regular supervised physiotherapy. Behavior changes were common, and all patients became cushingnoid; and so the high steroid dosage used for immunosuppression would appear to be responsible for most of the postoperative complications encountered.

In Case 3 at the time of heart transplant, a dissecting aneurysm of the ascending aorta had been repaired. At a second operation, the dissecting aneurysm was bypassed with an aorta-iliac graft, and a partial gastrectomy was performed for what was thought to be a benign ulcer but which histologically proved to be anaplastic carcinoma of the stomach. He was discharged 2 weeks after operation but was soon re-admitted with signs of intestinal obstruction. Laparotomy revealed extensive peritoneal metastases.

Only one of our three long-term survivors presented with the problem of rejection (Case 2).[6] Chronic subclinical, subacute rejection probably began at an early stage, but it was not until an acute exacerbation of rejection on the 25th day following transplant that clinical evidence became manifest. The salient feature at this stage was a rise in temperature, pulse, and sedimentation rate. There was also evidence of deterioration in cardiac function, with a rapid reduction in effort tolerance and a diminution in his feeling of well-being. Radiological examination showed enlargement of the cardiac silhouette. The most significant findings were the fall in ECG voltage and the rapid return to its previous level following treatment for rejection.

Another episode of acute rejection, occurring on the 135th day, was obscured by septicemia and *Listeria monocytogenes* meningitis, plus drug-related leukopenia. Again, voltage changes were the most helpful indications, and the patient improved after the administration of increased steroids and ALG. After his return home, this patient lived a restricted life, but the progressive evolution and persistence of ST-T wave changes indicated the presence of the chronic rejection process. Fifteen months after operation, several tests for return of cardiac innervation were made. His mean venous pressure was 14 mm. Hg with a cardiac index of 2 liters per min. per m². A persistent triple rhythm was present on auscultation. A pansystolic apical murmur had developed, suggestive of mitral incompetence. From here on, his course was downhill with more overt signs and symptoms of heart failure and attacks of acute paroxysmal cardiac dyspnea. He died more than 18 months following transplant.

NECROSCOPY FINDINGS

In Case 2, the main findings were gross atheroma and marked luminal narrowing of the coronary arteries.[7] The ventricular muscle appeared normal. Histology confirmed the deposition of atheroma in the intraventricular branches, but there was no lipid demonstrated in the intramuscular branches. The histology of the muscle showed areas of round cell infiltration suggestive of changes usually found in rejection (Fig. 37.1). All of these changes were generally found to be compatible with the diagnosis of chronic rejection.

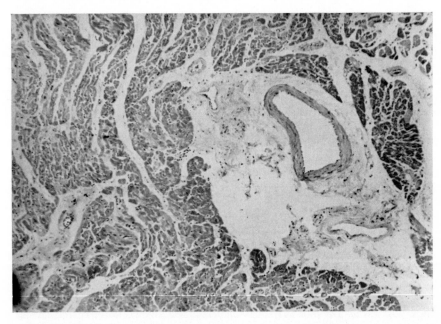

Fig. 37.1. Histology of heart muscle in Case 2, illustrating areas of round cell infiltration.

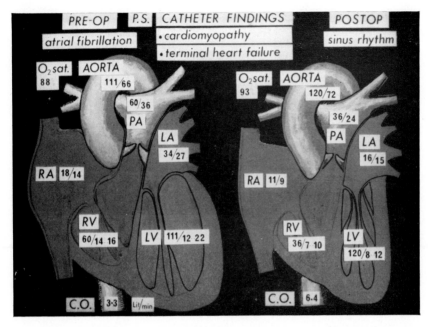

FIG. 37.2. Main catheter findings in Case 3 before and after operation.

At necropsy in Case 3, the heart was obviously atrophic, but no naked-eye abnormalities of the myocardium, valves, or coronary arteries were detected (Fig. 37.2). Histologically, very scanty minute foci of round cell infiltration were found and, apart from some atrophy, the myocardial fibers and small vessels appeared normal. The cause of death was widespread peritoneal metastases of the anaplastic carcinoma of the stomach. There was a complete aortic dissection entering from the site of the aortic anastomosis to below the iliac vessels, with multiple re-entry sites along the entire length of the aorta.

Endomyocardial biopsy of the other fatal case showed one small perivascular cell infiltrate of lymphocytes and plasma cells as the only evidence of rejection.

HEMODYNAMIC STUDIES

The two cases studied showed no clinical evidence of acute or chronic rejection at any stage in their postoperative course (Figs. 37.3 and 37.4). Both patients were in sinus rhythm with heart rates of 105. Mild elevation of right atrial and pulmonary artery pressures were present at rest, but the left ventricular end diastolic pressure in both patients was normal. Resting cardiac output was normal in Case 3, who was severely anemic

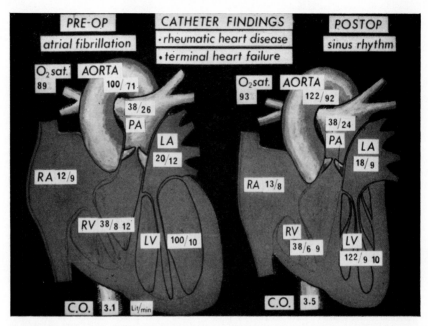

Fɪɢ. 37.3. Main catheter findings in Case 5 before and after operation.

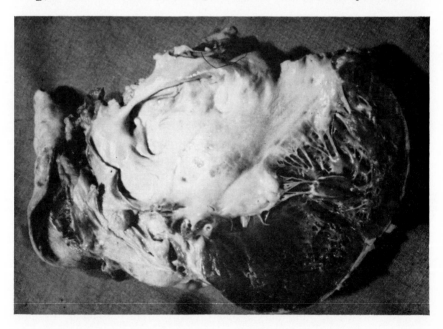

Fɪɢ. 37.4. Heart of Case 3. The heart is atrophic, but there are no naked-eye abnormalities of myocardium, valves, or coronary arteries.

at this stage (Hb. 7 g.%), but it was reduced in Case 5. Mild exercise caused a slight increase in heart rate, stroke volume, and cardiac output, with abnormal elevations of systemic and pulmonary artery pressures in Case 5. Normal ejection fractions of 80 and 57 per cent were found, but the end diastolic and end systolic volumes were smaller than normal in both cases. In both instances, there was no change in heart rate following acute changes in blood pressure after the inhalation of amyl nitrite or the infusion of phenylephrine. The coronary arteriograms were normal in Case 5.

The interpretation of any hemodynamic abnormalities in these cases is complicated by the high steroid dosage used for immunosuppression, the presence of cardiac denervation, pre-existing vascular changes in the lungs, and the presence of severe anemia in Case 3.

DISCUSSION

Up to October 1970, 165 transplants were performed on 162 recipients (Table 37.2). Only 21 are currently alive. Of the 162 recipients, only 57 survived after 3 months, 27 after 1 year, and 14 after 18 months, giving a survival rate of 35 per cent at 3 months, 17 per cent at 1 year, and 8 per cent at 18 months.[8] Ten recipients were still alive 21 to 25 months after their transplants. Three of our five patients survived more than 18 months, giving a 60 per cent survival for 3 months, 1 year, and 18 months. One was still alive 20 months later. Although it can be argued that our series is too small, it is very similar to that of Stinson and his group, who had a much larger reported series of 20 patients.[5] Their results showed 54 per cent survival at 3 months and 35 per cent at 1 year. Subdivision of their operative experience in the first two 1-year periods (1968 and 1969) reveals an increase in postoperative survival to 51 per cent at 1 year for the 2nd

Table 37.2. *Survival time in months after heart transplantation up to October 1970*

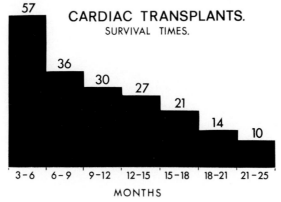

year (11 patients), as compared with 22 per cent at 1 year for the first interval (9 patients).[5] This compares very favorably with current results of cadaver renal transplants.

Two of our three long-term survivors died after 18 months. The death of Case 2 was clearly related to cardiac causes which were most probably due to the effects of chronic rejection, and this case must be considered a failure of immunosuppression. The cardiac function of Case 2 was normal except for slightly raised right heart pressures shortly before death. Case 5 continues to survive and is well 29 months after transplantation but has a subnormal cardiac output.

Long-term results are therefore possible in heart transplantation, especially if there is careful selection of patients, adequate immunosuppression, and the prompt and careful treatment of complications.

REFERENCES

1. Barnard, C. N.: Human heart transplantation. S. Afr. Med. J. (special edition) 41: No. 47 i, 1967.
2. Barnard, C. N.: Clinical heart transplantation. In proceedings of symposium, Organ Transplantation Today, June 1968. Excerpta Medica Foundation, Amsterdam.
3. Barnard, M. S., Bosman, S. C. W., and Barnard, C. N.: Immunosuppression in heart transplantation—1 year's experience. In *Book of Annals of the World Congress on Pharmacology*, Dec. 1969. Excerpta Medica, Amsterdam, 1192: 123.
4. Barnard, M. S.: The future of cardiac transplantation. Bull. Acad. Med. N. J. 16: 144, 1970.
5. Stinson, E. B., Griepp, R. B., Clark, D. A., and Shumway, N. E.: Cardiac transplantation in man. VIII. Survival and function. J. Thorac. Cardiovasc. Surg. 60: 303, 1970.
6. Schrire, V., and Barnard, C. N.: Title of article. Progr. Cardiovasc. Dis. 12: p no., 1969.
7. Thomson, J. G.: Production of severe atheroma in a transplanted heart. Lancet vol. no., 1088, 1969.
8. ACS/NIH Organ Transplant Registry. First report, October 1970.

Index